W0042418

Recent Developments in Prophylactic Immunization

RECENT DEVELOPMENTS IN PROPHYLACTIC IMMUNIZATION

IMMUNOLOGY AND MEDICINE SERIES

Biochemistry of Inflammation *Editors: J. T. Whicher and S. W. Evans*

Clinical Transplantation: Current Practice and Future Prospects *Editor: G. R. D. Catto*

Complement in Health and Disease *Editor: K. Whaley*

HLA and Disease *Authors: B. Bradley, P. T. Klouda, J. Bidwell and G. Laundy*

Immunodeficiency and Disease *Editor: A. D. B. Webster*

Immunoglobulins in Health and Disease *Editor: M. A. H. French*

Immunological Aspects of Oral Diseases *Editor: L Ivanyi*

Immunology of Endocrine Diseases *Editor: A. M. McGregor*

Immunology of ENT Disorders *Editor: G. Scadding*

Immunology of Eye Diseases *Editor: S. Lightman*

Immunology of Infection *Editors: J. G. P. Sissons, J. Cohen and L. K. Borysiewicz*

Immunology of Malignant Diseases *Editors: V. S. Byers and R. W. Baldwin*

Immunology of Pregnancy and its Disorders *Editor: C. Stern*

Immunology of Renal Diseases *Editor: C. D. Pusey*

Immunology of Sexually Transmitted Diseases *Editor: D. J. M. Wright*

Immunotherapy of Disease *Editor: T. J. Hamblin*

Lymphocytes in Health and Disease *Editors: G. Janossy and P. L. Amlot*

Lymphoproliferative Diseases *Editors: D. B. Jones and D. H. Wright*

Mast Cells, Mediators and Disease *Editor: S. T. Holgate*

Phagocytes and Disease *Editors: M. S. Klempner, B. Styrt and J. Ho*

Recent Advances in Prophylactic Immunization *Editor: A. J. Zuckerman*

IMMUNOLOGY
· SERIES · SERIES · SERIES · SERIES AND SERIES · SERIES · SERIES · SERIES ·
MEDICINE

Volume 12

Recent Developments in Prophylactic Immunization

Edited by
A. J. Zuckerman
Department of Medical Microbiology,
London School of Hygiene and Tropical Medicine
(University of London), London, UK

Series Editor: Professor K. Whaley

KLUWER ACADEMIC PUBLISHERS
DORDRECHT / BOSTON / LONDON

Distributors

for the United States and Canada: Kluwer Academic Publishers, PO Box 358, Accord Station, Hingham, MA 02018-0358, USA
for all other countries: Kluwer Academic Publishers Group, Distribution Center, PO Box 322, 3300 AH Dordrecht, The Netherlands

British Library Cataloguing in Publication Data

Zuckerman, A. J.
Recent developments in prophylactic immunization.
1. Medicine. Immunization
I. Title II. Series
614.4'7

ISBN-13: 978-94-010-6969-4 e-ISBN-13: 978-94-009-1067-6
DOI: 10.1007/978-94-009-1067-6

Published in the United Kingdom by Kluwer Academic Publishers, PO Box 55, Lancaster, UK

Kluwer Academic Publishers BV incorporates the publishing programmes of D. Reidel, Martinus Nijhoff, Dr W. Junk and MTP Press.

Contents

List of Contributors

J. W. Almond
Department of Microbiology
University of Reading
London Road,
Reading RG1 5AQ
UK

L. A. E. Ashworth
Pathology Division, PHLS Centre for Applied Microbiology and Research
Porton Down, Salisbury
Wilts. SP4 0JG
UK

J. E. Banatvala
Department of Virology
St Thomas' Hospital
Lambeth Palace Road
London SE1 7EH
UK

J. M. Best
Department of Virology
St Thomas' Hospital
Lambeth Palace Road
London SE1 7EH
UK

H. M. Dockrell
Department of Clinical Sciences
London School of Hygiene and Tropical Medicine
Keppel Street
London WC1E 7HT
UK

B. S. Drasar
Department of Clinical Sciences
London School of Hygiene and Tropical Medicine
Keppel Street
London WC1E 7HT
UK

R. W. Ellis
Department of Cellular and Molecular Biology
Merck Sharp & Dohme Research Labs
Sumneytown Pike
West Point PA 19486
USA

M. A. Epstein
Nuffield Department of Clinical Medicine
University of Oxford
John Radcliffe Hospital
Oxford OX3 9DU
UK

P. J. Greenaway
Pathology Division, PHLS Centre for Applied Microbiology and Research
Porton Down, Salisbury
Wilts. SP4 0JG
UK

R. B. Heath
Department of Virology
St Bartholomew's Hospital
51/53 Bartholomew Close
London EC1A 7BE
UK

K. P. W. J. McAdam
Department of Clinical Sciences
London School of Hygiene and Tropical Medicine
Keppel Street
London WC1E 7HT
UK

A. J. Morgan
Department of Pathology
University of Bristol Medical School
University Walk
Bristol BS8 1TD
UK

A. R. Neurath
The New York Blood Center
310 E 67th Street, New York
NY 10021
USA

K. G. Nicholson
Infectious and Tropical Diseases Unit
Groby Road Hospital
Groby Road
Leicester LE3 9QE
UK

J. E. Pennington
University of California, San Francisco
Cutter Biological
Berkeley
CA 94701
USA

P. J. Provost
Department of Virus and Cell Biology
Merck Sharp & Dohme Research Labs
Sumneytown Pike
West Point PA 19486
USA

A. Robinson
Biologics Division, PHLS Centre for Applied Microbiology and Research
Porton Down, Salisbury
Wilts. SP4 0JG
UK

G. L. Smith
Sir William Dunn School of Pathology
Oxford University
South Parks Road
Oxford OX1 3RE
UK

M. G. Taylor
Department of Medical Parasitology
London School of Hygiene and Tropical Medicine
Keppel Street
London WC1E 7HT
UK

R. A. Wall
Microbial Pathogenicity Research Group and Dept of Microbiology
Northwick Park Hospital and Clinical Research Centre
Harrow
Middlesex HA1 3UJ
UK

G. Webbe
Department of Medical Parasitology
London School of Hygiene and Tropical Medicine
Keppel Street
London WC1E 7HT
UK

Series Editor's Note

The interface between clinical immunology and other branches of medical practice is frequently blurred and the general physician is frequently faced with clinical problems with an immunological basis and is often expected to diagnose and manage such patients. The rapid expansion of basic and clinical immunology over the past two decades has resulted in the appearance of increasing numbers of immunology journals and it is impossible for a non-specialist to keep apace with this information overload. The *Immunology and Medicine* series is designed to present individual topics of immunology in a condensed package of information which can be readily assimilated by the busy clinician or pathologist.

Professor Gordon Reeves recognized the need for such a series and it is to his credit that the previous volumes in this series have been so successful. It is with some trepidation that I accepted the invitation to take over the series editorship but I hope that I can continue the high standards established by my predecessor. I have indeed been fortunate to begin my career with the present volume which deals with a topic at the heart of immunology and which has been so ably edited by Professor Zuckerman.

Professor K. Whaley
Pathology Department
Western Infirmary
University of Glasgow, Glasgow

Introduction

It has been said that "never in the history of human progress has a better and cheaper method of preventing illness been developed than immunization". This is well illustrated by the WHO Expanded Programme on Immunization (EPI) which in developing countries is now preventing nearly a million deaths annually from measles, pertussis and neonatal tetanus, and for which there is a commitment by the WHO and UNICEF to protect all children by immunization by the end of the decade. This enormous undertaking will be facilitated by the rapid advances in molecular biology and recombinant DNA technology, in the understanding of immunological mechanisms and by the production and application of monoclonal antibodies so that the structure and location of important antigenic determinants or epitopes can be determined. Chemical synthesis of oligopeptides has been simplified, and computer programmes and X-ray crystallography provide the tools for the determination of three-dimensional structure of proteins, so that the structure and location of important antigenic determinants or epitopes can be predicted.

These techniques have opened the way to the improvement of existing vaccines and to the development and production of new vaccines against infections for which vaccines are not available.

New vaccines under development include vaccines against hepatitis B, hepatitis A, malaria, vaccines for typhoid, cholera, rotavirus infection and other diarrhoeal diseases, leprosy, rabies, the acquired immune deficiency syndrome (AIDS), rubella, EB virus, schistosomiasis and other infections. These recent developments are discussed in the volume by internationally recognized experts assembled from several countries.

Professor A.J. Zuckerman

1
Pertussis vaccines

L. A. E. ASHWORTH and A. ROBINSON

INTRODUCTION

Whooping cough (pertussis) is a serious disease of infancy, and although mortality due to the disease is now relatively low in developed countries, perhaps 1 million children die from this infection per year worldwide[1]. Improvements in living conditions and standards of hygiene have contributed greatly to reducing the incidence of the infection but effective vaccination has also had a marked effect and a continuing high level of vaccination has been shown to be necessary to prevent recrudescence of the disease in the population. Provided physicians are alert to the possibility of adult pertussis infection, the disease is found in adults[2,3].

Most countries are still using vaccines which consist of a suspension of the causative organism, *Bordetella pertussis*, killed and partially detoxified. These whole-cell vaccines were developed and subjected to efficacy trials in the 1940s and 1950s, and are still the subject of much study. It had been established over many years that infection of a child with *B. pertussis* leading to clinically diagnosed disease, in the majority of cases gave lasting protection even into adulthood. This apparently solid immunity provided considerable encouragement to those developing whole-cell vaccines, and the hopes for such vaccines have generally been fulfilled in that they are effective in preventing clinical pertussis. The efficacy of whole-cell pertussis vaccines has recently been reviewed[4] and it is only necessary to state here that most studies indicate efficacy for these vaccines of 80–90%, although the range of estimates is very wide. In contrast to natural infection, the protection afforded by vaccination may wane quite rapidly[5], although this has not been the uniform conclusion of efficacy studies.

At the time of the empirical development of whole-cell vaccines there was little detailed knowledge of the biochemistry of the organism or of its interaction with the human host, and understanding of the immune response was in its infancy We now have a vastly increased knowledge in all these areas, and this has been applied to the development of acellular vaccines which should eventually replace the cellular vaccines. The latter may carry a small risk of long-term vaccine-induced damage and do give rise to a range of unwanted side-effects which, by discouraging vaccine uptake, undermine the protection which might otherwise be achieved. Acellular vaccines would be formulated to contain only those components of whole-cell vaccines responsible for protection and hence, it is hoped, will prove to be less reactive products. For some years Japan has been using acellular vaccines to immunize 2-year-old children routinely. Only recently have these vaccines been used to immunize infants under 1 year of age in Japan and in trials in Sweden. Further trials of Japanese and other vaccines are now taking place in the UK and elsewhere.

It is the aim of this chapter to review our understanding of the protective immune response to pertussis, particularly in the light of the more recent studies of vaccination and disease. There have been earlier reviews of this and associated fields to which the reader may wish to refer[6–9]. Firstly, however, it is necessary to review briefly the biochemical nature of the antigens of *B. pertussis* which play a role in pathogenesis of and immunity to pertussis.

ANTIGENS INVOLVED IN PATHOGENESIS AND IMMUNITY IN PERTUSSIS

The success of whole-cell pertussis vaccines in preventing pertussis in the child and the development of animal models for pertussis infection (in particular the mouse intracerebral challenge test) led to a search for 'the protective antigen' of *B. pertussis*. Indeed at some time most of the antigens described below have been given this title. It is now generally accepted that development of the disease pertussis in the child and resulting immunity to further infection, depends on the complex interaction of many bacterial virulence factors with the host. Any virulence factor will have one or more of several properties including toxicity, mediation of adherence or interference with the host's defence mechanism. All virulence factors play a distinct role in contributing to the infection which leads to the characteristic disease of pertussis[7–10]. The effective immune response represents to some degree a summation of the immune responses to the individual antigens. It is inappropriate to refer to one component as 'the protective antigen'.

The pathogenesis of pertussis can be considered as having four major stages in an overlapping sequence; (1) attachment of *B. pertussis* cells to the ciliated respiratory epithelium of the child, allowing the bacteria to resist the normal clearance mechanisms such as coughing and mucociliary flow; (2) growth and multiplication of the bacteria; (3) production of local disease effects such as ciliostasis and sloughing of cilia and ciliated cells into the lumen; and (4) production of systemic disease effects such as lymphocytosis and hyperinsulinaemia. By extrapolation of results of experiments involving animal models and *in vitro* cell cultures, the roles of individual virulence factors in the above scheme can now be assumed with some confidence[7–10]. Furthermore, examination of the immunogenic and protective potential of these virulence components in animals has provided evidence as to which antigens are likely to contribute to the protective immune response. The immune response of children to whole-cell vaccines has been of limited value in this regard (see below).

Filamentous haemagglutinin (FHA)

FHA is a high molecular weight surface component of *B. pertussis* which has been strongly implicated in the adhesion of the organism to mammalian cells, since antibodies to FHA will prevent this adhesion, bacteria deficient in FHA adhere less well to mammalian cells and the ability to adhere can be restored by the addition of exogenous FHA[11]. FHA is a highly immunogenic protein, but some controversy exists concerning its ability to protect animal species against experimental infection. Data from the mouse intracerebral protection test are unreliable for purified antigens or toxoid preparations because of the pronounced synergistic effect which traces of biologically active pertussis toxin (PT) have on their protective potency[12]. Nevertheless, protective activity has been shown for FHA in a number of animal respiratory infection studies (reviewed in refs 7 and 8). Because of its high immunogenicity, lack of intrinsic toxicity, ease of isolation and purification, and protective potency, FHA is widely considered to be a key component of acellular pertussis vaccines.

Agglutinogens (AGGs)

B. pertussis has three major AGGs designated 1, 2 and 3, and three minor AGGs, designated 4, 5 and 6, which in various combinations account for the serospecificity of different strains within the species. AGGs 2, 3 and 6 are fimbrial proteins[13–18] but it should be noted that there is no evidence for any of the *B. pertussis* AGGs acting as haemaglutinins. References in the literature to 'fimbrial haemagglutinin' are to FHA, and mostly pre-date the finding that, whilst antibodies to FHA do not interact with fimbriae, those to AGG2 and AGG3 do so[13,14]. The biochemical nature of AGG1 is not fully understood but it does not appear to be a fimbrial protein. A recent report[19], which is confirmed by unpublished data from our laboratory, indicates that certain monoclonal antibodies which react with lipopolysaccharide (LPS) can agglutinate most strains of *B. pertussis.* However, LPS, the O-somatic antigen, was specifically excluded from the typing scheme in which AGG1 was descrbed as the AGG common to all strains of *B. pertussis*[20]. AGG1 may consist of more than one surface antigen, though to be consistent with the original typing scheme these should not be found on other *Bordetella* species.

AGG2 has a subunit molecular weight, determined by SDS-PAGE, of 22 500[13–18] and its amino acid sequence has been deduced from the nucleotide sequence of the gene encoding the structural subunit[21]. AGG3 is also a fimbrial protein but its subunit molecular weight is 22 000[14,15,18]. Cowell and co-workers[22] have isolated a very similar (probably identical) protein to AGG3 and, on the basis of the agglutinating specificity of antisera raised against this protein, have concluded that it corresponds to AGG6. Since AGG6 usually occurs only in strains bearing AGG3 it is not possible at present to distinguish between AGG3 and AGG6. They may correspond to different epitopes on the same fimbrial subunit. A similar relationship may hold for AGG2 and AGGs 4 and 5. It can, however, be stated that there are two major fimbrial types in *B. pertussis*; the 22 500 subunit is isolated from cells of 1,2 or 1,2,3 serotype and the 22 000 subunit from cells of 1,3 or 1,2,3 serotype.

Historically the agglutinin response to vaccination in children has been considered to correlate with protection against pertussis (see later). It should be noted that the agglutinins measured in the 1950s MRC trials of whole-cell vaccines[23] could have encompassed antibodies to antigens other than the fimbrial AGG2 and AGG3. Nevertheless, the recommendation that whole-cell vaccines should contain both AGG2 and AGG3 in order to protect against all serotypes of pertussis should apply equally to acellular pertussis vaccines. This contention is supported by the fimbrial nature of these antigens which indicates their potential as adhesins in pathogenesis. To date the role of AGGs as adhesins has been inferred from the results of one study involving adherence of *B. pertussis* to Vero cells in tissue culture[24]. AGGs have, however, been found to protect mice against respiratory infections with *B. pertussis*[17,25]. Recent results from our laboratory indicate that the protection of mice is to some extent serotype-specific. Furthermore, immunization of mice with either purified AGG2 or AGG3 can result in selection of organisms of heterologous serotype in the lungs following subsequent infection with *B. pertussis* strains of known serotype. Thus mice were almost completely protected from infection with a strain of 1,3 serotype by prior immunization with AGG3 but not AGG2, and organisms that were recovered from the lungs of AGG3-immunized animals were mainly of 1,0,0 serotype. These experimental data are in agreement with the serotype-specific protection reported to occur in children immunized with whole-cell vaccine, which has been taken to indicate that acellular vaccines should contain both AGG2 and AGG3[26]. Experiments are under way to map immunochemically the AGG2 and AGG3 subunits, and to identify the conserved and variable epitopes.

Pertussis toxin (PT)

Research on PT has proceeded at an explosive rate compared to that on other pertussis antigens. The main reasons for this are the recent observations on the pharmacological activities of PT and the widely held view that PT is the major toxin of *B. pertussis*, and hence is the essential component of acellular pertussis vaccines. Recent reviews[27–29] have concerned the genetics, pharmacology, structure and isolation of PT. Of particular interest here are the intrinsic immunogenicity of PT, which is usually studied with detoxified or incomplete non-toxic forms of the protein, and its effects on the host's immune systems. PT conforms to an A–B toxin structure, where the A subunit (molecular weight 28 000) possesses NAD-glycohydrolase and ADP-ribosyltransferase activities and the binding or B oligomer consists of four smaller subunits, S2–S5, with molecular weights 23 000, 22 000, 11 700 and 9300, respectively. PT detoxified by glutaraldehyde or formaldehyde[7,8], hydrogen peroxide[30] or ethyl-dimethylaminopropyl carbodiimide[31] is immunogenic and protective against infection with *B. pertussis* in various systems.

Monoclonal antibodies to S1, S2 and S3 subunits have been shown to have toxin-neutralizing activity[32-34] and attempts have been made to map the protective epitope(s) on subunit S1[35]. The individual subunits have been expressed in *Bacillus subtilis*[36] or *Escherichia coli*, either directly[37] or as fused proteins[38], and found to be immunogenic, although they did not protect mice against intracerebral infection with *B. pertussis*. This lack of protection is not surprising because of the marked dependence of this test on active PT[12]. Immunization of mice with the B oligomer of PT did protect them against the toxic effects of PT[39]. No doubt PT subunits which induce a toxin-neutralizing immune response will eventually be synthesized in alternative bacterial hosts following genetic manipulation. If 'engineered' subunit preparations are to be included in acellular vaccines, then they should be produced in systems incapable of producing whole toxin to avoid the need for detoxification which will result if traces of active toxin are produced. The fine immunochemical mapping of PT is also being examined following synthesis of peptides corresponding to potential immunogenic epitopes[40].

PT can also have a marked effect on the immune response to other antigens. This has been observed following pertussis infection or immunization with whole-cell vaccines which contain active PT, but is unlikely to be found with acellular vaccines containing fully detoxified PT. The effects of PT on the host's immune system have recently been reviewed by Munoz[41] and include: (1) adjuvanticity for IgG, IgM and especially IgE antibodies; (2) induction of anaphylactic sensitivity; (3) promotion of delayed hypersensitivity reactions which correlated with the production of gamma interferon; (4) induction of experimentally induced autoimmune diseases, including allergic encephalomyelitis in mice and rats, allergic uveoretinitis in rats and allergic orchitis in mice; (5) promotion of lymphocytosis due to the failure of circulating lymphocytes to migrate back to the lymph nodes; (6) mitogenic effects on T-lymphocytes; and (7) inhibition of neutrophil function and of chemotactic migration of macrophages.

The murine encephalopathy which was proposed as a model of vaccine-induced neurological disorders of children[42] has been shown to be caused by PT[43,44] or by PT and LPS[45], and is considered to be due to anaphylactic shock[44]. It is clear that active PT has extremely complex effects on the immune system which are still being unravelled. A recent report has suggested that ADP-ribosyltransferase activity is required for the pathogenic action of PT and also for optimum immunoprotective capacity of the bacteria producing the toxin[46]. Incorporation of fully and irreversibly detoxified PT in acellular vaccines should mean that not only are the deleterious effects of active PT removed, but also that the adjuvanticity for other pertussis antigens and co-immunized toxoids is lost.

Adenylate cyclase (AC)

AC is an interesting protein because it is extracytoplasmic, activated by calmodulin and becomes internalized by a variety of mammalian cells causing intoxication due to unregulated cAMP production. The toxic effects of AC include the inhibition of a number of cellular activities including superoxide generation, chemiluminescence, phagocytosis, bactericidal activity and chemotaxis of phagocytic cells[47]. However, a precise role for AC in pathogenesis cannot readily be assigned because the reported toxic effects mostly relate to *in vitro* studies of crude toxin preparations and do not derive from *in vivo* studies as they do for PT. *B. pertussis* cells deficient in AC are avirulent in the mouse lung[48], although reasons for this loss of virulence are unclear. One of the problems of assessing toxicity and immunogenicity of AC is the difficulty in obtaining pure preparations. Different products which possess AC activity have been reported with extremely variant molecular weights[47], in keeping with a complex molecule appearing in different forms or a protein which adventitiously attaches to other bacterial proteins. Novotny *et al.*[49] found that an AC-associated protein with a molecular weight of 69 000 was immunogenic and possessed mouse protective activity. Unfortunately the relationship of this protein to AC is uncertain, and may have been fortuitous. A recent study[50] reported the neutralization of respiratory infection of mice with *B. pertussis* by polyclonal or monoclonal antibodies to AC. It is not known whether antibodies to AC are produced in children following immunization with whole-cell vaccines, although some vaccines possess AC activity[51]. The cloning and expression of AC in *Escherichia coli*[52] should help to resolve some of the problems concerning the role of this protein in pathogenesis and immunity.

Other pertussis antigens

Little is known of the involvement of other antigens in protection against pertussis. Heat-labile toxin (HLT) is an extremely potent toxin, very probably involved in pathogenesis of pertussis. In a toxoided form HLT can induce the formation of toxin-neutralizing antibodies[53]. HLT may interfere with the adjuvanticity of PT and suppress IgG1 production in mice[54]. A highly antigenic toxoided form of HLT is required for further immunogenicity studies.

Tracheal cytotoxin is a component of low molecular weight which is derived from released peptidoglycan fragments of *B. pertussis*[55], but nothing is known about its immunogenic properties. *B. pertussis* lipopolysaccharide (LPS) is immunogenic but the anti-LPS response has not been shown to be protective in animal studies. However, part of the adjuvant action of *B. pertussis* cells is due to LPS, and the effects of LPS on macrophage activation and in polyclonal B-cell activation should be borne in mind[56]. *B. pertussis* outer membrane proteins are immunogenic and protect mice against intracerebral and intranasal infections but their relevance to protection in the child is unknown[7,25].

IMMUNE RESPONSE TO PERTUSSIS INFECTION AND VACCINATION

Because of the apparent longevity of protection conferred on the child by pertussis infection, it might seem worthwhile to search for the basis of immune protection among the responses of pertussis cases. It should be remembered, however, that the infected child responds to a plethora of antigens of differing immunogenicities present at different concentrations. There is little possibility of discerning the features which provide protection within this complex response, and the presence of antibody of a particular specificity does not prove its relevance to protection; the absence of a response is more telling.

Because of this, and also because diagnostic techniques for pertussis have been unsatisfactory, most studies of the immune response to disease have been aimed at diagnosis. Unfortunately diagnosis based on antibody determinations, being largely retrospective, has been of limited clinical use but can be a valuable epidemiological tool. A further problem is that the spectrum of antibodies seen in disease has to be differentiated from maternal antibodies or those present due to vaccination. The latter may vary considerably from one country to another due to differences in immunization schedules and vaccine composition. With the advent of acellular vaccines diagnostic indicators may change again, although diagnosis may be simplified because antibodies to pertussis constituents absent from acellular vaccine would be indicative of infection. Ignoring the diagnostic implications we will now look at present information about immune responses to the pertussis antigens described above, beginning with antibodies in serum.

SERUM ANTIBODY RESPONSES

There are problems in comparing results from different laboratories because of the lack of standardization. This may soon be remedied if a reference serum (US Reference Pertussis Antiserum (human), Lot 3, Office of Biologics, Research and Review, US FDA, Bethesda) currently being evaluated is found to be satisfactory. Most groups are using ELISA techniques, which allow the classes of antibody to be determined. The purity of antigens used in these techniques is important, as are their biochemical credentials. FHA, for example, appears to be susceptible to degradation during purification and storage[57], and some epitopes might be destroyed preferentially. Also, different strains of *B pertussis* might conceivably make antigens with altered or missing epitopes. To date there is little evidence of this except for one example discovered using a monoclonal antibody (L10) to the S1 subunit of PT. L10 was found to react with PT from all strains except strain 18323[58] and this has since been shown to result from substitution of a single amino acid residue[35].

Antibodies to FHA

Functional assays for antibodies to FHA, i.e. tests which measure inhibition of adherence, will probably only become available for routine use when the relevant mammalian cell receptors for FHA are characterized. ELISAs have shown that anti-FHA antibodies are a feature of the response to both infection and vaccination. However, there are considerable differences between the levels of response to FHA reported by various groups. In a study of whooping cough in children and adults[59], IgG to FHA was detected after infection in the majority of cases. The response in unvaccinated subjects under 2 years of age was low, and a rapid decrease in titre was observed in these and other cases with low levels of IgG anti-FHA. Winsnes *et al.*[60] reported that although 80% of cases less than 1 year old had IgM anti-FHA and 50% had IgA anti-FHA, only 15% developed IgG antibodies to FHA. The proportion of cases with antibodies to FHA tended to increase with age, but it appears that the sensitivity of the IgG ELISA may have been poor compared to that for IgA and IgM anti-FHA. Alternatively the antigen preparation used in the ELISA may have contained LPS to which there were markedly similar responses of the type which might be expected for a relatively T-independent antigen. This possibility was stated recently in a review of these diagnostic serological methods[61]. It is worth noting that both the above studies used FHA prepared by the same method[62]. However, Nagel *et al.*[63] also concluded that 'antibodies against FHA are hardly induced by infection'.

In contrast to the above, Sato and Sato[64] also found IgG in convalescent sera from 195 infant pertussis cases. The proportion of these subjects that had been vaccinated was not stated, but was likely to have been low because of (a) the initial low mean titres of antibody and (b) the fact that Japan officially ceased vaccinating in 1975 prior to the reintroduction of vaccination for children over 2 years of age. A recent study[2] found that culture-confirmed pertussis infection induced a very similar mean serum IgG anti-FHA titre to that obtained 6 weeks after a third dose of whole-cell vaccine. Serum IgA anti-FHA was markedly higher after infection than after vaccine, which induced very little anti-FHA in this Ig class.

Antibodies to PT

A view of many, expressed by Pittman[65], is that whooping cough is a toxin-mediated disease. According to this view, and by analogy with tetanus and diphtheria, all that is required of immunization is that it should induce toxin-neutralizing antibody in serum. The *in vitro* Chinese hamster ovary (CHO) cell test for active PT provides a basis for the most widely used functional test for antibody which can inhibit PT toxicity[66]. However, antibodies which neutralize *in vivo* lymphocytosis-promoting or histamine-sensitizing activities, whilst being less amenable to routine use than neutralization of CHO cell activity, may be more relevant to protection. Granstrom *et al.*[67] used the CHO cell assay to measure serum anti-PT in 13 pertussis cases younger than 15 years. All these subjects seroconverted or, on paired samples, showed significant rises in titre. Only two had measurable anti-PT before day 20 of the disease but recent studies by these workers[61] found much poorer responses which were interpreted as being due to children in the earlier study having been vaccinated. The class of antibody acting in the CHO cell test was not investigated, and it would be difficult to do this routinely.

Other studies of anti-PT in infection have mainly used ELISA, which is more sensitive than the CHO cell assay. As for antibodies to FHA there is a wide variation in the findings from different studies. Nagel *et al.*[63] reported high levels of serum IgG anti-PT in about 70% of cases younger than 4 months and in 100% of cases aged 4-13 months. Winsnes *et al.*[60] found only 20% of pertussis cases less than 1 year old had detectable anti-PT IgG, whereas IgA and IgM were detected in 50% and 80%, respectively, of such cases. Only low levels of IgG anti-PT were induced by whole-cell vaccination in either of these two studies. In the study of Sato and Sato[64], appreciable levels of IgG anti-PT were found in convalescent sera from all of 195 infant pertussis cases. Somewhat lower levels of anti-PT were induced in children given whole-cell vaccine but only responses to two doses were reported. The more usual schedule of three vaccine doses has been compared with infection and found to give similar titres of serum IgG anti-PT[2]. Serum IgA to PT was markedly higher following infection than in vaccinees in this study.

Antibodies to agglutinogens

Antibodies to the AGGs have routinely been measured as agglutinins for many years, the main change in technique having been the introduction of microplate-based methods[68]. In studies prior to the formulation of the serotyping scheme[69,70] and in some later studies[71] the sera were not absorbed, so that the total agglutinins were measured. Despite this, only a proportion of pertussis cases had detectable agglutinins. Miller and Silverberg[69] found 15/17 children tested during the course of the disease had agglutinins compared to 36/67 tested after cessation of cough. The latter is very similar to the proportion of convalescent sera with detectable agglutinins in culture-confirmed cases in later studies[70,71]. In a study[72] in which sera were absorbed, 5/16 children from whom 1,0,3 serotype organisms were recovered had type 3 agglutinins by 1 month after onset of symptoms while 8/13 had these antibodies by 2 months. Serotype-specific responses to vaccination showed considerable variation with whole-cell vaccine used[72]. The majority of children responded to the better vaccines with agglutinins 2 and 3 detectable 1 month after a second injection. Preston *et al.*[73] confirmed this finding, although the type 3 agglutinin response was poorer than the type 2 with the vaccine used in this study.

As for FHA, routine tests for functional antibody able to prevent AGG-mediated adherence probably require characterization of the specific receptors with which the fimbriae interact. Only in the authors' laboratory has ELISA been used for titration of anti-AGGs 2+3. This fimbrial mixture has been available as it is one of the components of the acellular vaccine made at CAMR. Until now, practical difficulties in making purified AGG3 in sufficient quantity have prevented routine serotype-specific ELISA, a situation which may soon be remedied. In a recent study[2], individual serum IgG anti-AGG2+3 response to infection was very variable, and the mean response in unvaccinated children was modest. The mean ELISA titre of IgG anti-AGG2+3 after three doses of vaccine was much higher than after infection. Results from ELISA were therefore similar to those obtained by bacterial agglutination but with antibodies to the non-fimbrial AGG1 being excluded without the need for serum absorption. Serum IgA anti-AGG2+3 induced by infection was low but similar to that induced by vaccination[2].

ANTIBODY RESPONSE IN THE UPPER RESPIRATORY TRACT

In pertussis, antigens are produced by organisms colonizing the upper respiratory tract, and would be expected primarily to stimulate the local immune system. The latter is known to operate relatively independently of the systemic immune apparatus. Respiratory tract immunity has been reviewed generally[74] and as it relates to pertussis[6,7]. However, too little is known about the mechanisms of local immunity to allow predictions about host responses with anything approaching certainty. Antigens differing in hydrophobicity or molecular size are likely to gain entry to the lymphoid apparatus at different rates, with the possibility of different outcomes. Moreover, penetration of the mucosa by antigens is likely to be affected by any mucosal damage resulting from the local effects of *B. pertussis* components such as the heat-labile dermonecrotic toxin or tracheal cytotoxin. In view of the pathology of pertussis (reviewed in ref. 75) it is difficult to conceive of a role for specific cell-mediated immunity in eradication of the organism from the upper respiratory tract. The ability of *B. pertussis* cells to incapacitate phagocytes which ingest them (reviewed in ref. 47) would appear to have implications for events in the alveoli rather than the upper tract, where any phagocytes in the lumen will be expelled from the airways.

Although relatively little has been published on the local immune response either to pertussis infection or to vaccination, there is growing evidence that infection does induce the anticipated mucosal antibodies, and that parenteral vaccination can prime for local antibody production. Using the supernate of sonicated *B. pertussis* cells as antigen in ELISA, Goodman *et al.*[76] found that IgA antibody could be detected in nasal secretions of pertussis cases but not of vaccinees.

In collaboration with others, the authors have measured IgA antibodies to FHA, PT and AGG2+3 in nasal secretions of infants and adults in a study of whooping cough, in infants following whole-cell vaccination and in adults injected with one dose of CAMR acellular vaccine (see below). The nasal sampling was by means of a small cotton swab inserted in the nose and subsequently eluted in buffer. Preliminary results from these studies[77] indicated that IgA antibodies to all the test antigens could be detected in the secretions after infection, although the pattern of nasal response showed individual variation. Also the response, at least to FHA and AGG2+3, persisted for at least 6 months. This study has now been completed (manuscript in preparation) and the following are the broad findings with regard to nasal IgA responses. Of the unvaccinated culture-confirmed cases under 5 years of age, 70% had IgA antibodies to at least one of the test antigens in samples taken less than 2 weeks after onset of disease. All these subjects had a response to at least two of the antigens by 5–12 weeks after onset, with 83% having IgA to all the test antigens. Nasal IgA antibodies increased in the second sample compared to the first in all these subjects.

In a recently published study Granstrom *et al.*[78] studied IgA and IgG antibodies to FHA and PT in nasal aspirates and in saliva. They noted a rapid IgA response to PT in 100% of young unimmunized subjects, 70% of whom had detectable anti-FHA. In this study too the antibody levels increased between first and second samples. Granstrom *et al.* concluded that this early presence of anti-PT and anti-FHA IgA in the mucosal secretions of severe pertussis cases calls into question the role of these antibodies in protection. However, the onset of disease is some days after infection, and the decline in recoverable organisms, coincident with the paroxysmal stage of disease[75], could be due to these nasal antibodies. Moreover nasal antibodies, including those to AGG2+3, could signify a priming of the response in the respiratory tract which is responsible for the long-lasting protection. Where protection is maximal, antibodies in the primed mucosal tissue may act swiftly enough to stop colonization almost immediately, preventing the production of sufficient antigen(s) to cause any increase in antibody. This appeared to be the case when rabbits were immunized parenterally with purified FHA and challenged intranasally[79]. There was an inverse correlation between bacterial recoveries 18 and 28 days after challenge and nasal IgA anti-FHA levels at the time of challenge, but two of the best-protected animals showed subsequent decreases in this antibody. Hence, as for many diseases, the protection induced against reinfection, which vaccination may aim to mimic, could have a different time course than that which leads to eradication of the primary infection.

VACCINATION BY NASAL OR ORAL ROUTE

If protection against pertussis is indeed derived from local immunity then parenteral immunization may not be the optimal route for inducing such immunity. Thomas[80] administered killed whole-cell vaccine to adults by freeze-drying it and delivering it to the nose as an aerosol. This procedure gave rise to specific nasal IgA responses in eight subjects but no rise in serum antibodies, whereas one dose of the same vaccine given parenterally induced nasal antibodies in only three of six subjects, although all had rises in serum titres. Baumann *et al.*[81] administered a heat-inactivated whole-cell pertussis vaccine to over 11 000 infants by the oral route. The vaccine was given on days 2, 3, 4 and 5 after birth and, in comparison with a smaller control group vaccinated parenterally, no significant differences were found in pertussis morbidity for up to 1 year. A pertussis-specific IgA response developed in saliva, but unfortunately tests were not performed with individual antigens.

ACELLULAR PERTUSSIS VACCINES

Acellular vaccines is a term which includes preparations hardly less crude than the whole-cell vaccines, as well as those consisting of one or more purified pertussis components. The latter may be better termed defined-component vaccines[8], of which there are now several at various stages of development. Those manufactured in Japan, following the pioneering efforts of Dr Y. Sato and his co-workers, are the only preparations in routine use at present.

Japanese acellular vaccines

These vaccines consist largely of co-purified PT and FHA[82] and, because of differences in the fractionation procedures used by different manufacturers, they are essentially of two types: (1) Takeda (T)-type which has been described as containing FHA, PT and AGG2 in a ratio of 8:1:1[64] or in a ratio of 10:1:0.1[83] and (2) Biken (B)-type which has equal amounts of FHA and PT but which contains no measurable AGGs. Obviously much of the interest in defined-component vaccines lies in their promise of reduced toxicity, and field trials of the vaccines are concerned to a large extent with this aspect, which will not be considered in detail here, except to say that the Japanese vaccines appear to be well tolerated.

Use of T- and B-type vaccines in Japan has largely been confined to children over 2 years of age although there is a limited amount of data from younger children[84,85]. Estimates of efficacy for the vaccines lie within the range 77–95%[82,84,86–89]. The vaccines induced antibodies to both PT and FHA, the T-type also producing an agglutinin response[86,90] whereas the B-type did not[90]. Serum anti-FHA and anti-PT levels were similar to those seen in the convalescent stage of pertussis[82,86]. The lower dose of PT in the T-type vaccine resulted in a poorer anti-PT response than with the B-type after the first injection, although this difference probably became insignificant after further injections according to some data[82], but persisted according to results of other studies[88–90].

Humoral antibody responses to the T-type vaccines have also been examined in a number of studies in the USA. That of Anderson *et al.*[91] found children aged 2 months at the time of the first dose developed higher agglutinin titres to whole-cell vaccine than to a T-type vaccine. Anti-PT response to both vaccines was the same, but the T-type gave a significantly higher anti-FHA titre.

The reported efficacy of the Japanese component vaccines is evidence that protection can be induced by FHA and/or PT, at least to the extent provided by whole-cell vaccine. This does not undermine the case for inclusion of AGGs in a vaccine because these may be as effective as either or both of the other components. There is still no evidence as to whether the protection conferred by the Japanese vaccines lasts longer than that induced by whole-cell pertussis vaccine or whether it prevents colonization of the respiratory tract. Despite the large number of doses administered the immune mechanisms of protection have still not been identified, and no attempts have yet been made to examine the mucosal responses induced by the Japanese vaccines.

Swedish trials of Japanese acellular vaccines

General vaccination with whole-cell pertussis vaccine was discontinued in Sweden in 1979 because of low vaccine efficacy and the perceived risk of acute neurological illness associated with such vaccine. The incidence of pertussis remained high, providing a strong incentive to test acellular vaccine in infants at an age when the risks from infection are highest. Following the usual series of preliminary trials of reactogenicity and immunogenicity, a placebo-controlled trial of two acellular Japanese vaccines was carried out[92]. One vaccine was of the B-type, given at a dose of 3.75 μg protein nitrogen for each of the two antigens. The other was a monocomponent preparation consisting of purified PT detoxified with formaldehyde, given at a dose of 6 μg protein nitrogen. The inclusion of the latter meant that, for the first time, a basis of vaccine-induced protection might be conclusively demonstrated. Unfortunately this was not the outcome. The vaccines were given in a two-dose schedule because the preliminary trials had shown that serum antibody levels achieved with this schedule were not significantly increased by a third dose. Apparently the view was taken (see above – antibodies to PT) that induction of serum PT-neutralizing antibody was sufficient for protection, and hence was the primary aim of vaccination. A significantly higher anti-PT titre was achieved with the monocomponent vaccine, possibly due to the greater amount of PT per dose. However, the point estimate of efficacy (versus culture-confirmed pertussis) of the PT-only vaccine was 54% (95% confidence limits 26–72%), lower than that of the B-type vaccine which had an estimated efficacy of 69% (47-82%). If a more stringent case definition was applied (i.e. culture-confirmed pertussis with a cough lasting over 30 days) these estimates became 80% (59–91%) and 79% (57–90%), respectively. It is possible that the hoped-for level of efficacy (70% lower confidence limit[93,94]) would have been achieved had a three-dose schedule been used. Unfortunately, whole-cell vaccines could not be included in the trial for purposes of comparison, and it is inappropriate to compare the above estimates of efficacy with the 80–90% efficacy generally accepted for whole-cell vaccine.

Although the results of this trial were, in some respects, inconclusive and disappointing, not least for the Swedish public health authorities, they provide useful information.

1. Infants 5–11 months old respond well to the vaccines which are of low reactogenicity. The question of whether the vaccines reduce the risk of major neurological problems can only be addressed by further studies in this age range involving many more subjects.
2. The vaccines induce protection, but the degree of protection was found to depend markedly on the case definition applied. This could be interpreted as protection manifesting largely as a reduction in the severity of symptoms rather than as prevention of infection.
3. The post-vaccination levels of serum antibody to FHA and PT did not differ between vaccinees who subsequently had whooping cough and those who did not[92]. Therefore we now know that inactivated PT can indeed act alone as a protective antigen, but that it is unlikely that serum PT-neutralizing antibody provides the major mechanism of protection.

The last of these statements has major implications and is worth examining further. IgG antibodies to FHA and to PT were measured by ELISA and

PT-neutralizing antibodies by CHO-cell assay. It is possible that the latter assay of PT reflects properties of the toxin which are not relevant to its action in human disease. Alternatively, protection may correlate with levels of non-IgG serum antibodies measurable in ELISA, a possibility which is still being explored by the Swedish workers. The protection obtained may, however, have been due to antibodies induced in the respiratory tract, in which case these may have functioned either by neutralizing the PT locally or by blocking PT-mediated adherence. Unfortunately respiratory tract secretions were not sampled in this trial. According to our present understanding of the role of FHA (i.e. as an adhesin; see above), the lack of correlation between serum anti-FHA and protection does not decrease the likelihood that FHA in the B-type vaccine contributed to the protection observed.

OTHER ACELLULAR VACCINES AND FUTURE PROSPECTS

Vaccines which are currently undergoing phase 1 and 2 clinical trials in various countries are all similar to the T- or B-type products or are monocomponent PT preparations. In addition, the vaccine developed at CAMR[95], which contains equal amounts of PT, FHA and AGG2+3, is at present undergoing phase 2 clinical trials in the UK. All the vaccines appear to be immunogenic, inducing antibodies, at least in serum, to the constituent antigens.

Efficacy trials are now being planned in which acellular vaccines of different compositions will be compared and in which whole-cell vaccine will be run as a standard. Such trials could confirm which antigens are required for full protection but, because of ethical obstacles to testing monocomponent vaccines in a population for which an effective whole-cell vaccine is available, the results may not demonstrate meaningful correlates of protection. Such correlates would provide a basis for testing the next generation of vaccines which could contain genetically engineered antigens or synthetic peptides.

REFERENCES

1. Muller, A. S., Leeuwenburg, J. and Pratt, D. S. (1986). Pertussis epidemiology and control. *Bull. WHO*, **64**, 321–31
2. Thomas, M. G., Ashworth, L. A. E., Miller, E. and Lambert, H. P. (1988). Serum IgG, IgA and IgM responses to pertussis toxin, filamentous haemagglutinin and agglutinogens 2 and 3 following *Bordetella pertussis* infection. (Submitted for publication)
3. Trollfors, B. and Rabo, E. (1981) Whooping cough in adults. *Br. Med. J.*, **283**, 696–7
4. Fine, P. E. M. and Clarkson, J. A. (1987) Reflections on the efficacy of pertussis vaccines. *Rev. Infect. Dis.*, **9**, 866-83
5. Jenkinson, D. (1988). Duration of effectiveness of pertussis vaccine: evidence from a 10 year community study. *Br. Med. J.*, **296**, 612–14
6. Winsnes, R. (1988) Serological responses to pertussis. In Wardlaw, A. C. and Parton, R. (eds) *Pathogenesis and Immunity in Pertussis*, pp. 283–307. (Chichester: John Wiley & Sons)
7. Robinson, A., Irons, L. I. and Ashworth, L. A. E. (1985). Pertussis vaccine: present status and future prospects. *Vaccine*, **3**, 11–22
8. Robinson, A. and Ashworth, L. A. E. (1988). Acellular and defined-component vaccines

against pertussis. In Wardlaw, A. C. and Parton, R. (eds), *Pathogenesis and Immunity in Pertussis*, pp. 399–417. (Chichester: John Wiley & Sons)

9. Wardlaw, A. C. and Parton, R. (1988). The host–parasite relationship in pertussis. In Wardlaw, A. C. and Parton, R. (eds), *Pathogenesis and Immunity in Pertussis*, pp. 327–52. (Chichester: John Wiley & Sons)
10. Weiss, A. A. and Hewlett, E. L. (1986). Virulence factors of *Bordetella pertussis*. *Ann. Rev. Microbiol.*, **40**, 661–86
11. Tuomanen, E. (1988). *Bordetella pertussis* adhesins. In Wardlaw, A. C. and Parton, R. (eds), *Pathogenesis and Immunity in Pertussis*, pp. 75–94. (Chichester: John Wiley & Sons)
12. Robinson, A. and Irons, L. I. (1983). Synergistic effects of *Bordetella pertussis* lymphocytosis promoting factor on protective activities of *Bordetella* antigens in mice. *Infect. Immun.*, **40**, 523-48
13. Ashworth, L. A. E., Irons, L. I. and Dowsett, A. B. (1982). The antigenic relationship between serotype specific agglutinogens and fimbriae of *Bordetella pertussis*. *Infect. Immun.*, **37**, 1278–81
14. Ashworth, L. A. E., Dowsett, A. B., Irons, L. I. and Robinson, A. (1985). The location of surface antigens of *Bordetella pertussis* by immuno-electron microscopy. In *Proceedings of Fourth International Symposium on Pertussis. Develop. Biol. Standard*, **61**, 143–51
15. Irons, L. I., Ashworth, L. A. E. and Robinson, A. (1985). Release and purification of fimbriae from *Bordetella pertussis*. In *Proceedings of Fourth International Symposium on Pertussis, Dev. Biol. Stand.*, **61**, 153–63
16. Zhang, J. M., Cowell, J. L., Steven, A. C., Carter, P. H., McGrath, P. P. and Manclark, C. R. (1985). Purification and characterization of fimbriae isolated from *Bordetella pertussis*. *Infect. Immun.*, **48**, 422–7
17. Zhang, J. M., Cowell, J. L., Steven, A. C. and Manclark, C. R. (1985). Purification of serotype 2 fimbriae of *Bordetella pertussis* and their identification as a mouse protective antigen. In *Proceedings of Fourth International Symposium on Pertussis. Dev. Biol. Stand.*, **61**, 173–85
18. Mooi, F. R., van der Herde, H. G. J., ter Avest, A. R., Welinder, K. G., Livey, I., van der Zeijst, B. A. M. J. and Gaastra, W. (1987). Characterisation of fimbrial subunits from *Bordetella* species. *Microb. Pathogen.*, **2**, 473
19. Li, Z. M., Cowell, J. L., Brennan, M. J., Burns, D. L. and Manclark, C. R. (1988). Agglutinating monoclonal antibodies that specifically recognise lipooligosaccharide A of *B. pertussis*. *Infect. Immun.*, **56**, 699–702
20. Eldering, G., Hornbeck, C. and Baker, J. (1957). Serological study of *Bordetella pertussis* and related species. *J. Bacteriol.*, **74**, 133-6
21. Livey, I., Duggleby, C. J. and Robinson, A. (1987) Cloning and nucleotide sequence analysis of the serotype 2 fimbrial subunit gene of *Bordetella pertussis*. *Molec. Microbiol.*, **1**, 203–9
22. Cowell, J. L., Zhang, J. M., Urisu, A., Suzuki, A., Steven, A. C., Liu, T., Liu, Y. and Manclark, C. R. (1987). Purification and characterisation of serotype 6 fimbrae from *Bordetella pertussis* and comparison of their properties with serotype 2 fimbriae. *Infect. Immun.*, **55**, 916–22
23. MRC (1959). Vaccination against whooping cough – final report. *Br. Med. J.*, **1**, 994–1000
24. Gorringe, A. R., Ashworth, L. A. E., Irons, L. I. and Robinson, A. (1985). Effect of monoclonal antibodies on the adherence of *Bordetella pertussis* to Vero cells. *FEMS. Microbiol. Lett.*, **26**, 5–9
25. Robinson, A., Ashworth, L. A. E., Baskerville, A. and Irons, L. I. (1985). Protection against intranasal infection of mice with *Bordetella pertussis*. In *Proceedings of the Fourth International Symposium on Pertussis. Develop. Biol. Standard*, **61**, 165–72
26. Preston, N. W. (1988). Pertussis today. In Wardlaw, A. C. and Parton, R. (eds), *Pathogenesis and Immunity in Pertussis*, pp. 1–18. (Chichester: John Wiley & Sons)
27. Irons, L. I. and Gorringe, A. A. (1988) Pertussis toxin: production, purification, molecular structure and assay. In Wardlaw, A. C. and Parton, R. (eds), *Pathogenesis and Immunity in Pertussis*, pp. 95–120. (Chichester: John Wiley & Sons)
28. Ui, M. (1988). The multiple biological activities of pertussis toxin. In Wardlaw, A. C. and Parton, R. (eds), *Pathogenesis and Immunity in Pertussis*, pp. 121–45. (Chichester: John Wiley & Sons)
29. Furman, B. L., Sidey, F. M. and Smith, M. (1988). Metabolic disturbances produced by pertussis toxin. In Wardlaw, A. C. and Parton, R. (eds), *Pathogenesis and Immunity in Pertussis*, pp. 147–72. (Chichester: John Wiley & Sons)

30. Sekura, R. D., Schneerson, R. and Robbins, J. B. (1986). Safety and antigenicity of a pertussis toxoid vaccine evaluated in adult volunteers. In *Workshop on Acellular Pertussis Vaccines*; sponsored by the Interagency Group to Monitor Vaccine Development, Production and Usage, US Department of Health and Human Services and US Public Health Service, Bethesda. September, pp. 135–8
31. Christodoulides, M., Sidey, F. M., Parton, R. and Stewart-Tull, D. E. S. (1987). Acellular pertussis vaccine prepared by a simple extraction and toxoiding procedure. *Vaccine*, **5**, 199–207
32. Sato, H., Ito, A., Chiba, J. and Sato, Y. (1984). Monoclonal antibody against pertussis toxin: effect on toxin activity and pertussis infections. *Infect. Immun.*, **46**, 422–8
33. Sato, H., Sato, Y., Ito, A. and Ohishi, I. (1987). Effect of a monoclonal antibody to pertussis toxin on toxin activity. *Infect. Immun.*, **55**, 909–15
34. Anwar, H., Ashworth, L. A. E., Funnell, S., Robinson, A. and Irons, L. I. (1987). Neutralisation of the biological activities of pertussis toxin with a monoclonal antibody. *FEMS Microbiol. Lett.*, **44**, 141–5
35. Bartoloni, A., Pizza, M., Bigio, M., Nucci, D., Ashworth, L. A. E., Irons, L. I., Robinson, A., Burns, D., Manclark, C., Sato, H. and Rappuoli, R. (1988). Mapping of a protective epitope of pertussis toxin by *in vitro* refolding of recombinant fragments. *Biotechnology*, **6**, 709–12
36. Runeberg-Nyman, K., Engstrom, O., Lofdahl, S., Ylostalo, S. and Sarvas, M. (1987). Expression and secretion of pertussis toxin subunit S1 in *Bacillus subtilis*. *Microb. Pathogen.*, **3**, 461–8
37. Burnette, W. N., Mar, V. L., Cieplak, W., Morric, C. F., Kaljot, K. T., Marchito, K. S., Sachdev, R. K., Locht, C. and Keith, J. M. (1988). Direct expression of *Bordetella pertussis* toxin subunits to high levels in *Escherichia coli*. *Biotechnology*, **6**, 699-706
38. Nicosia, A., Bartoloni, A., Perugini, M. and Rappuoli, R. (1987). Expression and immunological properties of the five subunits of pertussis toxin. *Infect. Immun.*, **55**, 953–67
39. Arcinega, J. L., Burns, D. L., Garcia-Ortigoza, E. and Manclark, C. R. (1987). Immune response to the B oligomer of pertussis toxin. *Infect. Immun.*, **15**, 1132–6
40. Askelof, P., Rodmalm, K., Abens, J., Unden, A. and Bartfai, T. (1988). Use of synthetic peptides to map antigenic sites of *Bordetella pertussis* toxin subunit SI. *J. Infect Dis.*, **157**, 738–42
41. Munoz, J. J. (1988). Action of pertussigen (pertussis toxin) on the host immune system. In Wardlaw, A. C. and Parton, R. (eds), *Pathogenesis and Immunity in Pertussis*, pp. 173–92. (Chichester: John Wiley & Sons)
42. Steinman, L., Sriram, S., Adelman, N. E., Zamuip, S., McDevitt, H. O. and Urich, H. (1982). Murine model for pertussis vaccine encephalopathy: linkage to H-2. *Nature*, **299**, 738–40
43. Steinman, L., Weiss, A., Adelman, N., Lim, M., Ziniga, R., Oehlert, J., Hewlett, E., Falkow, S. (1985). Pertussis toxin is required for pertussis vaccine encephalopathy. *Proc. Natl. Acad. Sci. USA*, **82**, 8733–6
44. Munoz, J. J., Peacock, M. G. and Hadlow, W. J. (1987). Anaphylaxis or so-called encephalopathy in mice sensitised to an antigen with the aid of pertussigen (pertussis toxin). *Infect. Immun.*, **55**, 1004–8
45. Redhead, K., Robinson, A., Ashworth, L. A. E. and Melville-Smith, M. (1987). The activity of purified *Bordetella pertussis* components in murine encephalopathy. *J. Biol. Stand.*, **15**, 341–51
46. Black, W. J., Munoz, J. J., Peacock, M. G., Schad, P. A., Cowell, J. L., Burchall, J. J., Lim, M., Kent, A., Steinman, L. and Falkow, S. (1988). ADP-ribosyltransferase activity of pertussis toxin and immunomodulation by *Bordetella pertussis*. *Science*, **240**, 656–9
47. Hewlett, E. L. and Gordon, V. M. (1988). Adenylate cyclase toxin of *Bordetella pertussis*. In Wardlaw, A. C. and Parton, R. (eds), *Pathogenesis and Immunity in Pertussis*, pp. 193–209. (Chichester: John Wiley & Sons)
48. Weiss, A. A., Hewlett, E. L., Myers, G. A. and Falkow, S. (1984). Pertussis toxin and extracytoplasmic adenylate cyclase as virulence factors of *Bordetella pertussis*. *J. Infect. Dis.*, **150**, 219–22
49. Novotny, P., Chubb, A. P., Cownley, K., Montaraz, J. A. and Beesley, J. E. (1985). Bordetella adenylate cyclase: a genus specific protective antigen and virulence factor. In *Proceedings of the Fourth International Symposium on Pertussis. Dev. Biol. Stand.*, **61**, 27–41

50. Brezin, C., Gujiso, N., Ladant, D., Djavadi-Ohaniance, L., Megret, F., Onyeocha, I. and Alonso, J-M. (1987). Protective effect of *Bordetella pertussis* adenylate cyclase antibodies against lethal respiratory infection in the mouse. *FEMS Microbiol. Lett.*, **42**, 75–80
51. Wolff, J. and Cook, G. H. (1973). Activation of thyroid membrane adenylate cyclase by purine nucleotide. *J. Biol. Chem.*, **248**, 350–5
52. Glaser, P., Ladant, D., Sezer, O, Pichot, F., Ullman, A. and Danchin, A. (1988). The calmodulin-sensitive adenylate cyclase of *Bordetella pertussis*: cloning and expression in *Escherichia coli*. *Molec. Microbiol.*, **2**, 19–30
53. Nakase, J. and Endoh, M. (1988). Heat labile toxin of *Bordetella pertussis*. In Wardlaw, A. C. and Parton, R. (eds), *Pathogenesis and Immunity in Pertussis*, pp. 211–29. (Chichester: John Wiley & Sons)
54. Sekiya, K. (1983). Effects of *Bordetella pertussis* components on IgE and IgGI responses. *Microbiol. Immunol.*, **27**, 905–15
55. Rosenthal, R. S., Nogami, M., Cookson, B. T., Goldman, W. E. and Folkening, W. J. (1987). Major fragments of soluble peptidoglycan released from growing *Bordetella pertussis* is tracheal cytotoxin. *Infect. Immun.*, **55**, 2117–20
56. Chaby, R. and Caroff, M. (1988). Lipopolysaccharides of *Bordetella pertussis* endotoxin. In Wardlaw, A. C. and Parton, R. (eds), *Pathogenesis and Immunity in Pertussis*, pp. 247–71. (Chichester: John Wiley & Sons)
57. Irons, L. I., Ashworth, L. A. E. and Wilton-Smith, P. (1983). Heterogeneity of the filamentous haemagglutinin of *Bordetella pertussis* studied with monoclonal antibodies. *J. Gen. Microbiol.*, **129**, 2769–78
58. Perera, V. Y., Wardlaw, A. C. and Freer, J. H (1986). Antigenic heterogeneity in subunit S1 of pertussis toxin. *J. Gen. Microbiol.*, **132**, 553–6
59. Granstrom, M., Granstrom, G., Lindfors, A. and Askelof, P. (1982). Serologic diagnosis of whooping cough by an enzyme-linked immunosorbent assay using fimbrial hemagglutinin as antigen. *J. Infect. Dis.*, **146**, 741-5
60. Winsnes, R., Lonnes, T., Mogster, B. and Berdal, B. P. (1985). Antibody responses after vaccination and disease against leukocytosis promoting factor, filamentous hemagglutinin, lipopolysaccharide and a protein binding to complement-fixing antibodies induced during whooping cough. In *Proceedings of Fourth International Symposium on Pertussis. Dev. Biol. Stand.*, **61**, 353–65
61. Granstrom, G., Wretlind, B., Salenstedt, C-R. and Granstrom, M. (1988). Evaluation of serological assays for diagnosis of whooping cough. *J. Clin. Microbiol.*, **26**, 1818-23
62. Askelof, P., Granstrom, M., Gillenius, P. and Lindberg, A. A. (1982). Purification and characterization of a fimbrial hemagglutinin from *Bordetella pertussis* for use in an enzyme-linked immunosorbent assay. *J. Med. Microbiol.*, **15**, 73–83
63. Nagel, J., de Graaf, S. and Schiif-Evers, D. (1985). Improved serodiagnosis of whooping cough caused by *Bordetella pertussis* by determination of IgG anti-LPF antibody levels. In *Proceedings of Fourth International Symposium on Pertussis. Dev. Biol. Stand.*, **61**, 325–30
64. Sato, Y. and Sato, H. (1985). Anti-pertussis toxin IgG and anti-filamentous hemagglutinin IgG production in children immunized with pertussis acellular vaccine and comparison of these titers with the sera of pertussis convalescent children. In *Proceedings of Fourth International Symposium on Pertussis. Dev. Biol. Stand.*, **61**, 367–72
65. Pittman, M. (1985). The concept of pertussis as a toxin-mediated disease. *Paediatr. Infect. Dis.*, **3**, 467–86
66. Gillenius, P., Jaatmaa, E., Askelof, P., Granstrom, M. and Tiru, M. (1985) The standardisation of an assay for pertussis toxin and antitoxin in microplate culture of Chinese hamster ovary cells. *J. Biol. Standard*, **13**, 61-6
67. Granstrom, M., Granstrom, G., Gillenius, P. and Askelof, P. (1985). Neutralizing antibodies to pertussis toxin in whooping cough *J. Infect. Dis.*, **151**, 646–9
68. Manclark, C. R. and Meade, B. D. (1980). Serological response to *Bordetella pertussis*. In Rose, N. R. and Friedman, N. (eds), *Manual of Clinical Immunology*, pp. 497–9. (Washington, DC: American Society for Microbiology)
69. Miller, J. J. Jr and Silverberg, R. J. (1939). The agglutinative reaction in relation to pertussis and to prophylactic vaccination against pertussis with description of a new technic. *J. Immunol.*, **37**, 207–21
70. Winter, J. L. (1953). Development of antibodies in children convalescent from whooping cough. *Proc. Soc. Exp. Biol. Med.*, **83**, 866–70

71. Macauley, M. E. (1979). The serological diagnosis of whooping cough. *J Hyg. Camb.*, **83**, 95–102
72. Dolby, J. and Stephens, S. (1973). Pertussis antibodies in the sera of children exposed to *Bordetella pertussis* by vaccination or infection. *J. Hyg. Camb.*, **71**, 193-207
73. Preston, N. W., Mackay, R. I., Bamford, F. N., Crofts, J. E. and Burland, W. L. (1974). Pertussis agglutinins in vaccinated children: better response with adjuvant. *J. Hyg. Camb.*, **73**, 119–25
74. Bienenstock, J. (1986). Immunity in the gastrointestinal and respiratory tracts. In Tagliabue, A., Rappuoli, R. and Piazzi, S. E. (eds), *Bacterial Vaccines and Local Immunity. Ann. Sclavo. III*, **1-2**, 77–86
75. Linnemann, C. C. Jr (1979). Host–parasite interactions in pertussis. In Manclark, C. R. and Hill, J. C. (eds), *International Symposium on Pertussis*, pp. 3–18. (USDHEW Publication No. (NIH) 79–1830, Washington, DC)
76. Goodman, Y. E., Wort, A. J. and Jackson, F. L. (1981). Enzyme-linked immunosorbent assay for detection of pertussis immunoglobulin A in nasopharyngeal secretions as an indicator of recent infection. *J. Clin. Microbiol.*, **13**, 286–92
77. Ashworth, L. A. E., Day, A., Lambert, H. P., Lingham, S., Lissauer, T., Miller, E., Robinson, A., Rutter, D. A. and Thomas, M. G. (1986). Local and systemic immune responses to pertussis infection and cellular and acellular vaccines. In Tagliabue, A., Rappuoli, R. and Piazzi, S. E. (eds), *Bacterial Vaccines and Local Immunity. Ann. Sclavo. III*, **1-2**, 199–211
78. Granstrom, G., Askelof, P. and Granstrom, M. (1988). Specific immunoglobulin A to *Bordetella pertussis* antigens in mucosal secretion for rapid diagnosis of whooping cough. *J. Clin. Microbiol.*, **26**, 869–74
79. Ashworth, L. A. E., Fitzgeorge, R. B., Irons, L. I., Morgan, C. P. and Robinson, A. (1982). Rabbit nasopharyngeal colonization by *Bordetella pertussis*: the effects of immunization on clearance and on serum and nasal antibody levels. *J. Hyg. Camb.*, **88**, 475-86
80. Thomas, G. (1975). Respiratory and humoral immune response to aerosol and intramuscular pertussis vaccine. *J. Hyg. Camb.*, **74**, 233–7
81. Baumann, E., Binder, B. R., Falk, W., Huber, E. G., Kurz, R. and Rosanelli, K. (1984). Development and clinical use of an oral heat-inactivated whole cell pertussis vaccine. In *Proceedings of Fourth International Symposium on Pertussis. Dev. Biol. Stand.*, **61**, 511-16
82. Sato, Y., Kimura, M. and Fukumi, H. (1984). Development of a pertussis component vaccine in Japan. *Lancet*, **1**, 122–6
83. Shukuda, Y. (1986). Manufacturing methods for the Japanese acellular vaccines. In *Workshop on Acellular Pertussis Vaccines*, sponsored by the Interagency Group to Monitor Vaccine Development, Production and Usage, US Department of Health and Human Services and US Public Health Service, Bethesda, September, pp. 23-6
84. Aoyama, T., Murase, Y., Kato, T. and Iwata, T. (1985). Efficacy of an acellular pertussis vaccine in Japan. *J. Paediatr.*, **107**, 180–2
85. Isomura, S. (1986). Efficacy and adverse reactions associated with acellular pertussis vaccines in Japan. In *Workshop on Acellular Pertussis Vaccines*, sponsored by the Interagency Group to Monitor Vaccine Development, Production and Usage, US Department of Health and Human Services and US Public Health Service, Bethesda, September, pp. 47–50
86. Kimura, M. and Hikino, N. (1985). Results with a new DTP vaccine in Japan. In *Proceedings of Fourth International Symposium on Pertussis. Dev. Biol. Stand.*, **61**, 511-16
87. Isomura, S., Suzuki, S. and Sato, Y. (1985). Clinical efficacy of the Japanese acellular pertussis vaccine after intrafamilial exposure to pertussis patients. In *Proceedings of Fourth International Symposium on Pertussis. Dev. Biol. Stand.*, **61**, 531–7
88. Aoyama, T., Murase, Y., Gonda, T. and Iwata, T. (1988). Type-specific efficacy of acellular pertussis vaccine. *Am. J. Dis. Child.*, **142**, 40–2
89. Noble, G. R., Bernier, R. H., Esber, E. C., Hardegree, M. C., Hinman, A. R., Klein, D. and Saah, A. J. (1987). Acellular and whole-cell pertussis vaccines in Japan: report of a visit by US Scientists. *J. Am. Med. Assoc.*, **257**, 1351–2
90. Aoyama, T. (1986). Case contact studies of efficacy with the acellular pertussis vaccines in Japan. In *Workshop on Acellular Pertussis Vaccines*, sponsored by the Interagency Group to Monitor Vaccine Development, Production and Usage, US Department of Health and Human Services and US Public Health Service, Bethesda, September, pp. 50–3
91. Anderson, E. L., Belshe, R. B. and Bertram, J. (1988). Differences in reactogenicity and

antigenicity of acellular and standard pertussis vaccines combined with diphtheria and tetanus in infants. *J. Infect. Dis.*, **157**, 731–6

92. Kallings, L. O., Olin, P. and Storsaeter, J. *et al.* (1988). Placebo-controlled trial of two acellular pertussis vaccines in Sweden – protective efficacy and adverse events. *Lancet*, **1**, 955–60
93. Blackwelder, W. C. (1986). Design of clinical trials to demonstrate efficacy with the acellular pertussis vaccines. In *Workshop on Acellular Pertussis Vaccines*, sponsored by the Interagency Group to Monitor Vaccine Development, Production and Usage, US Department of Health and Human Services and US Public Health Service, Bethesda, September, pp. 81–5
94. Bernier, R. H., Onorato, I. A. and Romanus, V. (1986). The design of an efficacy trial of acellular pertussis vaccine in Sweden. In *Workshop on Acellular Pertussis Vaccines*, sponsored by the Interagency Group to Monitor Vaccine Development, Production and Usage, US Department of Health and Human Services and US Public Health Service, Bethesda, September, pp. 85–9
95. Rutter, D. A., Ashworth, L. A. E., Day, A., Funnell, S., Lovell, F. and Robinson, A (1988). Trial of a new acellular pertussis vaccine in healthy adult volunteers. *Vaccine*, **6**, 29-32

2
Meningoccal vaccines

R. A. WALL

INTRODUCTION

The first clinical descriptions of meningococcal disease were published in 1805[1] and 1806[2]. These highlighted the characteristic rash by which clinical infection can be suspected, and the ability of the organism to kill with dramatic speed, a feature which remains equally relevant today.

The predilection of disease for young children, and troops, particularly in wartime, and for most cases to occur in winter and spring was noted[3] before the causal organism was first described in cerebrospinal fluid[4]. It was soon appreciated, however, that the normal habitat of *Neisseria meningitidis* is the nasopharynx, with harmless commensalism the normal host–parasitic relationship. To cause disease a virulent organism must be transmitted to, acquired by, and invade, a susceptible host. These determinants of virulence, and the factors that generate susceptibility, are unclear in spite of more than 80 years of study.

Meningococcal infections remain an important and emotive cause of bacterial disease with significant morbidity and mortality. The recent upsurge in disease prevalence in the UK and elsewhere[5] has provided further impetus to produce effective intervention. Fundamental to achieving this goal is detailed knowledge of the complexity of surface antigens exposed *in vitro* and *in vivo*, and the way in which man, the only host, may respond.

THE CELL ENVELOPE – CLASSIFICATION AND STRUCTURE

N. meningitidis, one of the two recognized pathogens of the genus *Neisseria*, family Neisseriaceae, is a catalase-positive, oxidase-positive, Gram-negative coccus, distinguished from other members of the genus by sugar fermentation and aminopeptidase reactions.

Like other Gram-negative organisms the meningococcus has a complex cell envelope. An inner cytoplasmic membrane, containing the enzymes of the electron transport system and oxidative phosphorylation, systems for active transport of solutes and waste products, as well as synthetic apparatus for the production of external layers, is protected by a rigid peptidoglycan layer and an outer membrane. The latter is composed of proteins, phospholipids and lipo-oligosaccharide, and confers an important protective mechanism for the organism. When isolated from cases of invasive disease, meningococci are almost invariably encapsulated by polysaccharide material which provides an additional protective layer.

Capsules

Antigenic differences in polysaccharide capsular material form the basis of the current classification of *N. meningitidis* into serogroups A, B, C, D, X, Y, Z, 29E, W135, H, I and K. The nature and structure of these polysaccharides have been the subject of intensive study, and their composition has been defined[6].

Serogroup A strains have been responsible for the major epidemics of meningococcal disease worldwide. They were responsible for the major epidemics in all countries prior to and during World War II. Since then the prevalence of group A disease has been very low in the USA and UK, but such strains are responsible for the recurrent epidemics of disease in subsahelian Africa, epidemics in Finland, Russia and Brazil in the 1970s, and more recently epidemics focused on Mecca, Nepal, India and China.

Serogroup C strains are second in frequency in generating epidemic disease, as evidenced by outbreaks in São Paulo, Brazil, and northern Nigeria, and also contribute significantly to endemo-sporadic infection. Their contribution to disease in the UK is currently increasing[7].

Serogroup B strains are responsible for the majority of endemic disease. It has recently become appreciated, however, that certain group B strains, that are genetically closely related, appear to possess greater disease-generating potential than others, causing outbreaks, often prolonged, in many parts of the world, including Cuba, Norway, the UK and elsewhere in Western Europe[5,8].

Disease caused by other serogroups accounts for less than 10% of documented infection, while isolates of H, I, and K have been described only recently from China[9].

Strains isolated from asymptomatic nasopharyngeal carriers are often non-capsulate. This can result from the *in vivo* loss of capsule by capsulate strains[10], which could be relevant to the establishment of a long-term host–parasite relationship, and may contribute to the development of natural immunity by inducing antibodies to non-capsular antigens. In addition, such variation, and the variation in the quantity of capsule production, which can be induced *in vitro* by variation in growth conditions[11], complicates *in vitro* testing of immunity.

Non-capsular antigens

Major outer membrane proteins

Subdivisions based on differences in capsular polysaccharide alone are insufficiently discriminating for the analysis of epidemiology, virulence or protection.

It has long been appreciated that meningococci can be subdivided within serogroups on the basis of immunological differences in non-capsular antigens. Bactericidal assays were developed to produce a serotyping scheme for group C organisms[12] and a similar system[13] was subsequently applied to group B. The nature of the serotype determinants involved was investigated using mild acid extracts of organisms and agar double-diffusion[14]. The serotype antigens were found to consist of complexes of both protein and LPS[15]. Further studies showed that a number of different proteins and LPS antigens were involved in the serological reactivity seen in bactericidal or precipitation reactions[16]. These serotyping antigens could be shared across serogroups[17].

Because these reactions were based on absorbed sera, and the specificities of the antigenic determinants were unknown, these systems were not ideal and many strains were untypable. The application of SDS polyacrylamide gel electrophoresis to ultracentrifuged outer membrane vesicles, released as cell wall blebs during growth *in vitro*, demonstrated only a few proteins present in large amounts[18]. These major outer membrane proteins have been categorized by chymotrypsin ^{125}I-labelled peptide mapping into five different structural classes, that correlate with their apparent molecular weight on Laemmli gels[19]. Antigenic differences in these proteins now form the basis of classification into serotypes and subtypes[20].

Class 2,3 proteins

All meningococcal strains express either a class 2 (apparent molecular weight 40–42 kd) or class 3 (molecular weight 37–39 kd) major outer membrane protein, structurally related to the major outer membrane protein P1 of gonococci. Like the latter, they have a porin function, and the ability to insert into lipid bilayers[21] which may be important in the internalization of meningococci by host cells.

These proteins possess several common hydrophobic peptides embedded within the outer membrane, as well as a number of unique hydrophilic surface-exposed peptides[19]. Antigenic variations residing in the hydrophilic molecules, or related to tertiary conformations, have subsequently been shown to account for some of the previously designated serotype specifications[20].

Because of their stable expression in the outer membrane their invariant expression in epidemiologically related strains[22] and the antigenic variation seen in epidemiologically unrelated strains, these proteins now form the basis of serotyping using monoclonal antibodies[20,23].

Class 1 proteins

The class 1 proteins are a series of closely related trypsin-sensitive deoxycholate-insoluble outer membrane proteins with an apparent molecular weight of 44–46 kd. Serological diversity resides in surface-exposed hydrophilic peptides, while conserved peptides are probably embedded in the outer membrane[19].

Monoclonal antibody analysis of surface-exposed epitopes shows that antigenically related proteins may be shared across serogroups and serotypes[23], while the antigenic variation among epidemiologically unrelated strains, or strains of differing clonal origin as defined by isoenzyme typing[24] serves as an additional subtyping tool within a serotype. Strains can thus be classified on the basis of serogroup, serotype and subtype, i.e. group B, serotype 15, subtype P1.16 (B15 P1.16).

Unlike the class 2,3 proteins the expression of protein 1 in the outer membrane is not invariant. The protein may be either quantitatively diminished or absent in closely related isolates[25]. Although the frequency with which this occurs is unknown, approximately 8% of cases and carrier isolates, from a group A epidemic, failed to express the class 1 protein[26]. In addition group C isolates from the blood and pharynx of an individual patient expressed the class 1, while the isolate from the CSF did not[27]. Thus, although the function of this protein is unknown, expression would not appear to be essential for the organism's integrity or virulence.

Class 5 proteins

The class 5 proteins are a family of outer membrane proteins characterized by their molecular size of 26–30 kd, heat modifiability (protein solubilized at 37°C migrates faster than when solubilized at 100°C in SDS-PAGE) deoxycholate solubility, and sensitivity to proteolytic enzymes[20].

Chymotryptic I-peptide mapping of proteins from different strains shows similar or sometimes identical maps, with conserved hydrophobic, and unique hydrophilic peptides[19]. The occurrence of identical or nearly identical class 5 proteins in strains of different serotypes further explains some of the previously observed cross-reactions[28].

A single strain may produce none, one, or more than one class 5 protein[25], different isolates from the same individual may express different class 5 proteins[25,29] and different class 5 variants may be selected from a single isolate following *in vitro* subculture[30].

Monoclonal antibodies may be used to define these variants, and generate further type specificity, but the hypervariability of these proteins limits their use epidemiologically.

They may, however, have a significant role in pathogenesis. Phenotypically, structurally and genetically they are related to gonococcal PII's[31], proteins which may be involved in cellular attachment and susceptibility to serum killing[32,33]. Since they are highly immunogenic[25,34] variation in their expression may relate to host antibody modulation, or response to their microenvironment.

Class 4 proteins

The meningococcal class 4 proteins, molecular weight 33–34 kd, are resistant to trypsin and other proteolytic enzymes, suggesting only limited surface exposure. Because of their close association in the outer membrane with the class 2,3 protein, from which they are difficult to purify, and their apparent lack of antigenic diversity among strains, they do not contribute to current classification.

Gene cloning and DNA sequencing has demonstrated their close similarity to gonococcal PIII[35], a protein which has been shown to generate antibodies which are capable of blocking the bactericidal effect of antobodies directed against other antigens.

Lipopolysaccharides

Lipopolysaccharides are found exclusively in the outer membrane of Gram-negative organisms. Much of the current knowledge of these biologically potent molecules comes from studies of the family Enterobacteriaceae[36]. Three distinct regions are recognized: hydrophobic lipid A, a core region of complex oligosaccharides linked to lipid A by KDO, and polysaccharide side-chains which are responsible for antigenic diversity.

Neisserial glycolipids differ from those of the Enterobacteriaceae by lacking O side-chains, thus resembling enterobacterial R forms, and may more correctly be termed lipo-oligosaccharides[37]. Each strain of *Neisseria* may generate several, usually two to six, glycolipids, in the molecular weight range 3–7 kd when analysed by SDS-PAGE. Differences in the oligosaccharide, rather than the lipoidal moiety, account for the physical heterogeneity[38].

Monoclonal antibodies have defined a complex array of LOS epitopes reflecting variations in the oligosaccharides and the way they interact with the outer membrane[39]. Some epitopes are common to all LOS, not only in meningococci but also in gonococci and *N. lactamicus*; some are restricted and form the basis for additional serotyping. These serotyping antigens may also be shared both within and across species.

Epitope expression may vary depending on *in vitro* growth conditions[40,41] and the progeny of a single clone may generate several different variants each making a predominant LOS. Cell-to-cell variation has been demonstrated by immunogold electron microscopy[42,43]. While not influencing total antigenic or physicochemical properties such variation may be significant in pathogenesis, since different LOS molecules vary in their interaction with complement[44].

Pili

Meningococci are piliated when first isolated from cultures of cerebrospinal fluid, blood and nasopharynx[45]. Although their function is unclear, pili are expressed *in vivo*[46], and *in vitro* they are associated with attachment to human nasopharyngeal cells[47].

Meningococcal pili are polymers of a pilus polypeptide subunit, which may vary in size from 13 to 22 kd. Pili from some meningococci share structural, biochemical and immunological properties with those from gonococci[48,49]. There is both interstrain and intrastrain antigenic heterogeneity[50] and antigenic variation has been demonstrated during the course of infection[29].

By analogy with *N. gonorrhoeae* meningococcal pili may be involved in a variety of host–pathogen interactions, but their antigenic variation focuses attention on pathogenesis rather than use as an epidemiological tool.

SUSCEPTIBILITY AND IMMUNE RESPONSES

Although many facets are poorly understood, three factors are currently considered to contribute to susceptibility to meningococcal disease: the absence of relevant functional antibody, a failure of complement-dependent mechanisms, or diminished reticuloendothelial function.

Functional antibody

The concept that humoral immune mechanisms are intrinsic to host defence, has its origins in the following observations:

1. the inverse correlation between the age of maximal incidence of disease, and the age-related prevalence of antibody as measured by a bactericidal assay;
2. the successful application of serum therapy in the pre-antibiotic era;
3. that antibodies are produced in response to disease and second episodes are rare.

The currently considered keynote studies which support this concept were undertaken in the American Armed Forces[51]. Bleeding new recruits on entry to an army camp in which an outbreak of group C meningococcal disease was occurring provided a collection of pre-disease sera which were available for testing against their homologous infecting strain. Fifty-one of 54 pre-disease sera lacked antibodies to both the homologous and other disease-associated isolates when measured in a bactericidal assay or by immuno-fluorescence, whilst antibody was detectable in 82% of control sera.

In a further group of 492 basic recruits, 54 were found to lack bactericidal activity against the prevalent disease-producing strains; 44 of these presumed susceptibles acquired meningococci, but in only 13 were the organisms compatible with the case strains. Of these 13, five developed systemic disease.

Thus the presence of bactericidal antibody was correlated with protection from, and absence with susceptibility to, invasive disease.

A wide range of assays have since been used to investigate meningococcal immunology, using a variety of antigens[52]. Although the above investigators did not conclude that complement-dependent lysis is the protective function that antibody affords, bactericidal assays have become accepted as the yardstick by which to assess the critical issue of which antigens are relevant. Significant insight has been gained by investigating immune responses to disease, and the development of natural immunity.

Antigens involved in immune responses

Polysaccharides

The group C polysaccharide is immunogenic in adults and children over 2 years, convalescent from disease[53], and significantly contributes to bactericidal activity[54]. Data on infants are scant but a 4-month-old failed to develop anticapsular or bactericidal antibody[54].

Antipolysaccharide antibodies are thought to be responsible for the majority of bactericidal activity in normal adult sera[55]. This may result from carriage of group C organisms[56], although cross-reacting antigens from enteric organisms such as *Escherichia coli* K92 may contribute[57].

Both carriage of, and disease caused by, group A meningococci, generate specific anticapsular antibody[53] and such antibody has bactericidal activity. Children younger than 18 months serorespond, although the magnitude of the response is significantly less than in adults.

Children in the USA develop significant levels of anti-A antibody early in life, in the absence of disease or detection of circulating group A strains[58]. This has been interpreted as a response to other bacteria expressing cross-reacting antigens.

The role of the group B polysaccharide is less clear. Adults respond to group B disease by generating a four-fold or greater rise in anticapsular antibody as measured by haemagglutination[59] or a radioisotopic antigen-binding assay[54].

The anticapsular response in children may be more variable. Griffiss *et al.*[54] detected a response in only eight of 26 infants, and in these the response was of significantly lower magnitude than in adults. By contrast Leinonen and Frasch[60], using an ELISA assay to study children aged 6 months to 17 years, showed high levels of IgG and IgM in all acute-phase sera, with a significant rise in IgM but not IgG in convalescence, irrespective of age.

Whatever the anticapsular response, the contribution it makes to the bactericidal antibody that develops in most individuals following disease, or in normal adults, is more controversial. All the children studied by Griffiss *et al.*[54] developed bactericidal antibody but antipolysaccharide antibody contributed only 35%. Kasper *et al.*[61] showed that while anticapsular antibody developed during disease, convalescent sera and affinity-purified anticapsular antibody did not kill all group B strains. Similarly Holten *et al.*[62] demonstrated that carriage of group B meningococci did not generate antibodies bactericidal for heterologous group B strains. These findings thus suggest the importance of noncapsular antigens in bactericidal activity. Frasch[55], however, suggests that the majority of the bactericidal activity present in 95% of adults is directed against the capsule. This disparity may be methodological, and complement-dependent, since Zollinger and Mandrell[63] demonstrated that human antibody to group B polysaccharide was bactericidal with rabbit complement, but had little activity with human complement. Human antibodies that were bactericidal with human complement appeared to be primarily directed against noncapsular antigens.

Other antigens

Natural infection with meningococci of one serogroup induces bactericidal antibody with a broader spectrum than the capsular polysaccharide alone[51,56,61]. Initial studies using a haemagglutination assay[64] showed that outer membrane proteins and lipopolysaccharides contributed to the immune response in both disease and carriage.

Outer membrane proteins

The development of further classification of meningococci into serotypes within serogroups led to the investigation of serotype antigens and immune responses[65]. Efforts concentrated on serotype 2 strains, which were the major cause of disease at this time. The serotype antigen was shown by an ELISA technique to be immunogenic in disease, irrespective of age, and during carriage in army recruits. Normal sera had detectable antibody which increased with age.

Jones and Eldridge[66] demonstrated that carriage of serogroup W135, serotype 2 meningococci generated antiserotype antibody, and that this was associated with the development of bactericidal antibody against a group B serotype 2 strain. These antibodies are not, however, protective against other serotypes.

The precise nature of the antigens involved was unclear because of the problems separating different components of the outer membrane. The advent of improved methods of protein separation and purification, accompanied by the use of monoclonal antibodies and immunoblotting, has helped to resolve antigenic specificities and has further highlighted the complexities of the immune response.

Poolman *et al.*[67] examined immune responses by the direct application of acute and convalescent sera to outer membrane complexes separated by SDS-PAGE, or by an ELISA. Strong reactions were detected in convalescent sera against class 5 proteins and pili, although individual sera recognized LPS and other (minor) proteins. Class 5 proteins induced strain-specific immune responses. Cross-reactions were seen in minor proteins, LPS, and pili, these accounting for more than 50% of the activity detected in ELISA. The denaturing effect of SDS-PAGE limited recognition of antibodies to class 2,3 proteins. These and other proteins are immunogenic in some sera when analysed by a competitive solid-phase radioimmunoassay[68]. Using an outer membrane complex from a serotype 2a subtype P1.2 strain, 35 acute and convalescent sera were investigated for their ability to inhibit monoclonal antibody binding to the class 1, 2, and 5 proteins. Few of the acute sera, but most of the convalescent sera, inhibited all three monoclonals, greatest activity being demonstrable against the class 5 protein. Three convalescent sera were tested against group B15 P1.16 membranes. In two of the three no antibodies to the P1.16 epitope were seen, while only one serum recognized both epitopes.

This lack of response to both antigens has been confirmed in larger studies using purified proteins in a competitive ELISA[69,70]. Thirty-nine per cent of cases and 53% of carriers of B15 P1.16 meningococci failed to make detectable antibody to the class 3 protein, while 55% of cases and 78% of carriers failed to make detectable antibody to the class 1 protein. Although monoclonal antibodies to the class 1, 3 and 5 proteins are bactericidal *in vitro*, the above findings do not support their suitability as vaccine candidates.

ELISA assays[71,72] and immunoblotting[73,74] show that in convalescence antibodies are induced to other, cross-reacting, protein antigens, the nature of which requires investigation.

Lipopolysaccharides (LOS)

Homologous and heterologous responses have been detected in sera from patients convalescent from B and C disease[64,67] and carriers[64,66]. These anti-LOS antibodies contribute to the bactericidal activity demonstrable in children with group B disease[54]. The precise determinants involved have proven difficult to resolve because of the complex immunochemical structure of neisserial LOS, but have recently been assigned to LOS of defined molecular weight[75].

These antigenic determinants are not confined to *N. meningitidis*. Several studies have shown that children who become colonized with *N. lactamicus* may develop cross-reactive bactericidal antibodies against meningococci[56,76].

An analysis of LOS from *N. lactamicus* and group A meningococci using SDS-PAGE and monoclonal antibodies suggests that shared LOS epitopes may play an important role in such natural immunity[77].

Blocking antibodies

Theoretically, absent functional antibody could result from lack of appropriate antigenic exposure, or factors that block normal humoral defence. Sera from patients with meningococcal disease have been shown to inhibit the bactericidal activity of normal sera[78]. Griffiss[79] demonstrated that strain-specific IgA inhibited the bactericidal activity of IgG and IgM in sera taken 12–33 days after the onset of meningococcal disease. Subsequently[80] 24 of 28 individuals whose acute phase sera lacked bactericidal activity against their infecting strain, had this restored by removal of IgA. The bactericidal antibody was largely IgM. IgA can block IgG depending on the relative ratios, but blocking of IgM is non-competitive and depends on the ratio of IgA to target antigen[81]. While the nature of these putatitve antigens is unknown, the high levels of antipolysaccharide IgA present in 16% of the acute-phase sera studied by Kahyty *et al.*[53], suggest that capsular antigens may be involved. LOS has also been suggested[82]. The origin of such determinants is also unknown. One hypothesis suggests cotemporal mucosal colonization with cross-reacting enteric bacteria[82]. Equally plausible is variation in an individual's response to the meningococcus alone, with a subset of the population responding by a preferential increase in IgA.

Antibody-mediated blocking may also arise by antibodies to non-protective antigens hindering the access of protective antibody. Such a mechanism has been shown with *N. gonorrhoeae*, in which the target of blocking antibody is PIII[83]. The epitopes responsible have been shown by monoclonal antibodies to be expressed on the meningococcal class 4 protein[84]. This suggests not only a further mechanism by which susceptibility could be induced, but also a potential problem with vaccines containing this protein.

Complement deficiencies

Late complement component deficiency (LCCD)

The concept of the importance of complement-dependent lysis as a major host defence mechanism against meningococcal infection gained support by the recognition of the striking correlation of terminal complement pathway deficiencies and neisserial disease[85–89]. A review of 242 individuals with any abnormality of the complement cascade[90] revealed 61 who had suffered 90 episodes of invasive meningococcal disease and 23 with DGI. The majority of these patients lacked C_5, C_6, C_7 or C_8, and in these, invasive neisserial infection occurred to the virtual exclusion of other bacteria.

Such patients tended to be older, had a lower mortality and a higher frequency of group Y disease than the general population. About half of these individuals suffered multiple episodes. Since LCCD serum supports opsonization–phagocytosis[91], yet individuals develop disease in spite of antibody to their infecting strain[92], it seems that impaired complement-dependent lysis permits invasive disease but unimpaired phagocytosis reduces mortality. The relative contribution of lysis and phagocytosis may, however, be organism-dependent, as evidenced by the high frequency of group Y disease. Using C8-depleted and pooled human sera (PHS) Ross *et al.*[93] showed that serogroups B and 29E, but not A, C, Y or W135, were ingested and killed by human neutrophils in C8-depleted PHS. Conversely group B meningococci were resistant to complement-dependent bactericidal activity whereas group Y were susceptible. Non-correlation of killing by phagocytosis or lysis of a single strain suggested that these defence mechanisms may be initiated by different antigens. Of importance, vaccinating a C8-deficient individual with AC vaccine increased the phagocytic killing of these serogroups.

The frequency of LCCD deficiencies in the general population is very low (<0.03%)[94]. While deficiency is high in those with recurrent disease, the precise frequency in patients presenting with a first episode of meningococcal disease is unclear, with limited studies giving frequencies of 1% in epidemic disease in childhood[95] to 15% in sporadic cases in adults[96].

Other complement deficiencies

The association of meningococcal infection with complement deficiencies is not confined to the terminal pathway but may be seen in other deficiencies as part of a more general susceptibility to pyogenic bacteria.

Because of the central role of C_3 in the complement cascade, individuals with C_3 deficiency[97] or uncontrolled C_3 activation by C_3 nephritic factor[98], or factor I deficiency[99] may suffer severe disease. C_1-, C_4-, C_2-deficient individuals may have an increased susceptibility to meningococci, but are probably afforded some protection by an intact alternative pathway[90].

The critical importance of the alternative pathway is suggested by recent descriptions of properdin deficiency[100–102]. This disorder, exhibiting an X-linked mode of inheritance, is associated with rapidly fatal meningococcal infection. Shifting the burden of host defence to antibody-mediated classic pathway activation by vaccination has a theoretical role in such individuals[102] although a role in other proximal defects is less clear.

CURRENTLY/AVAILABLE VACCINES

Introduction

Early attempts to produce meningococcal vaccines were unsuccessful. A group A polysaccharide vaccine was non-immunogenic[103] probably because

Table 1 Geometric mean antibody levels (μg/ml) to groups A and C polysaccharide at different ages

Age	*Anti-A*	*Anti-C*
3 months	0.37	<0.11
7 months	0.19	<0.11
12 months	0.19	<0.11
18 months	0.23	<0.11
2–5 years	0.79	0.18
6–8 years	1.37	0.32
15–25 years	4.70	6.20

Adapted from ref. 58.

of its molecular size. The studies in the American armed forces in the 1960s led to the preparation of group-specific polysaccharides by a new method involving cetavlon precipitation which produced polysaccharide with a molecular weight above 100 kd. Those preparations were clearly immunogenic in adult volunteers, inducing both haemagglutinating and bactericidal antibody in 51 of 53 who received the group A vaccine, and all 145 who received group C.

Since then the polysaccharides have been standardized by chemical criteria, to exclude contaminating protein and LPS, and to confirm the critical molecular size.

Vaccine responses have been quantified mainly by a sensitive radioactive antigen binding assay[105] capable of detecting 0.08 μg of anti-C protein per millilitre and 0.13 μg of anti-A per millilitre[58]. While an accurate correlation between the level achieved and protection is not known, a level of 2 μg/ml has been suggested[106], based on the age-specific mean levels detected in the normal population (Table 1) and the vaccine-induced levels in children apparently protected.

Group A polysaccharide vaccine

Immunogenicity

Response to the group A polysaccharide is dependent on age, pre-existing antibody levels, dose and molecular weight. As long as the latter is above 100 000, age is the most important variable.

In immunogenicity studies[107] adults (with a mean pre-immunization level of 4.7 μg/ml) generated an eight-fold rise in antibody levels with 100% seroconversion. Primary immunization at age 3 months, however, did not result in a significant rise in antibody levels. By age 7 months a measurable response was detectable at a low level (mean level 0.39 μg/ml) with two-thirds of the recipients seroconverting. Increasing responses were detected with increasing age, those aged 6–8 years achieving one-quarter of the adult response, and the latter being seen by age 15 years.

Booster doses were given to infants[107] in an attempt to improve their response. Those receiving an initial dose at age 3 months showed a significant response to revaccination at 7 or 12 months, with geometric mean titres being eight-fold higher, and percentage seroconversions 50% higher than with primary immunizations at these ages.

In field trials in Finland infants aged less than 18 months therefore received two doses of vaccine 2 months apart[106]. Fifty per cent of children aged 3–5 months generated a two-fold rise in antibody after the first injection, but although a booster induced a further two-fold rise, the mean levels of antibody remained below 1 μg/ml.

In children aged 6–11 months, vaccination induced a five-fold increase after the first injection, and a seven-fold increase after the booster, the mean level post-booster being 2.47 μg/ml. The first injection in children aged 12–17 months induced a higher antibody response with the booster giving little further effect.

These responses seen in the period shortly after vaccination suggest that during an epidemic nearly all age groups can be afforded protection, including infants. How long the response lasts, however, is critical for determining its wider application and incorporation in standard immunization schedules. This has been followed in Finland and is clearly dependent on the age of the vaccinee and the height of the initial response[106].

In infants antibody levels after two doses remained elevated for 1 year in those under 12 months, and 2 years in those aged 12–17 months. The single dose given to children aged 18–23 months induced elevated levels for only 1 year. The higher post-vaccination levels of older children declined more slowly, with 67% of those aged 4 years, and 95% of those aged 13–14 years still having levels above 2 μg/ml after 3 years. These percentages compare with the 50% and 60%, respectively, for age-matched controls. The duration of elevated levels appears predictable for the IgM : IgG ratio of antipolysaccharide antibody detectable 14 days after vaccination[108], a high ratio indicating a short persistence, whereas a low ratio was associated with long persistence. These findings are consistent with the hypothesis that significant IgG responses are associated with prior priming of the immune system by naturally acquired antigens, whereas in those lacking such previous contacts shorter-lived IgM responses predominate.

The duration of antibody response is less clear in other geographical settings. Antibody levels measured by haemagglutination in a Nigerian population showed a rapid decline such that 2 years post-vaccination there was no difference in levels between vaccinees and age-matched controls[109]. This finding differs from those using haemagglutination assays in the USA[110]. When the same sera were pooled and tested by radioimmunoassay, however, higher levels of antipolysaccharide antibody were detected. It is thus unclear whether these observed differences are methodological or meaningful.

Efficacy

The first study of the group A vaccine, undertaken in 1971 in Nigeria, failed to show protection[111]. This was probably related to the low molecular weight of the polysaccharide and depolymerization at high ambient temperatures. Subsequent studies in Egyptian schoolchildren aged 6–15 years[112], in Sudanese under the age of 21 years[113], Finnish children[114], and Finnish army recruits[115] have affirmed that the vaccine is effective in aborting epidemics in all age groups.

Data are more limited on the duration of protection in a setting of ongoing exposure or re-exposure to group A organisms. In a case–control study in Burkino Faso[116] vaccine efficacy was shown to be 87% 1 year after vaccination; a figure comparable to the 89% protection shown in Finnish army recruits. Efficacy declined, however, to 70% at 2 years and 54% at 3 years. In keeping with immunogenicity data, protection was strongly related to age at the time of vaccination. In those aged over 4 years efficacy had fallen to 67% over 3 years, whilst in those under 4 years efficacy was 52% at 2 years and only 8% at 3 years.

Similar overall findings have been reported from China[117] and The Gambia[118].

An additional element of protection is afforded by vaccination if this reduces nasopharyngeal acquisition and thus interrupts transmission. The data available on the effects of group A vaccine on carriage are difficult to interpret. In Egyptian schoolchildren vaccination reduced meningococcal acquisition and shortened carriage[119], but did not appear to do so in northern Nigeria[120,121]; or The Gambia[122].

Group C polysaccharide vaccine

Immunogenicity

As with the group A vaccine, serological responses to group C vaccine are similarly dependent on dose, pre-existing antibody levels, and age. Adults with preimmunization levels of 6.2 μg/ml responded with a five-to-six-fold increase, whilst children, although responding to vaccination even at 3 months, produced significantly lower levels ranging from 0.42 μg/ml at this age, to 3.10 μg/ml at age 18 months[58,107,123,124]. Unlike group A vaccine no booster effect has been detected. On the contrary, it seems that, depending on the dose and timing of the second injection, there is evidence of depressed responsiveness to boosters compared to primary immunizations. Adults receiving 0.032–0.064 μg of C polysaccharide contaminating a group A vaccine failed to mount as high a response when given a standard dose of 50 μg of C polysaccharide 2 weeks later, as those receiving primary immunization[125]. A decreased antibody response was also observed in infants who had been immunized with 25 μg or more at age 3 months when they were reimmunized at 7 or 12 months compared with primary immunizations[107]. However, no such depression was seen with a 10 μg dose, hyporesponsiveness did not recur on revaccination at age 2 years, and such infants were not apparently more susceptible to disease[126].

Any vaccine response induced in children also declines rapidly[127]. Although infants who had been immunized at age 7 months produced significant peak antibody levels after reimmunization at 2 years and 5½ years such levels rapidly declined to below the 2 μg/ml associated with protection[128].

Efficacy of group C vaccine

Group C polysaccharide vaccines were developed under the impetus of outbreaks of disease in the US military. Field trials in the US army in 1969–

70 indicated that vaccination afforded 90% protection[129] and also reduced the nasopharyngeal acquisition of group C meningococci[130–132]. Since then the routine use of the vaccine in army recruits has essentially eliminated group C disease in this population. The vaccine is less successful in children. Approximately 67 000 Brazilians aged 6–35 months received 50 μg polysaccharide during the course of a group C epidemic in São Paulo[126]. By comparison with a control group the vaccine was 75% effective in those aged over 2 years, but showed no protection below this age.

Group Y, W135 polysaccharide vaccines

Although groups Y and W135 are uncommon causes of disease in the UK, relative increases in other populations[133] in particular the US military[134], have provided the impetus for developing vaccines. The two capsules are structurally similar. Immunogenicity studies of the vaccines given separately or together showed the induction of significant homologous and heterologous binding and bactericidal antibody[134] which declined only slowly over 6 months. Disease is too infrequent to demonstrate the efficacy of these preparations in field trials, but based on their immunogenicity they have been incorporated into a tetravalent ACYW135 vaccine.

Genetic control of immune response to polysaccharides

Although age of the vaccinee and molecular weight of the vaccine appear to be major determinants, basic knowledge of immune responses to polysaccharides, in particular their ontogeny, is relatively limited[135]. There is, however, increasing evidence that such responses may vary in relation to host genetics.

Whittle *et al.*[136] noted that patients recovered from serogroup A disease, and their siblings, showed a decreased response to group C polysaccharide compared with controls. An association between Km (1) allotype and response to group C polysaccharide in infants[137] and to group B polysaccharide in adults[138] was subsequently noted. Ig allotypes have been further investigated[139] concentrating on G2m(n) because of its location on the heavy chain of IgG2 and the predominance of this subclass in immune responses to polysaccharides[140]. Caucasian adults expressing G2m(n) developed higher anti-group C levels than those lacking G2m(n), although no effect was seen for group A.

The relative contribution of these, and other, variations in response to polysaccharides[141] to vaccine failure or host susceptibility are unknown but merit further study.

Vaccine use

Both groups A and C vaccines are capable of interrupting epidemic disease. In this setting group A vaccine may be given to all age groups with optimally two doses 2–3 months apart to those under 18 months. The age[114] and extent[120,142] of the target population may vary depending on financial, logistic, or geographical constraints. Group C vaccine may be used in similar settings for those over 2 years.

A/C vaccine should be offered to travellers to epidemic zones, while A, C, Y, W135 should be considered for those with complement pathway deficiencies or decreased splenic function.

Their use in endemic disease, or as part of a long-term strategy to prevent epidemics, is more controversial. In the former problems arise defining the population at risk and the delay in effecting protection. In the latter, although repeated vaccinations can induce protection throughout early childhood[128], the logistics may be prohibitive, and the need for repeated immunization in other age groups is not known.

DEVELOPMENT OF NEW VACCINES

Polysaccharides

Modifications to existing vaccines

The poor responses of children to the vaccines currently available clearly limits their wider application. One means to overcome this lack of immunogenicity is evident from studies on the other major pathogen of meningitis in childhood, *Haemophilus influenzae*, Covalent linking of *H. influenzae* type b polysaccharide to a protein carrier has generated a vaccine which elicits a response characteristic of T helper cell activation with enhanced immunogenicity in young infants, accompanied by a maturation of class-specific immunity with a predominance of IgG[143,144]. Such an approach has shown significant enhancement of immunogenicity in experimental animals immunized with groups A and C polysaccharides conjugated to tetanus toxoid[145,146], although greater attention has been given to other protein carriers (see below).

Group B polysaccharide

Group B polysaccharide prepared in the same way as groups A and C failed to elicit an immune response in volunteers, irrespective of its molecular weight or the use of adjuvants[147], and was non-immunogenic in tetanus toxoid conjugates[146].

The reasons for such poor immunogenicity in artificial or natural immunization remain unclear. The polysaccharide is a homopolymer of α(2–8)-linked sialic acid with structural similarities to the sialic acid oligomers found on human foetal glycopeptides[148]. A poor response could theoretically result from immune tolerance, with conformational determinants on the secondary or tertiary structure of the polysaccharide being more important in generating antibody than the primary structure[149]. One approach to developing a more immunogenic vaccine has been to stabilize the three-dimensional structure of the capsule in a non-covalent complex with outer membrane protein, either alone[150] or in conjunction with aluminium ions which, by binding strongly to the polysaccharide, inhibit internal esterification and neuraminidase degradation[151]. The former preparations have induced only short-lived IgM antibodies of low avidity. The latter are undergoing phase 1 trials.

An alternative approach has been to modify the polysaccharide structure by replacing *N*-acetyl groups with *N*-propionyl groups, and conjugating the modification to tetanus toxoid[152]. This preparation was immunogenic in experimental animals.

Outer membrane proteins

Because of the poor immunogenicity of, and theoretical objections to, the group B polysaccharide, considerable attention has been given to exploring the potential of other surface antigens. The demonstrable immune response to the major outer membrane proteins, in both disease and carriage, has generated a series of studies on their safety, immunogenicity and efficacy in animals and man.

Frasch and Robbins[153] extracted a serotype 2 strain in lithium chloride and used ultracentrifugation to yield 60 nm outer membrane vesicles. LPS was removed by detergent, and protein recovered by ethanol precipitation. This particulate preparation, consisting mainly of the class 2 protein, was immunogenic in guinea pigs[153], and a mouse bacteraemia model[154] showed protection for more than 4 months which was serotype-specific. Subsequent studies in man, however, showed that while these insoluble vaccines were safe, they were poorly immunogenic[55].

Outer membrane proteins were subsequently shown to be made soluble by the addition of group B polysaccharide[55]. Such non-covalent complexes of polysaccharides and proteins were more immunogenic and demonstrated greater protection in animal models than particulate vaccines.

Zollinger *et al.*[150] demonstrated that a group B serotype 2 complex containing four or five proteins including the major outer membrane protein, elicited a greater than four-fold increase in antipolysaccharide antibodies in six of eight adult volunteers, and serotype-specific antibodies in seven of eight. By comparison with previous preparations the serotype response had been improved by the presence of polysaccharide.

Several different methods of preparing the outer membrane proteins have now been developed, including their direct solubilization by sodium deoxycholate[155] the use of LPS depleted membrane vessicles[156], solubilization in Empigen BB[157], and extraction with Zwittergent 4–14[158].

Group B serotype 2 outer membrane vesicle preparations induced binding and bactericidal antibodies in adults[55]. A clinical trial of such a preparation was undertaken in children and adults in South Africa[159]. Seventy per cent of adults and older children generated bactericidal antibody, but the response was significantly less in young children, and any bactericidal response lasted less than a year. The study did not have the power to document efficacy. Similar vaccine adsorbed onto aluminium hydroxide had improved immunogenicity, although no polysaccharide-specific antibody was detected[160].

A group B 2a outer membrane vesicle vaccine trial was carried out in Norway in 1981–82. Responses have been evaluated by bactericidal reactions and immunoblotting[161]. SDS-PAGE of the preparation revealed class 1, 2, 4 and 5 proteins. Considerable individual heterogeneity in the antibody response was seen 6 weeks after vaccination, some individuals recognizing only one component, others multiple. Major immunoreactive components were the class 1 and class 5 proteins, but detecting reactions with the class 2 protein would not be expected in this system. Antipilus antibody was detected in individuals identified as meningococcal carriers, highlighting the problems of concomitant carriage in such studies. There was some correlation between high bactericidal antibody titres and immunoreactivity in the class I protein. The antibody responses of adult volunteers given a vaccine containing A, C, Y, W135 polysaccharides non-covalently complexed with serotype 2b P1.2 and 15 P1.16 outer membrane proteins prepared with Empigen have also been studied in Norway[72]. The vaccine contained the class 1 and 3 proteins of the 15 P1.16 strain, the class 1, class 2, and class 5 proteins of the 2b P1.2, and unspecified proteins of 60–70 kd. Although 70% of vaccinees responded by binding and bactericidal assays, the results are again complicated by concomitant meningococcal carriage, since antibody levels were significantly higher in carriers.

While these studies demonstrate that protein–polysaccharide complexes can be immunogenic, they also highlight the many probelms that such vaccines pose, related either to their formulation or to the method of their assessment.

Firstly they are crude preparations with variable amounts of residual LPS, different amounts of the major outer membrane proteins, and sometimes other proteins. Not only could each of these variables influence immunogenicity and protection, but the contribution of each is not assessable and quality control problematic. They are largely serotype-specific vaccines requiring modification as epidemiological change dictates. Although some cross-protection may be exhibited by the class 1 protein[23] its variable expression[25] and poor induction of response in natural infection[70] are limitations. A vaccine containing the class 4 protein may induce blocking antibodies, while the class 5 proteins are not only hypervariable but also may divert responses from other antigens[162].

Secondly, unlike the situation with polysaccharide vaccines in which a measurable antipolysaccharide response can be correlated with efficacy, with these preparations the only relevant *in vitro* determinant of response is a functional assay. Complement-dependent lysis has been mainly used, but opsonizing antibody may be more relevant than previously appreciated[93]. However, whatever functional assay is studied, both the choice of strain, with its known antigenic repertoire, and its growth conditions, are critical. The expression of surface molecules may vary depending on growth rates[163] or nutrient limitation, including iron[74,164], glucose, cysteine and oxygen[165]. Such variables may be fundamental to protection but the *in vivo* expression of surface structures has only recently started to be explored[166].

Other potential antigens

The presence of antigenic heterogeneity among major proteins of different strains, and of antigenic hypervariability within the progeny of a single strain, has provided the impetus to demonstrate stable antigens which may be cross-reactive and therefore potentially cross-protective among strains of different serogroups and serotypes.

Neisserial H8 antigen

Cannon *et al.*[167] demonstrated a surface-exposed outer membrane protein, recognizable by its characteristic migration pattern in SDS-PAGE, molecular weight 22–30 kd, and staining with silver nitrate but not Coumassie blue, in pathogenic *Neisseria* but not in commensals. Further studies[168] demonstrated its immunogenicity in both invasive gonococcal and meningococcal disease. Early enthusiasm has waned, however, after monoclonals were shown to be lacking bactericidal activity *in vitro*, or in an animal model[169].

70 kd Common antigen

Mice immunized with live meningococci respond vigorously to an antigen of molecular weight 70 kd, which appears to be common to all pathogenic and most commensal *Neisseria*[170]. The antigen appears surface-exposed since purified antibody is bactericidal for gonococci and binds to the gonococcal surface in immunogold electron microscopy[171]. Meningococcal carriage is thought to generate antibodies against this protein[172], but its function and potential protective role are as yet unknown.

Iron-regulated proteins

Under conditions of iron limitation *in vitro* meningococci express new proteins in the outer membrane[74,164]. SDS-PAGE of the outer membrane proteins of *Pseudomonas aeruginosa* examined directly from patients without *in vitro* passage suggests that this organism grows *in vivo* under iron limitation[173]. While similar analyses of *N. meningitidis* have yet to be performed, Western blotting of sera from patients with invasive menginococcal disease suggests that iron regulated proteins of 37, 70 and 94 kd are both expressed *in vivo* and antigenic[74].

Their cross-reactivity and potential role in protection are being explored (Wall, unpublished).

CONCLUSION

The currently available groups A and C polysaccharide vaccines have proven efficacy but their use remains restricted, pending the availability of more immunogenic preparations. Group B vaccines, at a stage of development that permits field trials, are relatively crude and generate multiple problems in production and assessment. The ideal menginococcal vaccine should be safe, immunogenic in early infancy and produce prolonged immunity. The continued collaboration between clinical and basic science, focusing on molecules which are not subject to antigenic or phenotypic change, which are expressed *in vivo* and accessible to immune attack, may make this ideal achievable.

REFERENCES

1. Vieusseaux, M. (1805). Memoire sur le maladie qui a regne a Geneve au printemps de 1805. *J. Med. Chirurg. Pharmacie*, **II**, 163–5
2. Danielson, L. and Mann, E. (1806). Medical and agricultural register, vol. 1; no. 5; quoted in *Rev. Infect. Dis.*, (1983), **5**, 969–72
3. Hirsch, A. (1886). *Handbook of Geographical and Historical Pathology*, Vol. 3, p. 547 (London: New Sydenham Soc.) Pub. New Sydenham Soc. No. 117
4. Weichselbaum, A. (1887). Uber die aetiologie der akuten meningitis cerebrospinalis. *Fortschr. Med.*, **5**, 573–5
5. Poolman, J. T., Lind, I., Jonsdottir, K., Forholm, L. D., Jones, D. M. and Zanen, H. C. (1986). Meningococcal serotypes and serogroup B disease in North West Europe. *Lancet*, **2**, 555–8
6. Gotschlich, E. C. (1984). Meningococcal meningitis. In Germanier, R. (ed.), *Bacterial Vaccines*, pp. 237–55. (New York and London: Academic Press)
7. Jones, D. M. (1988). Epidemiology of meningococcal infection in England and Wales. *J. Med. Microbiol.*, **26**, 165–8
8. Caugant, D. A., Froholm, L. O., Borre, K., Holten, E., Frasch, C. E., Mocca, L. F., Zollinger, W. D. and Selander, R. K. (1986). Intercontinental spread of a genetically distinctive complex of clones of *Neisseria meningitidis* causing epidemic disease. *Proc. Natl. Acad. Sci. USA*, **83**, 4927–31
9. Shao-Qing, D., Ren-Bang, Y. and Huan-Chun, Z. (1981). Three new serogroups of *Neisseria meningitidis*. *J. Biol. Stand.*, **9**, 307–15
10. Wall, R. A., Borriello, S. P., Reid, P., Gupta, R., Evans, R. and Jones, D. M. (1988). Isoenzyme analysis of *Neisseria meningitidis* by polyacrylamide gel electrophoresis and its application to epidemiological studies in England. *J. Med. Microbiol.*, **27**, xiii
11. Masson, L. and Holbein, B. E. (1985). Influence of environmental conditions on serogroup B *Neisseria meningitidis* capsular polysaccharide levels. In Schoolnik, G. K. (ed.), *The Pathogenic Neisseria*, pp. 571–8. (Washington, DC: American Society for Microbiology)
12. Gold, R. and Wyle, F. A. (1970). New classification of *Neisseria meningitidis* by means of bactericidal reactions. *Infect. Immun.*, **1**, 479–84
13. Frasch, C. E. and Chapman, S. S. (1972). Classification of *Neisseria meningitidis* group B into distinct serotypes. I. Serological typing by a microbactericidal method. *Infect. Immun.*, **5**, 98–102
14. Frasch, C. E. and Chapman, S. S. (1972). Classification of *Neisseria meningitidis* group B into distinct serotypes. II. Extraction of type specific antigens for serotyping by precipitin techniques. *Infect. Immun.*, **6**, 127–33
15. Zollinger, W. D., Kasper, D. L., Veltri, B. J. and Artenstein, M. S. (1972). Isolation and characterisation of native cell wall complex from *Neisseria meningitidis*. *Infect. Immun.*, **6**, 835–51
16. Poolman, J. T., Hopman, C. T. P. and Zanen, H. C. (1980). Immunochemical characterisation of *Neisseria meningitidis* serotype antigens by immunodiffusion and SDS-polyacrylamide gel electrophoresis immunoperoxidase techniques and the distribution of serotypes among cases and carriers. *J. Gen. Microbiol.*, **116**, 465–73
17. Zollinger, W. D. and Mandrell, R. E. (1977). Outer membrane protein and lipopolysaccharide serotyping of *Neisseria meningitidis* by inhibition of a solid phase radioimmunoassay. *Infect. Immun.* **18**, 424–33
18. Frasch, C. E., McNelis, R. M. and Gotschlich, E. C. (1976). Strain specific variation in the protein and lipopolysaccharide composition of the group B meningococcal outer membrane. *J. Bacteriol.*, **127**, 973–81
19. Tsai, C. M., Frasch, C. E. and Mocca, L. F. (1981). Five structural classes of major outer membrane proteins in *Neisseria meningitidis*. *J. Bacteriol.*, **146**, 69–78
20. Frasch, C. E., Zollinger, W. D. and Poolman, J. T. (1985). Serotype antigens of *Neisseria meningitidis* and a proposed scheme for designation of serotypes. *Rev. Infect. Dis.*, **7**, 504–10
21. Lynch, E. C., Blake, M. S., Gotschlich, E. C. and Mawo, A. (1984). Studies on porins spontaneously transferred from whole cells and reconstituted from purified proteins of *Neisseria gonorrhoeae* and *Neisseria meningitidis*. *Biophys. J.*, **45**, 104–107

22. Frasch, C. E. and Mocca, L. F. (1982). Strains of *Neisseria meningitidis* isolated from patients and their close contacts. *Infect. Immun.*, **37**, 155–9
23. Abdillahi, H. and Poolman, J. T. (1988). *Neisseria meningitidis* group B serosubtyping using monoclonal antibodies in whole-cell ELISA. *Microbiol. Pathogen.*, **4**, 27–32
24. Crowe, B. A., Abdillahi, H., Poolman, J. T. and Achtman, M. (1988). Correlation of serological typing and cloning typing methods for *Neisseria meningitidis* sero-group A. *J. Med. Microbiol.*, **26**, 183–4
25. Poolman, J. T., De Marie, S. and Zanen, H. C. (1980). Variability of low molecular weight, heat modification outer membrane proteins of *Neisseria meningitidis. Infect. Immun.*, **30**, 642–8
26. Achtman, M., Crowe, B. A., Olyhoek, A., Strittmater, W. and Morlli, G. (1988). Recent results on epidemic meningococcal meningitidis. *J. Med. Microbiol.*, **26**, 172–7
27. Wall, R. A., unpublished
28. Poolman, J. T., Hopman, C. T. P. and Zanen, H. C. (1982). Problems in the definition of meningococcal serotypes. *FEMS Microbiol. Lett.*, **13**, 339–48
29. Tinsley, C. R. and Heckels, J. E. (1986). Variation in the expression of pili and outer membrane protein by *Neisseria meningitidis* during the course of meningococcal infection. *J. Gen. Microbiol.*, **132**, 2483–90
30. Poolman, J. T., Hopman, C. T. P. and Zanen, H. C. (1985). Colony variants of *Neisseria meningitidis* strain 2996 (B:2b:P1.2): Influence of class 5 outer membrane proteins and lipopolysaccharides. *J. Med. Microbiol.*, **19**, 203–9
31. Kawula, T. H., Aho, E. L., Barritt, D. S., Klapper, D. G. and Cannon, J. G. (1988). Reversible phase variation of expression of *Neisseria meningitidis* class 5 outer membrane proteins and their relationship to gonococcal proteins. II. *Infect. Immun.*, **56**, 380–6
32. Lambden, P. R., Heckels, J. E., James, L. T. and Watt, P. J. (1979). Variations in surface protein composition associated with virulence properties in opacity types of *Neisseria gonorrhoeae. J. Gen. Microbiol.*, **114**, 305–12
33. Virji, M. and Heckels, J. E. (1986). The effect of protein II and pili on the interaction of *Neisseria gonorrhoeae* with human polymorphonuclear leucocytes. *J. Gen. Microbiol.*, **132**, 503–12
34. Achtman, M., Neibert, M., Crowe, B. A., Strittmatter, W., Kusecek, B., Weyse, E., Walsh, M. J., Slawig, B., Morelli, G., Moll, A. and Blake, M. (1988). Purification and characterization of eight class 5 outer membrane protein variants from a clone of *Neisseria meningitidis* serogroup A. *J. Exp. Med.*, **168**, 507–25
35. Gotschlich, E. C. (1988). Molecular studies of Neisserial outer membrane proteins. Abstracts of the Sixth International Pathogenic Neisseria Conference, Atlanta Georgia, p. 152
36. Hitchcock, P. J., Leive, L., Makela, P. H., Rietschel, E. T., Strittmater, W. and Morrison, D. C. (1986). Lipopolysaccharide nomenclature – past, present and future. *J. Bacteriol.*, **166**, 699–705
37. Griffiss, J. M., Schneider, H., Mandrell, R. E., Yamasaki, R., Jarvis, G. A., Kim, J. J., Gibson, B. W., Hamadeh, R. and Apicella, M. A. (1988). Lipooligosaccharides: the principal glycolipids of the neisserial outer membrane. *Rev. Infect. Dis.*, **10**, S287–S295
38. Griffiss, J. M., O'Brien, J. P., Jamasaki, R., Williams, G. D., Rice, P. A. and Schneider, H. (1987). Physical heterogeneity of neisserial lipooligosaccharides reflects oligosaccharides that differ in apparent molecular weight, chemical composition, and antigenic expression. *Infect. Immun.*, **55**, 1792–1800
39. Mandrell, R., Schneider, H., Apicella, M., Zollinger, W., Rice, P. A. and Griffiss, J. M. (1986). Antigenic and physical diversity of *Neisseria gonorrhoeae* lipooligosaccharides. *Infect. Immun.*, **54**, 63–69
40. Poolman, J. T., Wientjes, F. B., Hopman, C. T. P. and Zanen, H. C. (1985). Influence of the length of lipopolysaccharide molecules on the surface exposure of class 1 and class 2 outer membrane proteins of *Neisseria meningitidis.* In Schoolnik, G. K., Brooks, G. F., Falkow, S., Frasch, C. E., Knapp, J. S., McCutchan, J. A. and Morse, S. A. (eds.), *The Pathogenic Neisseria: Proceedings of the Fourth International Symposium*, pp. 562–70. (Washington, DC: American Society of Microbiology)
41. Morse, S. A., Mintz, C. M., Sarafian, S. K., Bartenstein, L., Bertram, M. and Apicella, M. A. (1983). Effect of dilution rate on lipopolysaccharide and serum resistance to *Neisseria gonorrhoeae* grown in continuous culture. *Infect. Immun.*, **41**, 74–82

42. Apicella, M. A., Shero, M., Jarvis, G. A., Griffiss, J. M., Mandrell, R. E. and Schneider, H. (1987). Phenotypic variation in epitope expression of *Neisseria gonorrhoeae* lipooligosaccharide. *Infect. Immun.*, **55**, 1755–61
43. Schneider, H., Hammack, C. A., Apicella, M. A. and Griffiss, J. M. (1988). Instability of Expression of lipooligosaccharides and their epitopes in *Neisseria gonorrhoeae. Infect. Immun.*, **56**, 942–6
44. Schneider, H., Griffiss, J. M., Mandrell, R. E. and Jarvis, G. A. (1985). Elaboration of a 3.6 kilodalton lipooligosaccharide, antibody against which is absent from human sera, is associated with serum resistance of *Neisseria gonorrhoeae. Infect. Immun.*, **50**, 672–7
45. Devoe, I. W. and Gilchrist, J. E. (1978). Piliation and colonial morphology among laboratory strains of meningococci. *J. Clin. Microbiol.*, **7**, 379–84
46. Stephens, D. S., Edwards, K. M., Morris, F. and McGee, Z. A. (1982). Pili and outer membrane appendages on *Neisseria meningitidis* in the cerebrospinal fluid of an infant. *J. Infect. Dis.*, **146**, 568
47. Stephens, D. S. and McGee, Z. A. (1981). Attachment of *Neisseria meningitidis* to human mucosal surfaces: influence of pili and type of receptor cell. *J. Infect. Dis.*, **143**, 525–32
48. Virji, M. and Heckels, J. E. (1983). Antigenic cross reactivity of *Neisseria* pili: investigations with type and species specific monoclonal antibodies. *J. Gen. Microbiol.*, **129**, 2761–8
49. Stephens, D. S., Whitney, A. M., Rothbard, J. and Schoolnik, G. K. (1985). Pili of *Neisseria meningitidis.* Analysis of structure and investigation of structural and antigenic relationships to gonococcal pili. *J. Exp. Med.*, **161**, 1539–53
50. Diaz, J. L., Virji, M. and Heckels, J. E. (1984). Structural and antigenic differences between two types of meningococcal pili. *FEMS Microbiol. Lett.*, **21**, 181–4
51. Goldschneider, I., Gotschlich, E. C. and Artenstein, M. S. (1969). Human immunity to the meningococcus–I. The role of humoral antibodies. *J. Exp. Med.*, **129**, 1307–26
52. Sippel, J. E. (1981). Meningococci. *C.R.C. Critical Reviews in Microbiology*, **1**, 267–302
53. Kayhty, H., Jousimies-Somer, H., Peltola, H. and Makela, P. H. (1981). Antibody response to capsular polysaccharides of Groups A and C *Neisseria meningitidis* and *Haemophilus influenzae* type b during bacteremic disease. *J. Infect. Dis.*, **143**, 32–41
54. Griffiss, J. M., Brandt, B. L., Broud, D. D., Goroff, D. K. and Baker, C. J. (1984). Immune response to infants and children to disseminated infections with *Neisseria meningitidis. J. Infect. Dis.*, **150**, 71–9
55. Frasch, C. E. (1983). Immunisation against *Neisseria meningitidis.* In Easman, C. (ed.), *Medical Microbiology*, Vol. 2: *Immunisation Against Bacterial Disease*, pp. 115–44. (London and New York: Academic Press)
56. Goldschneider, I., Gotschlich, E. C. and Artenstein, M. S. (1969). Human immunity to the meningococcus–II. Development of natural immunity. *J. Exp. Med.*, **129**, 1327–48
57. Glode, M. P., Robbins, J. B., Liu, T. Y., Gotschlich, E. C., Orskov, I. and Orskov, F. (1977). Cross antigenicity and immunogenicity between capsular polysaccharides of Group C *Neisseria meningitidis* and of *Escherichia coli* K92. *J. Infect. Dis.*, **135**, 94–102
58. Gold, R. and Lepow, M. (1976). Present status of polysaccharide vaccines in the prevention of meningococcal disease. *Adv. Paediatr.*, **23**, 71–93
59. Artenstein, M. S., Brandt, B. L., Tramont, E. C., Branche, W. C., Fleet, H. D. and Cohen, R. L. (1971). Serologic studies of meningococcal infection and polysaccharide vaccination. *J. Infect. Dis.*, **124**, 277–88
60. Leinonen, M. and Frasch, C. E. (1982). Class-specific antibody response to Group B *Neisseria meningitidis* capsular polysaccharide: use of polylysine precoating in an enzyme-linked immunosorbent assay. *Infect. Immun.*, **38**, 1203–7
61. Kasper, D. L., Windelhake, J. L., Brandt, B. L. and Artenstein, M. S. (1973). Antigenic specificity to bactericidal antibodies in antisera to *Neisseria meningitidis. J. Infect. Dis.*, **127**, 378–87
62. Holten, E., Vaage, L. and Lyssum, K. (1970). Bactericidal activity in sera from carriers of sulphonamide resistant meningococci. *Scand. J. Infect. Dis.*, **2**., 201–4
63. Zollinger, W. D. and Mandrell, R. E. (1983). Importance of complement source in bactericidal antibody and murine monoclonal antibody to meningococci. *Infect. Immun.*, **40**, 257–64
64. Zollinger, W. D., Pennington, C. L. and Artenstein, M. S. (1974). Human antibody response to three meningococcal outer membrane antigens: Comparison by specific hemagglutination assays. *Infect. Immun.*, **10**, 975–84

65. Frasch, C. E. (1977). Role of protein serotype antigens in protection against disease due to *Neisseria meningitidis*. *J. Infect. Dis.*, **136**, S84–S90
66. Jones, D. M. and Eldridge, J. (1979). Development of antibodies to meningococcal protein and lipopolysaccharide serotype antigens in healthy carriers. *J. Med. Microbiol.*, **12**, 107–11
67. Poolman, J. T., Hopman, C. T. P. and Zanen, H. C. (1983). Immunogenicity of meningococcal antigens as detected in patient sera. *Infect. Immun.*, **40**, 398–406
68. Zollinger, W. D. and Mandrell, R. E. (1983). Studies of the human antibody response to specific meningococcal outer membrane proteins of serotype 2 and 15. *Med. Trop.*, **43**, 143–7
69. Bundell, K. R., Fox, A. J., Guiver, M., Jones, D. M. and Poolman, J. T. (1987). The development of an inhibition enzyme-linked immunosorbent assay to detect total antibody to the P1.16 subtype antigen of *Neisseria meningitidis* in human sera. *Serodiagn. Immunother.*, **1**, 353–61
70. Jones, D. M., Fox, A. J., Bundell, K. and Cartwright, K. A. V. (1988). The detection of antibody specific for *Neisseria meningitidis* class 3 type 15 and class 1 type 16 outer membrane protein antigens in human sera. In *Abstracts of the Sixth Pathogenic Neisseria Conference*, p. 125
71. Harthug, S., Rosenqvist, E., Hoiby, E. A., Gedde-Dahl, T. W. and Froholm, L. O. (1986). Antibody response in group B meningococcal disease determined by enzyme-linked immunosorbent assay with serotype 15 outer membrane antigen. *J. Clin. Microbiol.*, **24**, 947–53
72. Rosenqvist, E., Harthug, S., Froholm, L. O., Hoiby, E. A., Bovre, K. and Zollinger, W. D. (1988). Antibody responses to serogroup B meningococcal outer membrane antigens after vaccination and infection. *J. Clin. Microbiol.*, **26**, 1543–8
73. Sugasawara, R. J. (1985). Recognition of serogroup A *Neisseria meningitidis* serotype antigens by human antisera. *Infect. Immun.*, **48**, 23–8
74. Black, J. R., Dyer, D. W., Thompson, M. K. and Sparling, P. F. (1986). Human immune response to iron-repressible outer membrane proteins of *Neisseria meningititis*. *Infect. Immun.*, **54**, 710–13
75. Griffiss, J. M. and Kim, J. J. (1988). Antigenic specificity of natural bactericidal activity for serogroup B and C strains of *Neisseria meningitidis* in human sera. In Poolman, J. T. *et al.* (eds), *Gonococci and Meningococci*, pp. 523–7. (Dordrecht: Kluwer)
76. Gold, R., Goldschneider, I., Lepow, M. L., Draper, T. F. and Randolph, M. (1978). Carriage of *Neisseria meningitidis* and *Neisseria lactamicus* in infants and children. *J. Infect. Dis.*, **137**, 112–21
77. Kim, J. J., Mandrell, R. E., Zhen, H. U., Poolman, J. T. and Griffiss, J. M. (1988). Electromorphic characterisation of the lipooligosaccharides of Group A *Neisseria meningitidis*. In Poolman, J. T. *et al.* (eds.), *Gonococci and Meningococci*, pp. 563–7. (Dordrecht: Kluwer)
78. Thomas, L., Smith, H. W. and Dingle, J. H. (1943). Investigations of meningococcal infection. II. Immunological aspects. *J. Clin. Invest.*, **22**, 361–73
79. Griffiss, J. M. (1975). Bactericidal activity of meningococcal antisera: blocking by IgA of lytic antibody in human convalescent sera. *J. Immunol.*, **114**, 1779–84
80. Griffiss, J. M. and Bertram, M. A. (1977). Immunoepidemiology of meningococcal disease in military recruits—II. Blocking of serum bactericidal activity by circulating IgA early in the course of invasive disease. *J. Infect. Dis.*, **136**, 733–9
81. Griffiss, J. M. and Goroff, D. K. (1983). IgA blocks IgM and IgG initiated immune lysis by separate molecular mechanisms. *J. Immunol.*, **130**, 2882–5
82. Griffiss, J. M. (1982). Epidemic meningococcal disease: Synthesis of a hypothetical immunoepidemiologic model. *Rev. Infect. Dis.*, **4**, 159–72
83. Rice, P. A., Vayo, H. E., Tam, M. R. and Blake, M. S. (1986). Immunoglobin G antibodies directed against PIII block killing of serum-resistant *Neisseria gonorrhoeae* by immune serum. *J. Exp. Med.*, **164**, 1745–48
84. Heckels, J. E. and Virji, M. (1988). Immunobiology of gonococcal outer membrane proteins. In *Abstracts of Sixth Pathogenic Neisseria Conference*, p. 162.
85. Lim, D., Gewurz, A., Lint, T. F., Cihaze, M., Sepheri, B. and Gewurz, H. (1976). Absence of the sixth component of complement in a patient with repeated episodes of meningococcal meningitis. *J. Pediatr.*, **89**, 42–7

86. Lee, T. J., Utsinger, P. D., Snyderman, R., Yount, W. J. and Sparling, P. F. (1978). Familial deficiency of the seventh component of complement associated with recurrent bacteraemic infections due to *Neisseria*. *J. Infect. Dis.*, **138**, 359–68
87. Petersen, B. H., Graham, J. A. and Brooks, G. F. (1976). Human deficiency of the eighth component of complement. The requirement of C_8 for serum *Neisseria gonorrhoea* bactericidal activity. *J. Clin. Invest.*, **57**, 283–90
88. Haeney, M. R., Ball, A. P. and Thompson, R. A. (1980). Recurrent bacterial meningitis due to genetic deficiencies of the outer membrane antigen. *J. Clin. Microbiol.*, **24**, 947–53
89. Leddy, J. P., Frank, M. M., Gaither, T., Baum, J. and Klemperer, M. R. (1974). Hereditary deficiency of the sixth component of complement in man. *J. Clin. Invest.*, **53**, 544
90. Ross, S. C. and Densen, P. (1984). Complement deficiency states and infection. *Medicine (Baltimore)*, **5**, 243–73
91. Nicholson, A. and Lepow, I. (1979). Host defence against *Neisseria meningitidis* requires a complement dependent bactericidal activity. *Science*, **205**, 298–9
92. Lee, T. J., Snyderman, R., Patterson, J., Rauchbach, A. S., Folds, J. D. and Yount, W. J. (1979). *Neisseria meningitidis* bacteraemia in association with deficiency of the sixth component of complement. *Infect. Immun.*, **24**, 656–60
93. Ross, S. C., Rosenthal, P. J., Berberich, H. M. and Densen, P. (1987). Killing of *Neisseria meningitidis* by human neutrophils: implications for normal and complement-deficient individuals. *J. Infect. Dis.*, **155**, 1266–75
94. Hassig, A., Borel, J. R., Amman, P., Thoni, M. and Butler, R. (1964). Essentielle hypokomplementamie. *Pathol. Microbiol.*, **27**, 542–7
95. Beatty, D. W., Ryder, C. R. and Heese, H. de V. (1986). Complement abnormalities during an epidemic of Group B meningococcal infection in children. *Clin. Exp. Immunol.*, **64**, 465–70
96. Ellison, R. T., Kohler, P. F., Curd, J. G., Judson, F. J. and Reller, L. B. (1983). Prevalence of congenital or acquired complement deficiency in patients with sporadic meningococcal disease. *N. Engl. J. Med.*, **308**, 913
97. Grace, H. J., Brereton-Stiles, G. G., Vos, G. H. and Schonland, M. (1976). A family with partial and total deficiency of complement C3. *S. Afr. Med. J.*, **50**, 139
98. Thompson, R. A., Yap, P. L., Brettle, R. B., Dunmow, R. E. and Chapel, H. (1983). Meningococcal meningitidis associated with persistent hypocomplementemia due to circulating C3 nephritic factor. *Clin. Exp. Immunol.*, **52**, 153–6
99. Thompson, R. A. and Lachmann, P. J. (1977). A second case of human C3b inhibitor (KAF) deficiency. *Clin. Exp. Immunol.*, **27**, 23–9
100. Sjoholm, A. G., Braconier, J. H. and Soderstrom, C. (1982). Properdin deficiency in a family with fulminant meningococcal infection. *Clin. Exp. Immunol.*, **50**, 291–7
101. Neilsen, H. E. and Koch, C. (1987). Congenital properdin deficiency and meningococcal infection. *Clin. Immunol. Immunopathol.*, **44**, 134–9
102. Densen, P., Weiler, J. M., Griffiss, J. M. and Hoffman, L. G. (1987). Familial properdin deficiency and fatal meningococcaemia. *N. Engl. J. Med.*, **36**, 922–6
103. Kabat, E. A., Kaiser, H. and Silovski, H. (1945). Preparation of the type specific polysaccharide of the type 1 meningococcus and a study of its effectiveness as an antigen in human beings. *J. Exp. Med.*, **80**, 299–307
104. Gotschlich, E. C., Goldschneider, I. and Artenstein, M. S. (1969). Human immunity to the meningococcus–IV. Immunogenicity of Group A and Group C meningococcal polysaccharides in human volunteers. *J. Exp. Med.*, **129**, 1367–84
105. Brandt, B. L., Wyle, F. A. and Artenstein, M. S. (1972). A radioactive antigen-binding assay for *Neisseria meningitidis* polysaccharide antibody. *J. Immunol.*, **108**, 913–20
106. Kayhty, H., Karanko, V., Peltola, H., Sarna, S. and Makela, P. H. (1980). Serum antibodies to capsular polysaccharide vaccine of Group A *Neisseria meningitidis* followed for three years in infants and children. *J. Infect. Dis.*, **142**, 861–8
107. Gold, R., Lepow, M. L., Goldschneider, I., Draper, T. L. and Gotschlich, E. C. (1975). Clinical evaluation of Group A and C meningococcal polysaccharide vaccines in infants. *J. Clin. Invest.*, **56**, 1536–47
108. Beuvery, E. C., Leussink, A. B., Van Delft, R. W., Tiesjema, R. H. and Nagel, J. (1982). Immunoglobulin M and G antibody responses and persistence of these antibodies in adults after vaccination with a combined meningococcal group A and group C polysaccharide vaccine. *Infect. Immun.*, **37**, 579–85

109. Greenwood, B. M., Whittle, H. C. and Bradley, A. K. (1980). The duration of the antibody response to meningococcal vaccination in an African village. *Trans. Roy. Soc. Trop. Med. Hyg.*, **74**, 756–60
110. Brandt, B. L. and Artenstein, M. S. (1975). Duration of antibody responses after vaccination with Group C *Neisseria meningitidis* polysaccharide. *J. Infect. Dis.*, **131** (Suppl.), S69–S72
111. Sanborn, W. R., Benck, Z., Cvjetanovk, B., Gotschlich, E. C., Pollock, T. M. and Sippel, J. E. (1972). Trial of serogroup A meningococcus polysaccharide vaccine in Nigeria. *Prog. Immunobiol. Stand.*, **5**, 497–505
112. Wahdan, M. H., Rizk, F., El-Akkad, A. M., El Ghoroury, A. A., Hablas, R., Girgis, N. I., Amer, A., Boctar, W., Sippel, J. E., Gotschlich, E. C., Triau, R., Sanborn, W. R. and Cvjetanovic, B. (1973). A controlled field trial of a serogroup A meningococcal polysaccharide vaccine. *Bull. WHO.*, **48**, 667–73
113. Erwa, H. H., Haseeb, M. A., Idris, A. A., Lapeyssonnie, L., Sanborn, W. R. and Sippel, J. E. (1973). A serogroup A meningococcal polysaccharide vaccine. Studies in the Sudan to combat cerebrospinal meningitis caused by *Neisseria meningitidis* group A. *Bull. WHO.*, **49**, 301–5
114. Peltola, H., Makela, P. H., Kayhty, H., Jousimies, H., Herva, E., Hallstrom, K., Sivonen, A., Renkonen, O. V., Pettay, O., Karanko, V., Ahvonen, P. and Sarna, S. (1977). Clinical efficacy of meningococcus group A capsular polysaccharide vaccine in children three months to five years of age. *N. Engl. J. Med.*, **297**, 686–91
115. Makela, P. H., Kayhty, H., Weckstrom, P., Sivonen, A. and Renkonen, O. V. (1975). Effect of Group A meningococcal vaccine in army recruits in Finland. *Lancet*, Vol. 8, 883–6
116. Reingold, A. L., Hightower, A. W., Bolan, G. A., Jones, E. E., Tiendrebeogo, H., Broome, C. V., Ajello, G. W., Adamsbaum, C., Phillips, C. and Yada, A. (1985). Age specific differences in duration of clinical protection after vaccination with meningococcal polysaccharide A vaccine. *Lancet*, Vol. 20, 114–8
117. Hu, Z., Rou, Y. L., Chen, C., Chen, R. S., Wu, Q. K., Zhang, V. Y., Dong, C. M., Liu, B. K., Chang, P. Y., Yang, T. Y., Wei, R. T. and Chen, C. Z. (1988). An epidemiological and serological study on duration of protection after meningococcal Group A polysaccharide vaccination. In Poolman, J. T. (ed.), *Gonococci and Meningococci*, pp. 199–207. (Dordrecht: Kluwer)
118. Greenwood, B. M., Smith, A. W., Hassan-King, M., Bijlmer, H. A., Shenton, F. C., Hughes, A. S. B., Nunn, P. P., Jack, A. D. and Gowers, P. R. S. (1986). The efficacy of meningopolysaccharide vaccine in preventing group A meningococcal disease in The Gambia West Africa. *Trans. Roy. Soc. Trop. Med. Hyg.*, **80**, 1006–7
119. Wahden, M. H., Sallam, S. A., Hassan, M. N., Gawad, A. A., Rakha, A. S., Sippel, J. E., Hablas, R., Sanborn, W. R., Kassem, N. M., Riad, S. M. and Cvjetanovic, B. (1977). A second controlled field trial of a serogroup A meningococcal polysaccharide vaccine in Alexandria. *Bull. WHO.*, **55**, 645–51
120. Greenwood, B. M., Hassan-King, M. and Whittle, H. C. (1978). Prevention of secondary cases in household contacts by vaccination. *Br. Med. J.*, **1**, 1317–19
121. Blakebrough, I. S., Greenwood, B. M., Whittle, H. C., Bradley, A. K. and Gilles, H. M. (1983). Failure of vaccination to stop transmission of meningococci in Nigerian schoolboys. *Ann. Trop. Med. Parasitol.*, **77**, 175–8
122. Hassan-King, M. K. A., Wall, R. A. and Greenwood, B. M. (1988). Meningococcal carriage, meningococcal disease and vaccination. *J. Infect.*, **16**, 55–9
123. Monto, A. S., Brandt, B. L. and Artenstein, M. S. (1973). Response of children to *Neisseria meningitidis* polysaccharide vaccines. *J. Infect. Dis.*, **127**, 394–400
124. Gotschlich, E. C., Rey, M., Triau, R. and Sparks, K. J. (1972). Quantitative determination of the human immune response to immunization with meningococcal vaccines. *J. Clin. Invest.*, **51**, 89–96
125. Artenstein, M. S. and Brandt, B. L. (1975). Immunological hyporesponsiveness in man to Group C meningococcal polysaccharide. *J. Immunol.*, **115**, 5–7
126. Tauney, A. de E., Galvao, P. A., de Morais, J. S., Gotschlich, E. C. and Feldman, R. A. (1974). Disease prevention by meningococcal serogroup C polysaccharide vaccine in preschool children. *Pediatric Res.*, **8**, 429
127. Lepow, M. L., Goldschneider, I., Gold, R., Randolph, M. and Gotschlich, E. C. (1977). Persistence of antibody following immunisation of children with groups A and C meningococcal polysaccharide vaccines. *Pediatrics*, **60**, 673–80

128. Gold, R., Lepow, M. L., Goldschneider, I., Draper, T. F. and Gotschlich, E. C. (1979). Kinetics of antibody production to Group A and Group C meningococcal polysaccharide vaccines administered during the first six years of life; prospects for routine immunization of infants and children. *J. Infect. Dis.*, **140**, 690–7

129. Gold, R. and Artenstein, M. S. (1971). Meningococcal infections. 2. Field trial of Group C meningococcal polysaccharide vaccine in 1969–70. *Bull. WHO.*, **45**, 279–82

130. Gotschlich, E. C., Goldschneider, I. and Artenstein, M. S. (1969). Human immunity to the meningococcus–V. The effect of immunization with meningococcal Group C polysaccharide on the carrier state. *J. Exp. Med.*, **129**, 1385–95

131. Artenstein, M. S., Gold, R., Zimmerly, J. G., Wyle, F. A., Schneider, H. and Harkins, C. (1970). Prevention of meningococcal disease by Group C polysaccharide vaccine. *N. Engl. J. Med.*, **282**, 417

132. Devine, L. F., Pierce, W. E., Floyd, T. M., Rhode, S. L., Edwards, E. A., Siess, E. E. and Peckinpaugh, R. O. (1970). Evaluation of Group C vaccine in marine recruits, San Diego, California. *Am. J. Epidemiol.*, **92**, 25–32

133. Galaid, E. I., Cherubin, C. E., Marr, J. S., Schaefler, S., Barone, J. and Lee, W. (1980). Meningococcal disease in New York City, 1973–1978. Recognition of groups Y and W135 as frequent pathogens. *J. Am. Med. Assoc.*, **244**, 2167–71

134. Griffiss, J. M., Brandt, B. L., Altieri, P. L., Pier, G. B. and Berman, S. L. (1981). Safety and immunogenicity of group Y and Group W135 meningococcal capsular polysaccharide vaccines in adults. *Infect. Immun.*, **34**, 725–32

135. Griffiss, J. M., Apicella, M. A., Greenwood, B. and Makela, P. H. (1987). Vaccines against encapsulated bacteria: a global agenda. *Rev. Infect. Dis.*, **9**, 176–88

136. Whittle, H. C., Oduloju, A., Evans-Jones, G. and Greenwood, B. M. (1976). Evidence for a familial immune defect in meningococcal meningitis. *Br. Med. J.*, **1**, 1247–50

137. Pandey, J. P., Fudenberg, H. H., Virella, G., Kyong, C. U., Loadholt, C. B., Galbraith, R. M., Gotschlich, E. C. and Parke, J. C. (1979). Association between immunoglobulin allotypes and immune responses to *Haemophilus influenzae* and meningococcus polysaccharides. *Lancet*, **1**, 190–2

138. Pandey, J. P., Zollinger, W. D., Fudenberg, H. H. and Loadholt, C. B. (1981). Immunoglobulin allotypes polysaccharide vaccine in children three months to five years of age. *N. Engl. J. Med.*, **297**, 686–91

139. Ambrosino, D. M., Schiffman, G., Gotschlich, E. C., Schur, P. H., Rosenberg, G. A., DeLange, G. G., van Loghem, E. and Siber, G. R. (1985). Correlation between G2m(n) immunoglobulin allotype and human antibody response and susceptibility to polysaccharide encapsulated bacteria. *J. Clin. Invest.*, **75**, 1935–42

140. Siber, G. R., Schur, P. H., Aisenberg, A. C., Weitzman, S. A. and Schiffman, G. (1980). Correlation between serum IgG2 concentrations and the antibody response to bacterial polysaccharide antigens. *N. Microbiol.*, **1**, 267–302

141. Ambrosino, D. M., Siber, G. R., Chilmonczyk, B. A., Jernberg, J. B. and Finberg, R. W. (1987). An immunodeficiency characterised by impaired antibody responses to polysaccharides. *N. Engl. J. Med.*, **316**, 790–3

142. Greenwood, B. M. and Wali, S. S. (1980). Control of meningococcal infection in the African meningitis belt by selective vaccination. *Lancet*, **1**, 729–32

143. Robbins, J. B. and Schneerson, R. (1987). *Haemophilus influenzae* type b: the search for a vaccine. *Pediatr. Infect. Dis. J.*, **6**, 791–4

144. Ward, J. (1987). Newer *Haemophilus influenzae* type b vaccines and passive prophylaxis. *Pediatr. Infect. Dis. J.*, **6**, 799–803

145. Beuvery, E. C., Miedema, F., Delft, R. W. van, and Nagel, J., (1982). Meningococcal group C polysaccharide/tetanus toxoid conjugate as immunogen. In Robbins, J. B. *et al.* (eds), *Seminars in Infectious Disease, Bacterial Vaccines*, pp. 268–74. (New York: Stratton)

146. Jennings, H. J. and Lugowski, C. (1982). Tetanus toxoid conjugates of the meningococcal polysaccharide. In Robbins, J. B. *et al.* (eds.), *Seminars in Infectious Diseases, Bacterial Vaccines*, pp. 247–53. (New York: Stratton)

147. Wyle, F. A., Artenstein, M. S., Brandt, B. L., Tramont, E. C., Kasper, D. L., Altieri, P. L., Berman, S. L. and Lowenthal, J. P. (1972). Immunologic response of man to Group B meningococcal polysaccharide vaccines. *J. Infect. Dis.*, **126**, 514–22

148. Finne, J., Leinonen, M. and Makela, P. H. (1983). Antigenic similarities between brain

components and bacteria causing meningitis: implications for vaccine development and pathogenesis. *Lancet*, **2**, 355–7

149. Lifely, M. R. and Moreno, C. (1986). Vaccine against meningococcal Group B disease. *Lancet*, **1**, 214–15
150. Zollinger, W. D., Mandrell, R., Griffiss, J. M. and Altieri, P. (1979). Complex of meningococcal Group B polysaccharide and type 2 outer membrane protein immunogenic in man. *J. Clin. Invest.*, **63**, 836–48
151. Moreno, C., Lifely, M. R. and Esdaile, J. (1985). Effect of aluminium ions on the chemical and immunological properties of Group B polysaccharide. *Infect. Immun.*, **49**, 587–92
152. Jennings, H. J., Roy, R. and Gamian, A. (1986). Induction of meningococcal group B polysaccharide specific IgG antibodies in mice by using an N-propionylated B polysaccharide-tetanus toxoid conjugate vaccine. *J. Immunol.*, **137**, 1708–13
153. Frasch, C. E. and Robbins, J. D. (1978). Protection against Group B meningococcal disease. *J. Exp. Med.*, **147**, 629–44
154. Craven, D. E. and Frasch, C. E. (1979). Protection against group B meningococcal disease; evaluation of serotype 2 protein vaccines in a mouse bacteremia model. *Infect. Immun.*, **26**, 110–17
155. Helting, T. B., Guthohrlein, G., Blackkolb, F. and Ronneberger, H. (1981). Serotype determinant protein of *Neisseria meningitidis*. *Acta. Pathol. Microbiol. Scand., J. Infect. Dis.*, **2**, 201–4
156. Frasch, C. E. and Peppler, M. S. (1982). Protection against Group B meningococcal disease: preparation of soluble protein and protein–polysaccharide immunogens. *Infect. Immun.*, **37**, 271–80
157. Zollinger, W. D., Boslego, J. W., Brandt, B., Moran, E. E. and Ray, J. (1986). Safety and antigenicity studies of a polyvalent meningococcal protein-polysaccharide vaccine. *Antonie van Leeuwenhoek*, **52**, 255–8
158. Beuvery, E. C., Witvliet, M., Timmermans, J. A. M., Poolman, J. T., Hopman, C. T. P., Teerlink, T., Speijers, G. J. A. and Danse, L. H. J. C. (1986). Characteristics of an alternative meningococcal type 15 P1.16 outer membrane protein vaccine. *Antonie van Leeuwenhoek*, **52**, 232–5
159. Frasch, C. E., Coetzee, G., Zahradnik, J. M. and Wang, L. Y. (1985). New developments in meningococcal vaccines. In Schoolnik, G. K. (ed.), *The Pathogenic Neisseria*, pp. 633–9. (Washington, DC: American Society for Microbiology)
160. Frasch, C. E., Zahradnik, J. M., Wang, L. Y., Mocca, L. F. and Tsai, C. M. (1988). Antibody response of adults to an aluminium hydroxide-adsorbed *Neisseria meningitidis* serotype 2b protein group B polysaccharide vaccine. *J. Infect. Dis.*, **158**, 710–18
161. Wedege, E. and Froholm, L. O. (1986). Human antibody response to a Group B serotype 2a meningococcal vaccine determined by immunoblotting. *Infect. Immun.*, **51**, 571–8
162. Poolman, J. T. (1988). Meningococcal vaccines. *J. Med. Microbiol.*, **26**, 170–2
163. Van Putten, J. M. P., Linders, M. T., Wheel, J. F. L. and Poolman, J. T. (1987). Differential expression of Fe-repressible and growth rate sensitive proteins in *Neisseria meningitidis* and *Neisseria gonorrhoeae*. *Antonie van Leeuwenhoek*, **53**, 557–64
164. Mietzner, T. A., Luginbuhl, G. H., Sandstrom, E. and Morse, S. A. (1984). Identification of an iron-regulated 37,000 Dalton protein in the cell envelope of *Neisseria gonorrhoeae*. *Infect. Immun.*, **45**, 410–16
165. Keevil, C. W., Davies, D. B., Spillane, B. J. and Mahenthiralingam, E. (1988). Influence of iron-limited and excess continuous culture on the virulence properties of *Neisseria gonorrhoeae*. In Poolman, J. T. (ed.), *Gonococci and Meningococci*, pp. 727–9. (Dordrecht: Kluwer)
166. Davies, H. A., Wall, R. A., Borriello, S. P., Patterson, S. and Gaunt, N. (1988). Immunogold electronmicroscopy of the outer membrane proteins of *Neisseria meningitidis* B.15.P1.16. examined directly from cerebrospinal fluid. *J. Med. Microbiol.*, **27**, vi
167. Cannon, J. G., Black, W. J., Nachamkin, I. and Stewart, P. W. (1984). Monoclonal antibody that recognises an outer membrane antigen common to the pathogenic Neisseria but not to most non pathogenic Neisseria species. *Infect. Immun.*, **43**, 994–9
168. Black, J. R., Black, W. J. and Cannon, J. G. (1985). Neisserial antigen H.8 is immunogenic in patients with disseminated gonococcal and meningococcal infections. *J. Infect. Dis.*, **151**, 650–7

169. Woods, J. P., Aho, E. L., Barritt, D. S., Black, J. R., Connell, T. D., Kawula, T. H., Spinola, S. M. and Cannon, J. G. (1988). The H8 antigen of pathogenic Neisseriae. In Poolman, J. T. (ed.), *Gonococci and Meningococci*, pp. 613–16. (Dordrecht: Kluwer)

170. Martin, P. M. V., Lavitola, A., Aoun, L., Ancelle, R., Cremieux, A. C. and Riou, J. Y. (1986). A common neisserial antigen evidenced by immunisation of mice with live *Neisseria meningitidis*. *Infect. Immun.*, **53**, 229–33

171. Lavitola, A., Aoun, L., Ohayon, H., Cremieux, A. C., Ancelle, R. and Martin, P. M. V. (1987). The 70 kd neisserial common antigen is a surface exposed antigenically stable peptidic structure. *Ann. Inst. Pasteur/Microbiol*, **138**, 333–42

172. Aoun, L., Lavitola, A., Aubert, G., Prere, M. F., Cremieux, A. C. and Martin, P. M. V. (1988). Human antibody response to the 70 kd common neisserial antigen in patients and carriers of meningococci or non pathogenic *Neisseria*. *Ann. Inst. Pasteur/Microbiol.*, **139**, 203–12

173. Brown, M. R. W., Anwar, H. and Lambert, P. A. (1984). Evidence that mucoid *Pseudomonas aeruginosa* in the cystic fibrosis lung grows under iron-restricted conditions. *FEMS Microbiol Lett.*, **21**, 113–17

3
Vaccines for the protection of the gastrointestinal tract against bacterial infection

B. S. DRASAR

INTRODUCTION

Infections of the gastrointestinal tract are among the major causes of morbidity and mortality. The exact number of cases of diarrhoea and dysentery is unknown, but it has been estimated that about 1500 million cases of infective diarrhoea occur yearly worldwide. Bacterial infection is thought to be the cause of about half this number. Prevention of these infections depends on the provision of clean water and adequate excreta disposal systems, and the inculcation of high standards of food hygiene. If they were available vaccines could also play a major role.

The study of bacterial vaccines has concentrated on the historically prominent serious gastrointestinal diseases, cholera, typhoid and dysentery. More recently elucidation of pathogenic mechanisms and success in control of animal disease has raised hopes for a vaccine against enterotoxigenic *Escherichia coli*. However, many important intestinal pathogens remain as the subject of current and future research.

Bacterial vaccines were reviewed in 1984 by Germinier[1]. This chapter reviews the recent advances that have been made in the development of vaccines for protection of the gastrointestinal tract from bacterial infection, and sets them in the context of our knowledge of the pathogenesis of these infections.

THE PATHOGENESIS OF GASTROINTESTINAL INFECTION

The development of diarrhoea or dysentery is a common symptom of intestinal infection. Studies over the past 25 years have elucidated many of the mechanisms important in the development of diarrhoea and have resulted in a new understanding of many aspects of intestinal physiology. Fundamental insights resulted from the study of weaning diarrhoea in piglets by H. W. Smith and his co-workers, who demonstrated the importance of specific attachment to the intestinal mucosa in the initiation of the infection caused by enterotoxigenic *E. coli* in piglets. In order for infection to occur in this system three necessary conditions must be satisfied:

1. the production of an adhesin, the K88 antigen, by the bacteria;
2. the production of a specific mucosal receptor by the pig;
3. the production of enterotoxin by the bacteria.

It is now realized that even in pigs the situation may be more complex than appears from this idealized system. Other receptors and toxins may be produced by the bacteria while strains of pig differ in their ability to produce receptors. Nevertheless this system serves as the paradigm on which our understanding of intestinal infection is based. The normative value of this system was enhanced by studies on an analogous system based on the K99 adhesin in calves.

From the viewpoint of the investigation, these well-understood systems have the major advantage of being related to diseases of farm animals. Thus they were demonstrated on the basis of studies and experiments performed on infections of the natural host, and further on a population of the natural host that has been subject to considerable selective breeding.

The diseases discussed here – cholera, typhoid, dysentery and human enterotoxic *E. coli* infection – have man as their natural host, and this limits the range of experiments that can be undertaken. Further, the human population is more heterogeneous than farm animal populations and thus the scope for the range of specific interactions is much greater. The specificity of the host/bacteria interactions involved in these gastrointestinal infections has important consequences in terms of the development of animal models. Though particular aspects of these interactions can be reproduced in animal models it is not possible in these diseases to infect other animals with bacteria isolated from humans and reproduce the mechanisms of disease and the host response in all its aspects. This has had important consequences for the testing of oral vaccines against *Vibrio cholerae.*

The pathogenesis of bacterial intestinal infections has been reviewed from the viewpoint of vaccine development[2]. In this section the relevant features of the infections are outlined.

Cholera

Vibrio cholerae adheres to the intestinal mucosa and secretes a toxin which causes the watery diarrhoea typical of cholera (Table 1). *V. cholerae* is a non-invasive pathogen and the infection is localized in the intestinal lumen.

Cholera toxin is among the best-understood of biologically active molecules and its activity provides an explanation for the physiological changes that accompany the disease. However, the very detail of our knowledge of the toxin has tended to obscure our ignorance of other aspects of the disease, particularly the mechanism of attachment. Adherence of *V. cholerae* to the

Table 1 Pathogenesis of intestinal infections caused by bacteria

	Mucosal attachment	*Toxin production*	*Mucosal invasion*	*Systemic spread*
Vibrio cholerae 01	+	+	−	−
Enterotoxigenic *Escherichia coli*	+	+	−	−
Shigellae	+	±	+	−
Salmonella typhi	+	−	+	+

brush-border membrane is not well understood. The model of lectin–ligand interactions which was developed from studies of enterotoxigenic *E. coli* in which specific adhesins, e.g. K88, K99, CFAI, CFAII, are associated with specific mucosal receptors, is unable to explain the attachment of *V. cholerae*. The major cell-associated haemagglutinins, fucose-sensitive for classical strains and fucose- and mannose-sensitive for El Tor strains, have been thought of as analogous to *E. coli* adhesins[3]. Undoubtedly, specific cell-associated receptors, perhaps H substance, are involved in cell–bacterium interactions mediated by these haemagglutinins, but other factors such as secretor status may modulate this interaction. Attempts to find fimbrial adhesins on *V. cholerae* have not all been successful. A variety of outer membrane proteins may be involved. Motility is also important[4,5]; indeed the flagellum may act as an adhesin. The picture is further complicated by the observation that cholera toxin increases the efficacy of colonization in experimental animals.

Thus it can be seen that a variety of virulence-related factors (Table 2) may be important in attachment. These may include fimbriae, flagellum, outer membrane proteins, the lipopolysaccharide (LPS) responsible for serological reactions of strains (O1, Ogawa and Inaba serotypes) as well as the functionally described haemagglutinins[6].

Studies on candidate vaccine strains (see below) have revealed that cholera toxin is not the only physiologically active molecule produced by *V. cholerae* that may influence intestinal absorption. A variety of other toxins may be produced. Nevertheless it is certain that attachment to the intestinal mucosa and the production of physiologically active toxins are the crucial stages in

Table 2 Virulence factors and vaccine targets of bacteria causing intestinal infections

	Mucosal adhesion/invasion	*Heat-labile toxin (LT); cholera toxin*	Shigella-*like toxin, VTI, VTI*	*Other toxins*
Vibrio cholerae	LPS flagellar sheath protein haemagglutinins, outer membrane proteins	+	+	+
Enterotoxogenic *Escherichia coli*	CFA/I CFA/II E8775 and other fimbrae	+	+*toxin (St)	Heat-stable
Shigellae	Smooth LPS invasins	?	+	−
Salmonella typhi	Vi antigen?: invasins	?	?	?

*VTI and VTII most usual in absence of LT.

the pathogenesis of cholera. Recent studies have added to our knowledge but decreased the certainty of our understanding.

Diarrhoea caused by enterotoxigenic *E. coli*

Enteropathogenic strains of *Escherichia coli* have long been identified on the basis of epidemiological associations in outbreaks of diarrhoea among children. The investigation of weanling diarrhoea or scours in pigs and calves led to the identification of enterotoxigenic *E. coli.* A worldwide search for these organisms showed that they produce a major childhood illness, particularly in developing countries.

These bacteria produce diarrhoea as a result of colonization of the small intestine and the elaboration of toxins. Like that caused by *V. cholerae*, the infection by enterotoxigenic *E. coli* is restricted to the intestinal lumen. Two aspects of pathogenicity have been demonstrated: adhesion to the intestinal mucosa and production of toxins (Table 1). A number of host-specific adhesins have been demonstrated[7], and these enable a variety of toxins to produce the illness.

The most notable toxin in the present context is the heat-labile toxin (LT). Structurally, functionally and immunologically the toxin is very similar to cholera toxin. As would be expected, there is a very high degree of nucleotide sequence and amino acid sequence homology between these molecules[8–10]. Cholera toxin and LT belong to a family of similar toxins that include enterotoxins from a range of Enterobacteriaceae producing gastrointestinal disease in man and other animals. Unlike cholera toxin, LT is coded for a plasmid-borne gene (ENT^+), and this has been a great help in studies of both of these toxins.

This family of toxins consists of six subunits. There are five B subunits and one A subunit. The B subunits bind to the mucosal membrane of the intestinal cell and cause a conformation change in the membrane that inserts the A subunit into the enterocyte. Individual B subunits are good antigens but a complex of the five B subunits is even more highly antigenic. The A subunit stimulates the production of cyclic AMP, which results in enhanced electrolyte secretion by the cell. The A subunits are not good antigens.

The heat-stable (ST) toxins of *E. coli* are also known to be of major importance in the production of diarrhoea. Again this is a family of toxins which share some common amino acid sequence receptors and modes of action. Enhancement of electrolyte secretion is mediated by cyclic GMP. These toxins are not effective antigens and have to be coupled to carrier molecules to stimulate antibody production. This technique has been used in the development of assays. As more investigations of *E. coli* strains are undertaken the number and variety of toxins detected increases[11–13]. Though our understanding of these bacteria is based on LT (now LTI) and ST (now STa) the various Vero cell cytoxins and Shiga-like toxins[12] must not be forgotten. They must also be candidates for inclusion in vaccines. Further, a new family of heat-labile toxins, LTII, that do not share amino acid homology with LT, have been described, as have a new series of heat-stable toxins (STb)[13].

Invasive pathogens: Shigellae and *Salmonella typhi*

Attachment to the small intestine and toxin production are probably the best-understood of the infective strategies employed by bacteria. Gastrointestinal disease is also caused by organisms able to invade the intestinal mucosa. Though these processes can be described in similar ways it is doubtful if the same type of virulence factors are involved.

Salmonellae, including *Salmonella typhi*, are able to invade the small intestinal mucosa, probably in the ileum. Shigellae invade the mucosa of the colon. Invasion by *S. typhi* is followed by systemic spread. Shigellae grow intracellularly in the colonic mucosa. This results in mucosal ulceration but systemic spread does not occur (Table 1).

The virulence factors involved in this process are not well defined. Attachment to the intestinal mucosa is an essential part of the process, but it is unclear if this is analogous to the adhesion that is demonstrated with toxigenic pathogens.

Invasion results from receptor-mediated endocytosis (RME). Binding of ligands on the bacteria to receptors on the enterocyte membrane induces engulfment of bacterium. Salmonellae in endocytic vacuoles migrate to the lamina propria where the bacteria are extruded. In contrast, Shigellae, after uptake by RME, leave the endocytic vacuole and invade the cytoplasm of the enterocytes[14]. The nature of the ligands that stimulate RME is unknown, though existence of a class of invasins, analogous to adhesins, has been postulated (Table 2). The ability to invade cells is plasmid-encoded in at least some species of Shigellae. However, transconjugants with *E. coli* do not grow intracellularly, indicating that both plasmid-borne and chromosomal genes are needed for full virulence.

Shigella dysenteriae type I produce Shiga toxin. It has been reported that this or similar toxins are produced by other Shigellae. Indeed, Shigellae may produce a range of cytotoxins. Production of toxins by Salmonellae other than *S. typhi* has also been reported[13]. The importance of these substances to the diseases caused by invasive enteropathogens is unclear.

VACCINES FOR GASTROINTESTINAL INFECTION

The brief description of the pathogenesis of gastrointestinal infection that is set out above indicates the many targets against which protective immunity could be directed (Table 2). The object of a vaccine rationally conceived must be to block those crucial aspects of the pathogenesis of the infection or to neutralize those substances producing the pathological effects. Thus, it is clear why the current vaccines are unsatisfactory. Parenteral vaccines against cholera and typhoid, consisting of killed bacterial cells, are widely used, but these vaccines are undefined in terms of the known virulence mechanisms of organisms. Historically similar vaccines have been produced against Shigellae and *E. coli*, but they proved to be without value. The adhesins, toxins and invasins present rational targets for vaccine development and this goal is being actively pursued.

The major difficulty is the definitive identification of important virulence factors. These are human diseases for which there are, in some instances, equivalent animal infections, but in no case is there an animal model that reproduces the pathological features of the disease. The major advantage in these studies results from the relative ease with which these organisms can be subject to genetic manipulation. Many of the genes coding for virulence factors are plasmid-borne. Indeed, plasmids were originally recognized in *Shigella dysenteriae*. Well-established plasmid vector systems such as pBR322 have been used successfully for cloning of virulence factors.

Thus, although problems remain, it is likely that the bacterial enteropathogens will be controlled by designer vaccines.

Cholera vaccines

The discovery of cholera toxin gave a major impetus to the study of the pathogenesis of the disease, which in turn led to the reassessment of the vaccine. The parenteral vaccine provides 40–80% protection during the first 2–3 months after administration, but no significant protection after 6 months. Some evidence suggests that the vaccine may be more effective when administered to the inhabitants of highly endemic areas.

The low level of protection afforded by the conventional parenteral vaccine has reawakened interest in oral vaccination. This seemed particularly appropriate in view of the limitation of the infection to the intestinal lumen.

Establishment of toxin as a major virulence factor made this a natural target for investigation. The toxin genes were cloned[15,16] and shown to be expressed in a biologically active form in *E. coli*[17]. These studies were greatly assisted by the knowledge of the relationship of cholera toxin and *E. coli* LTI. Plasmids encoding LT toxins were used as probes to detect the cholera toxin genes in restriction digests of chromosomal DNA from *V. cholerae*.

This success was rapidly followed by further advances in the study of the molecular biology of *V. cholerae*. Particular attention was focused on the haemolysins as possible accessory virulence factors. Haemolysin genes were cloned and characterized from both El Tor[18,19] and Classical[20,21] biotypes. The genes that determine the biosynthesis of Inaba and Ogawa serotypes of the lipopolysaccharide cell wall O antigen have also been cloned into and expressed by *E. coli*[22]. These advances resulted from attempts by several groups to understand the molecular biological basis of the virulence of *V. cholerae* and to develop a vaccine. The relative isolation of the infection from systemic immunity, and the lack of success of parenteral vaccines, means that cholera is a prime candidate for the development of an oral vaccine. Studies have focused on the development of a live oral vaccine, though killed vaccines have also been investigated. Considerable advances have been made and several candidate oral vaccines have been developed and shown to protect against challenge in volunteer studies[23,24].

The first new vaccines to reach the field trial stage were killed oral vaccine. These were tested in an extensive controlled trial in Bangladesh. A mixture of heat-killed and formalin-killed cells of *V. cholerae* O1 of both Ogawa and Inaba subtypes formed the basic vaccine. The second formulation consisted of killed cells as in the basic vaccine, together with the B subunit of cholera toxin. An *E. coli* K12 preparation was administered to the control group. These vaccines provided good short-term protection against clinical cholera, both in the trial[25] (Table 3) and in adult volunteers[26].

The vaccines stimulate production of vibriocidal antibodies and, in the case of the B subunit vaccine, an antitoxic response. These vaccines seem to be free of side-effects[27]. Further, the results obtained with the B subunit–containing vaccine underline the value of antitoxic immunity (Table 3).

The success of the killed oral vaccines demonstrates the possibilty of a successful vaccination campaign. However, these vaccines needed to be administered and boosted twice by further vaccine. In theory at least, a live vaccine should overcome this problem. Several candidate vaccine strains have been developed and tested (Table 4).

These studies have concentrated on the development of a strain attenuated by deletion or mutation in the genes encoding for cholera toxin. This approach led to the development and testing of the prototype candidate vaccine strain Texas Star SR. This strain, isolated after nitrosoguanidine mutagenesis, produces B subunits only. Texas Star SR may be considered as establishing the principles by which the development and testing of candidate vaccine are governed, but more recent strains have had more sophisticated methods employed in their production[28,29]. A range of strains have been developed and tested (Table 4)[30,31].

Candidate vaccine strains have been tested in volunteers as part of a vaccine development programme. These studies have included examination of the response to wild-type *V. cholerae*. Volunteers are assessed in terms of their vibriocidal and antitoxic antibody responses, their physiological response and, where appropriate, their resistance to challenge by virulent *V. cholerae*[30,31].

Table 3 Field trial of oral *Vibrio cholerae* vaccine[25]

Vaccine	*Number of subjects*		*Percentage effectiveness*
	Vaccinees	*Controls*	
Killed bacteria cells	21 137	21 220	58
Killed bacterial cells plus B subunit of cholera toxin	21 141	21 220	85

Table 4 Candidate vaccine strains of *Vibrio cholerae*[30,31]

Strain number	*Toxigenic status*	*Parent strain*		
		Number	*Biotype*	*Serotype*
Texas Star SR	A^-B^+	3083	El Tor	Ogawa
JBK 70	A^-B^-	N16961	El Tor	Inaba
CVD 101	A^-B^+	395	Classical	Ogawa
CVD 102*	A^-B^+	CVD 101	Classical	Ogawa
CVD 104	$A^-B^{-\dagger}$	JBK 70	El Tor	Inaba
CVD 105	$A^-B+\dagger$	CVD 101	Classical	Ogawa

*Thymine-dependent mutant
†Genes encoding El Tor haemolysin deleted

Those strains which colonize the small intestine result in the development of vibriocidal and antitoxic responses comparable to those induced by wild-type strains. Further, though the number of subjects involved is small, the protection to challenge as judged by percentage effectiveness can also be high (Table 5).

Unfortunately, candidate vaccine strains also induced diarrhoea in many of the volunteers (Table 6). It has been suggested that some diarrhoea is a small price to pay for immunity to cholera, but it must be remembered that these studies were undertaken in well-nourished adults. Children would be the preferred target group for vaccine administration[32], and in a developing country some degree of malnutrition is likely. Our studies suggest that the effects of cholera toxin may be amplified by zinc deficiency. Undoubtedly, such oral vaccines would exacerbate the effects of malnutrition on absorption. The diarrhoea these candidate vaccine strains cause in adults renders them unacceptable for field use among children in developing countries.

The reasons for these side-effects is not clear; however, it is now recognized that *V. cholerae* has a range of accessory virulence factors (Table 2) whose effects may be unmasked by the disabling of cholera toxin[33]. The candidate

Table 5 Protection of volunteers to challenge with virulent *Vibrio cholerae* by oral immunization with candidate vaccine strains or infection with virulent organisms[30,31]

Immunogen	*Challenge*	*Number of subjects*		*Percentage effectiveness*
		Vaccinees	*Controls*	
Texas Star SR	E7946	7	10	59
	N16961	18	15	62
JBK 70	N16961	10	8	89
Wild-type strains				
Classical vibrios	Virulent *V. cholerae*	16	27	100
El Tor vibrios	Inaba and Ogawa	22	37	90

Table 6 Physiological response of volunteers to some pathogenic and candidate vaccine strains of *Vibrio cholerae*[30,31]

Strain	*Number of subjects*		*Percentage of subjects that developed diarrhoea*
	Tested	*With diarrhoea*	
Candidate vaccine strains			
Texas Star-SR	68	16	24
JBK 70	14	7	50
CVD 101	24	13	54
CVD 102	5	0	0
CVD 104	6	2	30
CVD 105	9	3	30
Wild-type strains			
3083	4	0	0
N16961	15	11	73
	38	35	92
395	36	33	92
E7946 (El Tor Ogawa)	10	7	70

vaccine strains listed in Table 4 probably produce a variety of such factors, including Shiga toxin or a similar cytotoxin. The role of haemolysin has also been recognized[34,35] but deletion of these genes as in strain CVD104 and CVD105 does not reduce the level of side-effects. Strain CVD103 lacks the Shiga-like toxin, and this may prove to be the solution to this problem.

It must be emphasized that the level of diarrhoea induced by these candidate vaccines can in no way be compared with clinical cholera. To well-informed adults the protection afforded may seem to far outweigh the minor discomfort caused, but it must be remembered that the emotional reaction to any vaccine side-effects in children can be very damaging to the whole concept of prevention.

Equally important for general acceptance of oral vaccines must be recognition of their long-term effectiveness. It has long been believed that the immunity conferred by an attack of cholera is short-lived, and that a clinical attack of the disease may occur within a few weeks of the first. Further, even when symptoms do not occur, re-infection of cholera cases is said to be common.

Aspects of the problem have been investigated in animal studies, in family contacts of cholera patients[36] and in vaccines[37]. A major difficulty results from the lack of definition of the protective antigen. Studies in mice[38], rabbits[39], and human volunteers[31] have all demonstrated that colonization of the intestine is a most important factor in determining the quality of the immune response.

However, as discussed above, in spite of major efforts the colonization factors of *V. cholerae* remain to be defined. It may well be that while colonization is important in animal models and man, different factors are involved.

Epidemiological studies have shown that vibriocidal antibody is associated with protection against both colonization and disease[36]. However, it is unclear how long these responses remain. Animal studies have raised questions concerning the existence of immunological memory in the intestinal secretory IgA system. Studies of volunteers in Sweden[37] have provided some evidence for long-lasting memory, but the importance of low-dose exposure for long-term immunity in endemic areas awaits elucidation. These questions need to be the subject of intensive long-term investigation in volunteer vaccinees in the developed world and among the populations of endemic areas. These studies will be assisted by the use of proxy measures of gut immunity[40].

The understanding of cholera, its pathogenesis and prevention has advanced rapidly during the past decade, but many further questions have been raised. However, how these problems might be solved is clear. It seems likely that the next decade will see the arrival of a safe effective live oral vaccine.

Escherichia coli *(ETEC) vaccines*

Weanling diarrhoea caused by enterotoxogenic *E. coli* is an important disease of human and animal infants. However, there has been a concerted effort to develop protective vaccines only for animals of commercial significance, such as pigs and cattle. Successful approaches have included vaccination of dams with enterotoxin toxoid or killed vaccines, and the addition of antigens to weaning food to stimulate gut immunity. In this way considerable protection against weanling diarrhoea can be conferred on piglets and calves.

The infections of piglets and calves are much better understood and more open to experimental investigation than those of human infants, and these advances must give hope of a successful human vaccine. It is notable that pilus antigens have been shown to be protective in pigs[41], and that the use of colonization factors (CFAI, CFAII) has been attempted in human beings[42]. Studies on these animal infections have also demonstrated what may prove to be the major problem with enteric vaccines. Studies in both calves and piglets have apparently shown that the intestinal secretory immune system responds by means of a series of primary responses and that secondary boosting does not occur[43]. The relevance of this finding to long-term immunological memory needs to be clarified. The problems with the development of *E. coli* vaccine were reviewed by Levine[44]. Parenteral, killed oral and live oral vaccines have all been considered as conferring particular advantages. Vaccines directed against colonization factors have been most successful in test systems. Orally administered purified CFAI is able to stimulate pre-existing immunity in volunteers, but not to prime newly exposed subjects. However, SIgA responses result when it is coated on bacterial cells[42].

Rabbits have been considered to be a suitable model for human ETEC infection, largely on the basis of the responses obtained to toxins in ligated ileal loops. Successful oral immunization of rabbits has been achieved using live oral vaccine strains[45], and this model has been suggested as a suitable screening system.

Antitoxic immunity seems to play a much greater protective role in ETEC infection than with cholera. Indeed, it had been hoped that cholera toxoid would protect against LT. Should it be found that the antitoxins have a major protective role in infants as well as animal models, an antitoxic vaccine could readily be developed. Genes coding for LT, and Shiga-like toxin have been cloned[46] and STa has been produced as a synthetic peptide vaccine[47].

Enterotoxigenic *E. coli* have been the subject of an imaginative attempt at passive immunoprophylaxis. The immunoglobulin concentrate was prepared from colostrum and milk of dairy cows immunized with ST, LT, cholera toxin and a number of *E. coli* serogroups. In a double-blind volunteer study protection was achieved against challenge with an enterotoxigenic strain of *E coli*[48]. Thus we have every reason to believe that diarrhoea caused by ETEC could be prevented by vaccination, but the problem has not received the same concentrated scientific attention as cholera.

Shigellae vaccines

At the present there is no useful vaccine against Shigellae. The various attempts that have been made employing a wide range of techniques were reviewed by Formal[49]; indeed, he and his co-workers have come closest to success. There is no evidence that parenteral administration of killed vaccines can prevent the disease. A variety of live oral vaccines have been studied, these include: (1) spontaneous non-invasive mutants of Shigellae, (2) *E. coli–Shigella* hybrids, (3) streptomycin-dependent strains of Shigellae.

The major problem results from the specificity of the immune response. Vaccines can be tested in man or monkeys, and confer significant protection against disease, though colonization may still occur. If for example, the vaccine is directed against *Shigella flexneri* 2a, protection will be limited to this type of this species[50].

Salmonella typhi

Alone among the bacteria causing intestinal disease an effective vaccine is available for protection against infection caused by *S. typhi.* This killed parenteral vaccine is widely available and has been shown in controlled field trials to provide about 80% protection. However, in volunteer challenge studies the vaccine does not perform as well. Further, the vaccine produces transient fever in many recipients.

Many aspects of typhoid vaccine were reviewed by Germanier[51]. This review outlines the reasons for, and the development of, the live oral vaccine Ty21a. An innovative aspect of this study was the use of the mouse/*S. typhimurium* system to overcome the problems that result from the lack of an animal model for *S. typhi* infections. In this case a natural animal infection was studied to allow the conceptual and practical tools needed to be developed.

The final outcome was the development of a UDP-galactose-4-epimerase (gal.E) mutant of *S. typhi* that retains the ability to invade and spread systemically but is unable to grow in the absence of galactose. Thus, the growth of Ty21a can be readily limited. In effect this vaccine behaves as though it were fully virulent and delivers antigen in the same way as a natural infection with *S. typhi.* The genetic characteristics of the strain have recently been analysed[52].

As a live oral vaccine it has many advantages and has performed well in controlled field trials in Egypt[53], but less well in later trials in Chile[54] (Table 7). Further trials are now under way[55]. The efficacy of the vaccine seems to be very dependent on the formulation in which it is delivered. This needs to be sorted out before full advantage can be taken of this exciting development.

In addition to its importance as a typhoid vaccine *S. typhi* Ty21a has great potential as a delivery system for other vaccines. Use of the techniques

Table 7 Field trials of live oral vaccine *Salmonella typhi* Ty21a

Country	*Reference*	*Number of subjects*		*Percentage effectiveness*
		Vaccinees	*Controls*	
Egypt 1978–81	53	16486	15902	96
Chile 1983–86	54	22170	21906	67

Table 8 *Salmonella typhi* Ty21a hybrid strains

Hybrid	*Reference*	*Antigens expressed*
Ty21a – *Shigella flexneri* 2a	56	*S. flexneri* type, group antigens
S. typhi SE12	57	B subunit heat-labile enterotoxin
Ty21aS – *E. coli*	58	CFI fimbriae heat-stable enterotoxin

Immunization against leprosy

of recombinant DNA technology has enabled restriction fragments of DNA from other organisms to be transferred into Ty21a and to be expressed. *S. typhi* is related to Shigellae, *E. coli* and other Enterobacteriaceae. Further it is known that *V. cholerae* genes can express in *E. coli.* Thus, all bacterial intestinal pathogens, in theory at least, are able to express antigens and virulence factors in Ty21a. This has resulted in the development of a series of Ty21a hybrid strains that express other antigens[56–58] (Table 8). In model systems these result in the development of circulating antibody directed against the expressed antigens. The value of such immunity remains to be demonstrated. *V. cholerae* and ETEC infections are limited to the lumen of the gut and Ty21a hybrids may not be good stimulators of the secretory immune system in the gut. Nonetheless, these studies open up new vistas in vaccine development.

S. typhi Ty21a is not the sole mutant vaccine strain considered for use in typhoid fever. Temperature-sensitive vaccine strains have also been developed[59] and are used for the same function as Ty21a. They may have major advantages in terms of reduced shedding and environmental survival.

CONCLUSION

The application of the techniques of genetic engineering to the development of vaccines against the bacterial infection of the gastrointestinal tract has resulted in many exciting advances. Lack of complete success can be attributed to the problem of deficiency of virulence factors and protective antigens. These bacteria only cause natural infections in man and some other primates. This limits the range of experimentation.

REFERENCES

1. Germanier, R. (1984). *Bacterial Vaccines.* (London: Academic Press)
2. Levine, M. M., Kaper, J. B., Black, R. E. and Clements, M. L. (1983). New knowledge on pathogenesis of bacterial enteric infections as applied to vaccine development. *Microbiol. Rev.*, **47**, 510–50
3. Jones, G. W. and Freter, R. (1976). Adhesive properties of *Vibrio cholerae*: nature of the interaction with isolated rabbit border membranes and human erythrocytes. *Infect. Immun.*, **14**, 240–5
4. Bhattacharjee, J. W. and Srivastava, B. S. (1979). Adherence of wild-type and mutant strains of *Vibrio cholerae* to normal and immune intestinal tissue. *Bull. WHO*, **57**, 123–8
5. Freter, R. and Jones, G. W. (1976). Adhesive properties of *Vibrio cholerae*: Nature of the interaction with intact mucosal surface. *Infect. Immun.*, **14**, 246–56

6. Manning, P. A. (1987) Involvement of cell envelope components in the pathogenesis of *Vibrio cholerae*: targets for cholera vaccine development. *Vaccine*, **5**, 83–7
7. Gaastra, W. and Graaf, F. K. (1982). Host-specific fimbrial adhesions of non-invasive enterotoxigenic *Escherichia coli* strains. *Microbiol. Rev.*, **46**, 129–61
8. Dallas, W. S. and Falkow, S. (1980). Amino acid sequence homology between cholera toxin and *Escherichia coli* heat-labile toxin. *Nature*, **228**, 499–501
9. Gill, D. M. and Richardson, S. H. (1980). Heat-labile enterotoxin of *Escherichia coli*. *J. Infect. Dis.*, **141**, 64–70
10. Moseley, S. L. and Falkow, S. (1980). Nucleotide sequence homology between the heat-labile enterotoxin gene of *Escherichia coli* and *Vibrio cholerae* deoxyribonucleic acid. *J. Bacteriol.*, **144**, 444–6
11. Law, D. (1988). Virulence factors of enteropathogenic *Escherichia coli*. *J. Med. Microbiol.*, **26**, 1–10
12. Smith, H. R. and Scotland, S. M. (1988). Vero cytotoxin producing strains of *Escherichia coli*. *J. Med. Microbiol.*, **26**, 77–85
13. Scotland, S. M. (1988). Toxins. *J. Appl. Bacteriol.*, **65**, (Symposium supplement), 109S–129S
14. Williams, P. H., Roberts, M. and Hensen, G. (1988). Stages in bacterial invasion. *J. Appl. Bacteriol.*, **65** (Symposium supplement), 131S–147S
15. Kaper, J. B. and Levine, M. M. (1981). Cloned cholera enterotoxin genes in study and prevention of cholera. *Lancet*, **2**, 1162–3
16. Gennaro, M. L., Greenaway, P. J. and Broadbent, D. A. (1982). Expression of cloned cholera enterotoxin gene in *Escherichia coli* and possibilities of vaccine development. *Lancet*, **1**, 1239–40
17. Gennaro, M. L., Greenaway, P. J. and Broadbent, D. A. (1982). The expression of biologically active cholera toxin in *Escherichia coli*. *Nucl. Acids Res.*, **10**, 4883–90
18. Manning, P. A., Brown, M. H. and Heuzenroeder, M. W. (1984) Cloning of the structural gene (hly) for the haemolysin of *Vibrio cholerae* el Tor strain 017. *Gene*, **31**, 225–31
19. Goldberg, S. L. and Murphy, J. R. (1984). Molecular cloning of the haemolysin determinant from *Vibrio cholerae* el Tor. *J. Bacteriol.*, **160**, 239–44
20. Goldberg, S. L. and Murphy, J. R. (1985). Cloning and characterization of the haemolysin determinants from *Vibro cholerae* el Tor. *J. Bacteriol.*, **162**, 35–41
21. Richardson, K., Michalski, J. and Kaper, J. B (1986). Haemolysin production and cloning of two haemolysin determinants from classical *Vibrio cholerae*. *Infect. Immun.*, **54**, 415–20
22. Manning, P. A, Heuzenroeder, M. W., Yeadon, J., Leavesley, D. I., Reebes, P. R. and Rowley, D. (1986). Molecular cloning and expression in *Escherichia coli* K-12 of the O antigens of the Inaba and Ogawa serotypes of the *Vibrio cholerae* O1 lipopolysaccharides and their potential for vaccine development. *Infect. Immun.*, **53**, 272–7
23. Levine, M. M., Black, R. E., Clements, M. L. and Kaper, J. B. (1984). Present status of cholera vaccines. *Biochem. Soc. Trans.*, **12**, 200–2
24. Finkelstein, R. A. (1984). Cholera. In Germanier, R. (ed.), *Bacterial Vaccines*, pp. 107–36. (London: Academic Press)
25. Clemens, J. D., Sack, D. A., Harris, J. R., Chakrabarty, J., Khan, M. R., Stanton, B. F., Kay, B. A., Khan, M. U., Yunus, M., Atkinson, W., Svennerholm, A. and Holgren, J. (1986). Field trial of oral vaccine in Bangladesh. *Lancet*, **2**, 124–7
26. Black, R. E., Levine, M. M., Clements, M. L., Young, C. R., Svennerholm, A M. and Holmgren, J. (1987) Protective efficacy in humans of killed whole-vibrio oral cholera vaccine with and without the B subunit of cholera toxin. *Infect. Immun.*, **55**, 1116–20
27. Clemens, J. D., Stanton, B. F., Chakraborty, J., Sack, D. A., Khan, M. R., Huda, S., Ahmed, F., Harris, J. R., Yunus, M., Khan, M. U., Svennerholm, A. M., Jertborn, M. and Holmgren, J. (1987). B subunit-whole cell and whole cell-only oral vaccines against cholera: studies on reactogenicity and immunogenicity. *J. Infect. Dis.*, **155**, 79–85
28. Mekalanos, J., Goldberg, I., Miller, V., Pearson, G., Swartz and Taylor, R. (1985). Genetic construction of cholera vaccine prototypes. In *Vaccines*, Vol. 85, pp. 101–5. (Cold Spring: Cold Spring Harbor Laboratory)
29. Kaper, J. B., Levine, M. M., Lockman, H. A., Baldini, M. M., Black, R. E., Clements, M. L. and Morris, J. G. (1985). Development and testing of a recombinant live oral cholera vaccine. In *Vaccines*, Vol. 85, pp. 107–11. (Cold Spring: Cold Spring Harbor Laboratory)
30. Levine, M. M., Black, R. E., Clements, M. L., Lanata, C., Sears, S., Honda, T., Young, C.

R. and Finkelstein, R. A. (1984). Evaluation in humans of attenuated *Vibrio cholerae* el Tor Ogawa strain Texas star-SR as a live oral vaccine. *Infect. Immun.*, **43**, 515–22

31. Levine, M. M., Kaper, J. B., Herrington, D., Losonsky, G., Morris, J. G., Clements, M. L., Black, R. E., Tall, B. and Hall, R. (1988). Volunteer studies of deletion mutants of *Vibrio cholerae* O1 prepared by recombinant techniques. *Infect. Immun.*, **56**, 161–7
32. de Zoysa, I. and Feachem, R. G. (1985). Interventions for the control of diarrhoeal diseases among young children: rotavirus and cholera immunization. *Bull. WHO*, **63**, 569–83
33. Harley, V., Tomkins, C. A. and Drasar, B. S. (1987). Extracellular products of mutant strains of *Vibrio cholerae*: physiological response. *Biochem. Soc. Trans.*, **15**, 550–1
34. Mann, G. F. and Drasar, B. S. (1986). Monoclonal antibodies against *Vibrio cholerae* haemolysin: positive selection and use. *Biochem. Soc. Trans.*, **14**, 119
35. Miller, C. J., Foxall, P. A., Harrison, T. J. and Drasar, B. S. (1988). *Vibrio cholerae* haemolysin: genetic constitution and biotype. *Biochem. Soc. Trans.*, **16**, 638–9
36. Glass, R. I., Svennerholm, A. M., Khan, M. R., Huda, S., Huq, I. and Holmgren, J. (1985). Seroepidemiological studies of el Tor cholera in Bangladesh: Association of serum antibody levels with protection. *J. Infect. Dis.*, **151**, 236–42
37. Jertborn, M., Svennerholm, A. M. and Holmgren, J. (1988). Five-year immunologic memory in Swedish volunteers after oral cholera vaccination. *J. Infect. Dis.*, **157**, 374–7
38. Bloom, L. and Rowley, D. (1979). Persistence in the mouse gut as an important factor in oral immunogenicity of strains of *V. cholerae. Austral. J. Exp. Biol. Med. Sci.*, **57**, 325–33
39. Pierce, N. F., Cray, W. C., Kaper, J. B. and Mekalonos, J. J. (1988). Determinants of immunogenicity and mechanisms of protection by virulent and mutant *Vibrio cholerae* O1 in rabbits. *Infect. Immun.*, **56**, 142–8
40. Jertborn, M., Svennerholm, A. M. and Holmgren, J. (1986). Saliva, breast milk, and serum antibody responses as indirect measures of intestinal immunity after oral cholera vaccination or natural. *J. Clin. Microbiol.*, **24**, 203–9
41. Runnels, P. L., Moseley, S. L. and Moon, H. W. (1987). F41 Pili as protective antigens of enterotoxigenic *Escherichia coli* that produce F41, K99, or both pilus antigens. *Infect. Immun.*, **55**, 555–8
42. Evans, D. G., Evans, D. J., Opekun, A. R. and Graham, D. Y. (1986). Oral whole cell vaccine protective against enterotoxigenic *Escherichia coli* diarrhoea. *Bacterial Vaccines and Local Immunity – Annali Sclavo III*, pp. 155–6
43. Porter, P. and Allen, W. D. (1979). Antibody response in pigs and calves to antigens from the intestinal lumen and the efficacy of oral immunoprophylaxis against post-weaning enteric infection. In Hennings, W. A. (ed.), *Antigen Absorption by the Gut*, pp. 81–92. (Lancaster: MTP Press)
44. Levine, M. M. (1984). *Escherichia coli* infections. In Germanier, R. (ed.), *Bacterial Vaccines*, pp. 187–235. (London: Academic Press)
45. Sack, R. B., Kline, R. L. and Spira, W. M. (1988). Oral immunization of rabbits with enterotoxigenic *Escherichia coli* protest against intraintestinal challenge. *Infect. Immun.*, **56**, 387-94
46. Newland, J. W., Strockbine, N. A., Miller, S. F., Brien, A. D. and Holmes, R. K. (1985). Cloning of shiga-like toxin structural genes from a toxin converting phage of *Escherichia coli. Science*, **230**, 179–81
47. Klipstein, F. A., Engert, R. F. and Houghton, R. A. (1986). Immunisation of volunteers with a synthetic peptide vaccine for enterotoxigenic *Escherichia coli. Lancet*, **1**, 471–3
48. Tacket, C. O., Losonsky, G., Link, H., Hoang, Y., Guesry, P., Hilpert, H. and Levine, M. M. (1988). Protection by milk immunoglobulin concentrate against oral challenge with enterotoxigenic *Escherichia coli. N. Engl. J. Med.*, **318**, 1240–3
49. Formal, S. B. (1984). Shigellosis. In Germanier, R. (ed.), *Bacterial Vaccines*, pp. 167–86. (London: Academic Press)
50. Formal, S. B., Hale, T. L., Kaper, C., Cogan, J. P., Snoy, P. J., Chaug, Wingfield, M. E., Elisberg, B. L. and Baron, L. S. (1984). Oral vaccination of monkeys with an invasive *Escherichia coli*-12 hybrid expressing *Shigella flexneri 2a* somatic antigen. *Infect. Immun.*, **6**, 465–9
51. Germanier, R. (1984). Typhoid fever. In Germanier, R. (ed.), *Bacterial Vaccines*, pp. 137–65. (London: Academic Press)
52. Silva, B. A., Gonzalez, C., Mora, G. C. and Cabello, F. (1987). Genetic characteristics of the *Salmonella typhi*, strain Ty21a vaccine. *J. Infect. Dis.*, **155**, 1077–8

53. Wahdan, M. H., Serie, C., Cerisier, Y., Sallam, S. and Germanier, R. (1982). A controlled field trial of live *Salmonella typhi* strain Ty21a oral vaccine against typhoid: three-year results. *J. Infect. Dis.*, **145**, 292–5
54. Levine, M. M., Ferreccio, C., Black, R. E. and Germanier, R. (1987). Large-scale field trial of Ty21a live oral typhoid vaccine in enteric-coated capsule formulation. *Lancet*, **1**, 1049–52
55. Germanier, R. and Levine, M. M. (1986). The live oral typhoid vaccine Ty21a: recent field trial results. *Annali Sclavo III*, 19–22
56. Baron, L. S., Kopecko, D. J., Formal, S. B., Seid, F., Guerry, P. and Powell, C. (1987). Introduction of *Shigella flexneri* 2a type and group antigen genes into oral typhoid vaccine strain *Salmonella typhi* Ty21a. *Infect. Immun.*, **55**, 2797-801
57. Clements, J. D. and El-Morshidy, S. (1984) Construction of a potential live oral bivalent vaccine for typhoid fever and cholera–*Escherichia coli*-related diarrhoeas. *Infect. Immun.* **46**, 564–9
58. Yamamoto, T., Tamura, Y. and Yokota, T. (1985). Enteroadhesion fimbriae and enterotoxin of *Escherichia coli*: genetic transfer to a streptomycin-resistant mutant of the galE oral-route live-vaccine *Salmonella typhi* Ty21a. *Infect. Immun.*, **50**, 925–8
59. Hooke, A., Wang, Z., Cerquetti, C. and Bellanti, J. A. (1986). Temperature-sensitive vaccine strains of *Salmonella typhi*. *Annali Sclavo III*, pp. 23–30

4
Immunization against leprosy

H. M. DOCKRELL and K. P. W. J. McADAM

In 1978 the WHO Committee on the Immunology of Leprosy, IMMLEP, defined the development of a prophylactic vaccine against leprosy as an objective of high priority. Ten years later, trials are under way of the approaches they identified, namely, vaccines based on antigenically similar cultivatable mycobacteria, killed *Mycobacterium leprae*, or of a mixture of killed *M. leprae* with BCG. This chapter will discuss the rationale for such vaccines, together with the possibility of a second-generation vaccine, based on protective antigens produced either by molecular biology or as synthetic peptides.

WHY VACCINATE AGAINST LEPROSY?

There are estimated to be between 10 and 12 million cases of leprosy worldwide; the highest incidence (1–5 per 1000) is found in Asia and some areas of Africa and South America. Although these figures are low in comparison to many other diseases, and the disease is chronic and not fatal, the deformities which can result are responsible for the stigma attached to leprosy. Drug treatment with dapsone alone was so inefficient that cases of multibacillary disease were treated for life, but the introduction of a new multidrug regimen recommended by WHO has shortened the duration of therapy to 6 months for paucibacillary cases and to 2 years for multibacillary cases. However, in many areas the incidence of leprosy is not falling. This is due to the long incubation period before clinical disease develops, and to delays in diagnosing highly infectious multibacillary cases who are often not identified until the disease has been active for many years. Therefore to control leprosy, a protective vaccine is needed. As human–human contact is thought to be responsible for infection, and there is no identified animal reservoir in most endemic areas (the exception is natural infection in armadillos in the southern US[1] and there are recent reports of transmission in certain strains of monkey[2]) it has been stated that leprosy could be eradicated within one generation if a suitable vaccine were found[3].

WHAT IS PROTECTIVE IMMUNITY?

Clinical leprosy presents as a continuous spectrum of disease, ranging from the paucibacillary tuberculoid to the multibacillary lepromatous forms. When classified according to the Ridley and Jopling scale[4], the polar forms (polar tuberculoid, TT, and polar lepromatous, LL) are generally stable, while the borderline cases (borderline tuberculoid, BT, borderline BB, and borderline lepromatous, BL) are unstable and may upgrade or downgrade towards the tuberculoid or lepromatous poles, respectively. At the tuberculoid pole the skin lesions contain very few bacteria, but the patients show strong cell-mediated immunity as measured by skin testing or lymphocyte transformation tests with leprosy antigens. Lepromatous patients may contain up to 10^{10} bacilli per gram of tissue, but fail to make cell-mediated responses to leprosy antigens, although they do make a range of antibodies to *M. leprae* as well as to unrelated antigens. Thus it is assumed that cell-mediated immune responses are important in immunity, presumably due to the activation of macrophages to kill the *M. leprae* by cytokines such as gamma-interferon, which are produced by activated T cells. Recent studies in which gamma-interferon has been injected directly into lesions[5], resulting in a decrease of acid-fast bacilli, support this view, although with other mycobacteria such as *M. tuberculosis* there have been reports that macrophages activated by gamma-interferon become less microbicidal for the mycobacteria[6]. It is also generally assumed that antibodies are not important for protection. It is, however, worth noting that the initial interaction of an invading *M. leprae* with the immune system, in the first minutes or hours, may be controlled by mechanisms unrelated to those involved in maintaining a bacterial load in the chronic stage of the disease years later.

It is also questionable whether patients with tuberculoid leprosy have the sort of immunity that a protective vaccine should mimic. Despite the successful control of the overall bacterial load in these patients, considerable nerve damage can occur due to immunopathological responses.

Many individuals are thought to become infected with *M. leprae* but to self-cure without any apparent clinical signs. At present there are no tests which can identify such individuals within a population, but healthy contacts of leprosy patients can be assumed to have developed effective immunity against leprosy. Staff working with patients or household members of patients have been used in a number of studies on immunity. In Ethiopia, staff arriving from non-endemic areas to work in a Leprosy Centre showed an increased lymphocyte transformation response within 6 months to a year[7], suggesting that they had been infected and were mounting an immune response. Ideally, the small number of individuals in such groups who will subsequently develop clinical disease should be identified and excluded, but this is not possible at present. However, despite the limitations of working with such groups, the sort of immunity shown by healthy contacts is what a successful protective vaccine should mimic.

BCG AS A VACCINE AGAINST LEPROSY

BCG (Bacillus Calmette-Guérin) is a live attenuated strain of *M. bovis*. Its potential use as a vaccine against leprosy stems from the observation that

BCG vaccination could induce a positive Mitsuda skin test to leprosy antigens[8]. Early work in the mouse footpad model of leprosy also demonstrated that vaccination with BCG induced protection[9]. It is interesting that in this model addition of killed *M. leprae* did not increase the protection[10].

There have been four major trials of BCG vaccination against leprosy[11], in which the protection has varied from approximately 20% in Burma[12] to 80% in Uganda[13]. Many explanations have been suggested for these differences. These include the strain of BCG used – for example, in Malawi Glaxo BCG was found to cause larger ulcers and a greater conversion to skin test positivity than Copenhagen BCG[14] – although the same Glaxo freeze-dried vaccine was used in both the Uganda and Burma trials. Other variables which might contribute to the differences include the age at which vaccination was given, the existence of different atypical mycobacteria in the different areas, and differences in the natural history of infection and disease in the different areas[11]. BCG vaccine is, however, very widely used, and accepted as a cheap and safe vaccine, so that in spite of the variable results in these trials it has been used in combination with *M. leprae* in a number of newer trials.

PRODUCTION OF *M. LEPRAE* FOR VACCINE STUDIES

Research into leprosy has lagged behind many other diseases, as the bacteria cannot be grown *in vitro*. Limited growth can be achieved in the mouse footpad in a model developed by Shepard[15] and viability of organisms and their sensitivity to drugs can be tested in this way. The main source of material comes from the nine-banded armadillo, found by Kirchheimer and Storrs[16] to support growth of the bacteria.

Armadillo-derived *M. leprae*, purified from the spleens and liver of infected animals, was shown to induce similar lymphocyte transformation[17] and skin test responses in humans[18] to human-derived bacteria. It was also found that irradiation did not decrease immunogenicity[19]. Yields of up to 10^9–10^{10}/g tissue can be obtained, and Draper[20] has established standardized protocols for the production of irradiated whole *M. leprae* and of soluble sonicates of the bacteria.

USE OF IRRADIATED *M. LEPRAE* VACCINE

The vaccine was first tried in a group of non-endemic controls. Doses of 5×10^7–5×10^8 irradiated *M. leprae* vaccine, given intradermally, induced delayed-type hypersensivity, measured at 72 h, to a soluble *M. leprae* skin-test antigen, while there was little effect on the reactivity to PPD[21]. Doses of 1.5×10^8-5×10^8 also induced a significant increase in lymphocyte proliferation to *M. leprae* when tested 3 months after vaccination, which persisted for the study period of 1 year[22]. Some enhancement of responses to PPD, an antigen expected to show cross-reactivity, was observed, as well as to unrelated antigens such as tetanus toxoid, suggesting that the vaccine also caused some non-specific immune enhancement. The same doses of vaccine also induced a humoral response to *M. leprae*, measured by an enzyme-linked immunosorbent test (ELISA) or a serum antibody competition test[23].

A panel of 42 human T cell clones were raised from the vaccinated volunteers[24]. Eleven out of 42 were *M. leprae*-specific, not responding to BCG or to PPD. Ten of the clones were tested for the ability to recognize recombinant antigens from *M. leprae*, and 4 out of 10 responded to the recombinant 18 kd antigen, suggesting that it might be an immunodominant antigen in the human T cell response to the vaccine.

VACCINATION WITH A COMBINATION OF BCG WITH *M. LEPRAE* VACCINE

The rationale for using a combination of BCG with *M. leprae* in immunoprophylaxis has been largely as a result of extensive studies by Convit and his group in Venezuela, using this combination in immunotherapy[25,26].

A mixture of heat-killed, armadillo-derived *M. leprae* with BCG was used in lepromatous and indeterminate leprosy to stimulate the immune system. In initial studies *M. leprae* (6.4×10^7) and 0.1 ml BCG vaccine were injected intradermally into individuals who failed to show skin test responses to leprosy antigens[25]. An immune granuloma developed, with rapid elimination of both organisms. Immunotherapy was then started in larger groups of patients. The results of giving 8–10 vaccinations over a period of 18–30 months to 531 patients were striking[26]. Patients with BL/LL leprosy showed a marked reduction in the number of lesions present, over 70% of the patients having no detectable lesions after immunotherapy. There was also a reduction in the bacterial index, a measure of the number of bacteria present in the skin. Reversal reactions, another indication of increased immune competence, were seen in 54% of LL and 83.1% of BL patients. Patients with indeterminate leprosy, an early stage of the disease, were also treated, and after treatment 87.5% showed no evidence of disease. Histologically the most striking changes observed in the skin after vaccination were the accumulations of small macrophages and lymphoid cells within the lesions[27]. One potential danger of increasing immune responsiveness is that reactions in the nerves might also be induced; however, out of a total of 354 lepromatous patients only 4 developed severe, and 19 moderate, neuritic reactions which were controlled by thalidomide and steroids[27]. Lepromatous patients given the combined immunotherapy also showed increased lymphocyte transformation to *M. leprae*, to a level similar to tuberculoid patients[28]. In addition the combined vaccine reduced the suppression of a concanavalin A mitogen response induced by Dharmendra lepromin.

COMBINED BCG AND *M. LEPRAE* VACCINATION FOR IMMUNOPROPHYLAXIS

A number of studies have now been set up to test the protection given by the BCG and *M. leprae* combination. In Venezuela, a group of contacts who failed to give a positive skin test to *M. leprae* were vaccinated and 98% converted to a positive skin test, 85% remaining positive after 8 months[26]. A much larger trial of 65 000 contacts was then started in 1984. Another study is under way in the Karonga district of northern Malawi, in an area previously surveyed epidemiologically. Started in 1986, this trial has been designed to compare whether the combination of BCG with *M. leprae* gives better protection than BCG alone, and to determine if repeat BCG vaccinations can increase the 50% protection against clinical leprosy given by a first vaccination in the same area[29].

CULTIVATABLE MYCOBACTERIA AS VACCINES

Although *M. leprae* cannot be cultivated *in vitro*, there have been a number of reports describing the cultivation of mycobacteria from leprosy patients. The relationship of these organisms to *M. leprae* is not always clear, but the presence of cross-reactive antigens, and the ease with which they can be grown, has led to their use as vaccines against leprosy.

The ICRC Bacillus

The ICRC bacillus was isolated in 1969 from a lepromatous leprosy patient, by scientists at the Indian Cancer Research Campaign laboratories. It can be grown *in vitro* and belongs to the *M. avium–intracellulare* group of mycobacteria. It has been shown to share cross-reactive antigens with *M. leprae*, detected by a range of tests including delayed hypersensitivity in guinea pigs and mice[30], and skin testing in man[31]. A vaccine of irradiated ICRC bacilli was found to induce lepromin conversion in about 55% of lepromatous patients and in 95% of lepromin-negative healthy subjects[32,33]. Some patients developed a reversal reaction associated with conversion to lepromin positivity[34]. The vaccine produced ulceration, simîlar to that seen with BCG vaccination. The lepromin conversion induced by vaccination in leprosy contacts or normal schoolchildren was stable over 3 years, and was not associated with any increase in antibodies to phenolic glycolipid (PGL-1)[35]. More recently, an immunogenic subunit has been isolated from the ICRC vaccine; this is a high molecular weight glycolipoprotein which contains both T- and B- cell epitopes[36]. At present a large-scale phase III trial of the ICRC vaccine is under way in which the vaccine is being given to healthy volunteers irrespective of their lepromin status.

Mycobacterium w

Another fast-growing cultivatable atypical mycobacterium, *Mycobacterium w*, has also been selected for vaccine trials, based on its antigenic cross-reactivity with *M. leprae*[37]. When BL/LL leprosy patients were immunized with autoclaved *Mycobacterium w*, about 60% converted to lepromin positivity[38]. This vaccine is now undergoing phase II/phase III trials in India, where patients on drug therapy are given the vaccine or a placebo every 3 months. The preliminary results show a promising improvement in the clinical and bacteriological status of the patients receiving the vaccine[39].

PROBLEMS ASSOCIATED WITH THE USE OF WHOLE MYCOBACTERIAL VACCINES

There are a number of problems associated with the use of vaccines containing whole *M. leprae*. Firstly, there is a need to obtain larger numbers of bacteria, involving large colonies of armadillos which unfortunately do not breed in captivity. Secondly, there are problems associated with the extraction of the bacteria from the armadillo tissues, which can result either in the loss of leprosy antigens due to the extraction procedures, or to contamination of the bacteria with armadillo proteins. More worrying, however, is the potential inclusion of antigens which are involved in immunopathology, for example, in nerve damage, or which in some individuals may trigger a suppressive rather than a beneficial immune response, leading to lepromatous disease. Obviously, a vaccine based on one or more purified antigens, and which could be obtained using molecular biology techniques, or as a synthetic peptide, would be preferable.

ROLE OF INDIVIDUAL *M. LEPRAE* ANTIGENS IN IMMUNITY

So far, only one antigen from *M. leprae* has been shown to be *M. leprae*-specific. This is PGL-1, which has a unique terminal trisaccharide[40]. PGL has been purified from *M. leprae* and synthetic disaccharide–BSA conjugates synthesized. Lepromatous patients in particular have high levels of antibodies to PGL[41]. In mice, PGL failed to stimulate cell-mediated immune responses, such as delayed-type hypersensitivity and lymphocyte proliferation[42], although delayed-type hypersensitivity granulomas were detected at 21 days when armadillos were given PGL[43]. In fact PGL may be immunosuppressive, inhibiting both T- cell[44] and macrophage function[45], a further reason why it is not a vaccine candidate.

IDENTIFICATION OF ANTIGENS BY MOLECULAR BIOLOGY

Work on *M. leprae* protein antigens has focused on the protein antigens identified by Young and colleagues[46] in a λgt11 recombinant DNA expression library of *M. leprae*. Mouse monoclonal antibodies directed to proteins of 65, 36, 28, 18 and 12 kd were used to probe the library and recombinant DNA clones encoding the antigens isolated. A clone encoding an antigen of 70 kd has also been isolated[47]. With the exception of the 65 kd protein which is produced under its own promoter, the proteins are expressed as fusion proteins with β-galactosidase. Similar approaches have been used to identify genes encoding antigens from *M. tuberculosis*[48–50] and *M. bovis* BCG[51]. Antigens so far identified include a *M. bovis* 64 kg protein[51], and *M. tuberculosis* 35 and 53 kd[49] and 71, 65 and 14 kg antigens[50].

T CELL RECOGNITION OF RECOMBINANT ANTIGENS

A number of approaches have been used to investigate the recognition of these recombinant proteins by T cells. Many workers have used T cell clones, isolated from the peripheral blood or from skin lesions, which are screened for their ability to recognize the recombinant proteins. The relevant epitopes can then be mapped using sublibraries encoding portions of the protein, and synthetic peptides[52]. Another approach has been to use fractionated mycobacterial antigens separated by sodium dodecyl sulphate polyacrylamide electrophoresis and blotted onto nitrocellulose to screen for antigens of interest[53,54].

The 65 kd antigen of *M. leprae* is very similar to that of other mycobacteria, showing greater than 95% homology with the 65 kd antigens of *M. tuberculosis* or *M. bovis* BCG[55]. Testing with a panel of monoclonals showed that there are at least 14 separate epitopes[56]; many of the epitopes recognized by mouse monoclonal antibodies are cross-reactive, although there are also unique epitopes[57]. The positions of the dominant epitopes were identified using a gene sublibrary and synthetic peptides[58,59]. The 65 kd antigen is also important in the T cell response to mycobacteria. Studies in mice have shown that the *M. leprae* 65 kd protein stimulates lymphocyte proliferation and delayed-type hypersensitivity[60].

The 64/65 kd protein is also important in the immune response to tuberculosis: approximately one in five *M. tuberculosis*-reactive mouse T cells recognized the 64 kd protein[61], and it can also be recognized by human T cells[62]. Two out of four cross-reactive T cell clones from a tuberculoid leprosy patient responded to the 64 kd protein from *M. bovis* BCG[63]. In a larger panel of clones, 9/38 T cell clones isolated from two tuberculoid leprosy patients recognized the 65 kd antigen, and two individual epitopes, one cross-reactive and one specific, were identified[64].

The 65 kd antigen was initially thought to be a major cross-reactive antigen associated with the cell wall[65] or located in the 'periplasmic' space[66]. It has become of much wider general interest since it was recognized to be one of a family of heat-shock or stress proteins[67,68]. When extracts from clones containing recombinant DNA were screened on Western blots, an additional band was recognized in the control *E. coli* extracts. This cross-reactivity with the *E. coli* ams gene proved to be part of a much wider cross-reactivity between other bacteria[67]. The *M. leprae* 70 kd and 18 kd proteins also have homology with stress proteins[68].

Another antigen of interest is the 18 kd antigen of *M. leprae* which was shown to contain leprosy-specific epitopes stimulating human T cell clones[24]. The gene for the whole 18 kd antigen has been sequenced[69], but although the site recognized by the L5 mouse monolonal antibody is *M. leprae*-specific[70], T cell clones recognizing this protein have been isolated from a

BCG-vaccinated donor who has not been in contact with leprosy patients. This implies that the protein must also contain at least one cross-reactive epitope recognized by T cells (Dockrell, Lee, Stoker and McAdam, *Infect. Immun.*, 1989 in press).

Crude lysates of *E. coli* expressing recombinant antigens have been used to screen T- cell clones for reactivity (for example, see ref. 24) but purification of the proteins is usually required before they can be added to cell cultures *in vitro*. One problem with β-galactosidase fusion proteins is that they are frequently insoluble, which makes purification difficult. For this reason, other expression systems such as *Streptomyces lividans* are being used, in which the recombinant protein of interest is secreted into the culture medium[71]. Another advantage of expression in *S. lividans* is that sets of proteins involved in the synthesis of glycolipids, or polysaccharides, could be expressed.

A final objective is to introduce genes for specific *M. leprae* proteins of interest to a cultivatable mycobacterium such as BCG, which is already approved for human use[72]. A shuttle plasmid with which foreign DNA can be introduced into *M. smegmatis*, and which can integrate stably into the host chromosome, has been recently described[73]. Plasmid vectors which can be introduced into mycobacteria, including BCG, have also been developed[73,74].

ARE THERE MAJOR ANTIGENS AS YET UNIDENTIFIED?

The genome of *M. leprae* is estimated to be between 1.3×10^9 and 2.2×10^9 *M*r (daltons)[71] so that the few antigens so far isolated represent only a small proportion of the total complement of *M. leprae* proteins. In addition, many of the proteins have been identified by mouse rather than human antibodies, so that there has been a disproportionate emphasis on the antigens recognized by antibodies from one particular strain of mouse (Balb/c). Other candidate antigens recognized by human antibodies include proteins of 22 and 33 kd[35] and of 15 and 25 kd[76].

LIVE OR DEAD VACCINES?

A number of studies have shown that live bacilli can be more effective vaccines than dead bacteria[77]. For example, relatively few T-cell clones which have been isolated using a sonicate of *M. tuberculosis* can recognize live bacilli[78]. These observations have led to studies on proteins secreted by live mycobacteria, such as *M. bovis* BCG[79] and *M. tuberculosis*[80]. The antigens present in the culture filtrate from *M. tuberculosis* stimulated T-cell responses, even though they were not recognized by antibodies directed against dead mycobacterial antigens. Thus a live vaccine of a cultivatable mycobacterium into which additional genes for *M. leprae*-specific antigens have been cloned may prove to be the ideal vaccine. BCG has been proposed as the basis for such a vaccine[72]: it has been approved and well tried as a human vaccine, is approved as part of EPI by the WHO, to be given at birth, when there is the greatest chance of complete coverage, and has an excellent adjuvant already built in. The challenge for immunologists is to identify which additional leprosy antigens should be added to make BCG (or other live organisms such as vaccinia or salmonella) a protective vaccine against leprosy.

REFERENCES

1. Walsh, G. P., Meyers, W. M., Binford, C. H., Gerone, P. J., Wolf, R. H. and Leininger, J. R. (1981). Leprosy – a zoonosis. *Lepr. Rev.*. **52** (Suppl. 1), 77–83
2. Gormus, B. J., Wolf, R. H., Baskin, G. B., Ohkawa, S., Gerone, P. J., Walsh, G. P., Meyers, W. M., Binford, C. H. and Greer, W. E. (1988). A second sooty mangabey monkey with naturally acquired leprosy: first reported possible monkey-to-monkey transmission. *Int. J. Lepr.*, **56**, 61–5
3. Bloom, B. R. (1983). Rationales for vaccines against leprosy. *Int. J. Lepr.*, **51**, 505–9
4. Ridley, D. S. and Jopling, W. H. (1966). Classification of leprosy according to immunity; a five group system. *Int. J. Lepr.*, **34**, 255–73
5. Nathan, C. F., Kaplan, G., Levis, W. R., Nusrat, A., Witmer, M. D., Sherwin, S. A., Job, C. K., Horowitz, C. R., Steinman, R. M. and Cohn, Z. A. (1986). Local and systemic effects of intradermal recombinant interferon gamma in patients with lepromatous leprosy. *N. Engl. J. Med.*, **315**, 6-15
6. Douvas, G. S., Looker, D. L., Vatter, A. E. and Crowle, A. J. (1985). Gamma interferon activates human macrophages to become tumoricidal and leishmanicidal but enhances replication of macrophage-associated mycobacteria. *Infect. Immun.*, **50**, 1–8
7. Godal, T. and Negassi, K. (1973). Subclinical infection in leprosy. *Br. Med. J.*, **2**, 557-9
8. Doull, J. A., Guinto, R. S. and Mabalay, M. C. (1957). Effect of BCG vaccination, lepromin testing and natural causes in inducing reactivity to lepromin and to tuberculin. *Int. J. Lepr.*, **25**, 13–37
9. Shepard, C. C. (1965). Vaccination against experimental infection with *Mycobacterium leprae. Am. J. Epidemiol.*, **81**, 150–63
10. Shepard, C. C. (1976). Vaccination of mice against *M. leprae* infection. *Int. J. Lepr.*, **44**, 222–6
11. Fine, P. E. M. (1988). BCG vaccination against tuberculosis and leprosy. *Br. Med. Bull.*, **44**, 691–703
12. Lwin, K., Sundaresan, T., Gyi, M. M., Bechelli, L. M., Tamondong, C., Gallego Garbajosa, P., Sansarricq, H. and Noordeen, S. K. (1985). BCG vaccination of children against leprosy: fourteen-year findings of the trial in Burma. *Bull. WHO*, **63**, 1069–78
13. Stanley, S. J., Howland, C., Stone, M. M. and Sutherland, I. (1981). BCG vaccination of children against leprosy in Uganda: final results. *J. Hyg. (Camb).*, **87**, 233–48
14. Ponnighaus, J. M. and Fine, P. E. M. (1986). The Karonga prevention trial – which BCG? *Lepr. Rev.*, **57** (Suppl. 2), 285–92
15. Shepard, C. C. (1960). The experimental disease that follows the injection of human leprosy bacilli into footpads of mice. *J. Exp. Med.*, **112**, 445–54
16. Kirchheimer, W. F. and Storrs, E. E. (1971). Attempts to establish the armadillo (*Dasypus novemcinctus* Linn.) as a model for the study of leprosy. 1. Report of lepromatoid leprosy in the experimentally infected armadillo. *Int. J. Lepr.*, **39**, 693–702
17. Smelt, A. H. M., Rees, R. J. W. and Liew, F. Y. (1981). Induction of delayed-type hypersensitivity to *Mycobacterium leprae* in healthy individuals. *Clin. Exp. Immunol.*, **44**, 501–6
18. Bechelli, L. M., Haddad, N., Pagnano, P. M. G., Neves, R. G., Melchior, E. and Fregnan, R. C. (1980). Double blind trials to determine the late reactivity of leprosy patients and unaffected persons to different concentrations of armadillo lepromin in comparison to human lepromin. *Int. J. Lepr.*, **48**, 126–34
19. Shepard, C. C., Draper, P., Rees, R J. W. and Lowe, C. (1980). Effect of purification steps on the immunogenicity of *Mycobacterium leprae. Br. J. Exp. Pathol.*, **61**, 376–9

20. Draper, P. (1980). WHO report of the fifth meeting on the immunology of leprosy. *Annex 4, TDR-IMMLEP-SWG, (5)80.3*, 24–6
21. Gill, H. K., Mustafa, A. S. and Godal, T. (1986). Induction of delayed-type hypersensitivity in human volunteers immunized with a candidate leprosy vaccine consisting of killed *Mycobacterium leprae*. *Bull. WHO*, **64**, 121–6
22. Gill, H. K., Mustafa, A. S. and Godal, T. (1987). *In vitro* proliferation of lymphocytes from human volunteers vaccinated with armadillo-derived, killed *M. leprae*. *Int. J. Lepr.*, **55**, 30–5
23. Gill, H. K., Mustafa, A. S., Ivanyi, J., Harboe, M. and Godal, T. (1986). Humoral immune responses to *M. leprae* in human volunteers vaccinated with killed, armadillo-derived *M. leprae*. *Lepr. Rev.*, **57** (Suppl. 2), 293–300
24. Mustafa, A. S., Gill, H. K., Nerland, A., Britton, W. J., Mehra, V., Bloom, B. R., Young, R. A. and Godal, T. (1986). Human T-cell clones recognise a major *M. leprae* protein antigen expressed in *E. coli*. *Nature* (*Lond.*), **319**, 63–6
25. Convit, J., Pinardi, M. E., Rodriguez, Ochoa, G., Ulrich, M., Avila, J. L. and Goikmon-Yakr, M. (1974). Elimination of *Mycobacterium leprae* subsequent to local *in vitro* activation of macrophages in lepromatous leprosy by other mycobacteria. *Clin. Exp. Immunol.*, **17**, 821–6
26. Convit, J., Ulrich, M., Aranzazu, N., Castellanos, P. L., Pinardi, M. E. and Reyes, O. (1986). The development of a vaccination model using two microorganisms and its application in leprosy and leishmaniasis. *Lepr. Rev.*, **57** (Suppl. 2), 263–73
27. Convit, J., Aranzazu, N., Ulrich, M., Pinardi, M. E., Reyes, O. and Alvarado, J. (1982). Immunotherapy with a mixture of *Mycobacterium leprae* and BCG in different forms of leprosy and in Mitsuda-negative contacts. *Int. J. Lepr.*, **50**, 415-25
28. Rada, E. M., Convit, J., Ulrich, M., Gallinotto, M. E. and Aranzazu, N. (1987). Immunosuppression and cellular immunity reactions in leprosy patients treated with a mixture of *Mycobacterium leprae* and BCG. *Int. J. Lepr.*, **55**, 646–50
29. Fine, P. E. M., Ponnighaus, J. M., Maine, N., Clarkson, J A. and Bliss, L. (1986). The protective efficiency of BCG against leprosy in Northern Malawi. *Lancet*, **2**, 499–502
30. Gangal, S. G. and Khanolkar, S. R. (1974). Delayed hypersensitivity *in vitro* to an acid fast mycobacterium cultivated from human lepromatous leprosy. *Indian J. Med. Res.*, **62**, 290–6
31. Girdhar, B. K. and Desikan, K. V. (1978). Results of skin tests with five different mycobacteria. *Lepr. India*, **50**, 555–9
32. Deo, M. G., Bapat, C. V., Chullawalla, R. G. and Bhatki, W. S. (1981). Potential anti-leprosy vaccine from killed ICRC bacilli – a clinicopathological study. *Indian J. Med. Res.*, **74**, 164–77
33. Deo, M. G., Bapat, C. V, Bhalerao, V., Chaturvedi, R. M., Bhatki, W. S. and Chullawalla, R. G. (1983). Anti-leprosy potentials of ICRC vaccine: a study in patients and healthy volunteers. *Int. J. Lepr.*, **51**, 540–9
34. Bhatki, W. S. Chulawala, R. G., Bapat, C. V. and Deo, M. G. (1983). Reversal reactions in lepromatous patients induced by a vaccine containing killed ICRC bacilli – a report of five cases. *Int. J. Med.*, **51**, 466–72
35. Chaturvedi, R. M., Chirmule, N. B., Yellapurkar, M. V., Shaikh, S. U. and Deo, M. G. (1987). Effects of ICRC anti leprosy vaccine in healthy subjects. *Int. J. Lepr.*, **55**, 657–66
36. Chirmule, N. B., Chaturvedi, R. M. and Deo, M. G. (1988). Immunogenic 'subunit' of the ICRC antileprosy vaccine. *Int. J. Lepr.*, **56**, 27–35
37. Mustafa, A. S. and Talwar, G. P. (1978). Five cultivatable mycobacterial strains giving blast transformation and leukocyte migration inhibition of leukocytes analogous to *Mycobacterium leprae*. *Lepr. India*, **50**, 498–508
38. Chaudhuri, S., Fotedar, A. and Talwar, G. P. (1983). Lepromin conversion in repeatedly lepromin negative BL/LL patients after immunization with autoclaved *Mycobacterium w*. *Int. J. Lepr.*, **51**, 159-68
39. Zaheer, S. A., Talwar, G. P., Walia, R. and Mukherjee, R. (1988). Results of one year of phase II/phase III trials with the candidate antileprosy vaccine *Mycobacterium w*. *Health Cooperation Papers*, **9**, 245
40. Hunter, S. W. and Brennan, P. J. (1981). A novel phenolic glycolipid from *M. leprae* possibly involved in immunogenicity and pathogenicity. *J. Bacteriol.*, **147**, 728–35

41. Young, D. B. and Buchanan, T. M. (1983). A serological test for leprosy with a glycolipid specific for *M. leprae*. *Science*, **221**, 1057–9

42. Brett, S. J., Lowe, C., Payne, S. N. and Draper, P. (1984). Phenolic glycolipid-1 of *Mycobacterium leprae* causes non-specific inflammation but has no effect on cell-mediated responses in mice. *Infect. Immun.*, **46**, 802–8

43. Job, C. K., Sanchez, R. M., McCormick, G. T. and Hastings, R. C. (1987). Ability of the phenolic glycolipid-1 antigen of *M. leprae* to elicit a positive Mitsuda response in the armadillo (*Dasypus novemcinctus*). *Int. J. Lepr.*, **55**, 299–304

44. Mehra, V., Brennan, P. J., Rada, E., Convit, J. and Bloom, B. R. (1984). Lymphocyte suppression in leprosy induced by unique *M. leprae* glycolipid. *Nature*, **308**, 194–96

45. Neill, M. A. and Klebanoff, S. J. (1988). The effect of phenolic glycolipid-1 from *Mycobacterium leprae* on the antimicrobial activity of human macrophages. *J. Exp. Med.*, **167**, 30–42

46. Young, R. A., Mehra, V., Sweetser, D., Buchanan, T., Clark-Curtiss, J., Davis, R. W. and Bloom, B. R. (1985). Genes for the major protein antigens of the leprosy parasite *Mycobacterium leprae*. *Nature*, **316**, 450–2

47. Britton, W. J., Garsia, R. J., Hellqvist, L., Watson, J D. and Basten, A. (1986). The characterization and immunoreactivity of a 70 kd protein common to *Mycobacterium leprae* and *Mycobacterium bovis* (BCG). *Lepro. Rev.*, **57** (Suppl. 2), 67–75

48. Young, R. A., Bloom, B. R., Grosskinsky, C. M., Ivanyi, J., Thomas, D. and Davis, R. W. (1985). Dissection of *Mycobacterium tuberculosis* antigens using recombinant DNA. *Proc. Natl. Acad. Sci. USA*, **82**, 2583–7

49. Cohen, M. L., Mayer, L. W., Rumschlag, H. S., Yakrus, M. A., Jones, W. D. and Good, R. C. (1987). Expression of proteins of *Mycobacterium tuberculosis* in *Escherichia coli* and potential of recombinant genes and proteins for development of diagnostic reagents. *J. Clin. Microbiol.*, **25**, 1176–80

50. Young, D. B., Kent, L. and Young, R. A (1987). Screening of a recombinant mycobacterial DNA library with polyclonal antisera and molecular weight analysis of expressed antigens. *Infect. Immun.*, **55**, 1421–5

51. Thole, J. E. R., Dauwerse, H. G., Das, P. K., Groothuis, D. G., Schouls, L. M. and van Embden, J. D. A. (1985). Cloning of *Mycobacterium bovis* BCG DNA and expression of antigens in *Escherichia coli*. *Infect. Immun.*, **50**, 800–6

52. Lamb, J. R. and Rees, A. D. M. (1988). Antigen specificity and function of human T lymphocyte clones reactive with mycobacteria. *Br. Med. Bull.*, **44**, 600–10

53. Lamb, J. R. and Young, D. B. (1987). A novel approach to the identification of T-cell epitopes in *Mycobacterium tuberculosis* using T-lymphocyte clones. *Immunology*, **60**, 1–5

54. Abou-Zeid, C., Filley, E., Steele, J. and Rook, G. A. W. (1987). A simple new method for using antigens separated by polyacrylamide gel electrophoresis to stimulate lymphocytes *in vitro* after converting bands cut from Western blots into antigen-bearing particles. *J. Immunol. Meth.*, **98**, 5-10

55. Shinnick, T. M., Sweetser, D., Thole, J., van Embden, J. and Young, R. A. (1987). The etiologic agents of leprosy and tuberculosis share an immunoreactive protein antigen with the vaccine strain *Mycobacterium bovis* BCG. *Infect. Immun.*, **55**, 1932-5

56. Buchanan, T. M., Nomaguchi, H., Anderson, D. C., Young, R. A., Gillis, T. P., Britton, W. J., Ivanyi, J., Kolk, A. H. J., Closs, O., Bloom, R. and Mehra, V. (1986). Characterisation of mycobacterial species specificity of 14 separate epitopes which reacted with monoclonal antibodies to the 65,000 molecular weight protein molecule of *Mycobacterium leprae.*, *Lepr. Rev.*, **57** (Suppl. 2), 63-6

57. Husson, R. N. and Young, R. A. (1987). Genes for the major protein antigens of *Mycobacterium tuberculosis*: the etiological agents of tuberculosis and leprosy share an immunodominant antigen. *Proc. Natl. Acad. Sci. USA*, **84**, 1679–83

58. Mehra, V., Sweetser, D., Young, R. A. (1986). Efficient mapping of protein antigenic determinants. *Proc. Natl. Acad. Sci. USA*, **83**, 7013–17

59. Lamb, J. R., Ivanyi, J., Rees, A. D. M., Rothbard, J. B., Howland, K., Young, R. A. and Young, D. B. (1987). Mapping of T cell epitopes using recombinant antigens and synthetic peptides. *EMBO J.*, **6**, 1245–9

60. Lamb, F. I., Kingston, A. E., Estrada-G., I. and Colston, M. J. (1988). Heterologous expression of the 65-kilodalton antigen of *Mycobacterium leprae* and murine T-cell responses to the gene product. *Infect. Immun.*, **56**, 1237-41

61. Kaufmann, S. H. E., Vath, U., Thole, J. E. R., van Embden, J. D. A. and Emmrich, F. (1987). Enumeration of T-cells reactive with *Mycobacterium tuberculosis* organisms and specific for the recombinant mycobacterial 64-kDa protein. *Eur. J. Immunol.*, **17**, 351–7
62. Oftung, F., Mustafa, A. S., Husson, R., Young, R. A. and Godal, T. (1987). Human T-cell clones recognise two abundant *Mycobacterium tuberculosis* protein antigens expressed in *Escherichia coli*. *J. Immunol.*, **138**, 927–31
63. Emmrich, F., Thole, J., van Embden, J. and Kaufmann, S. H. E. (1986). A recombinant 64 kilodalton protein of *Mycobacterium bovis* Bacillus Calmette-Guerin specifically stimulates human T4 clones reactive to mycobacterial antigens. *J. Exp. Med.*, **163**, 1024–9
64. Van Schooten, W. C. A., Ottenhoff, T. H. M., Klatser, P. R., Thole, J., de Vries, R. R. P. and Kolk, A. H.. J. (1988). T cell epitopes on the 36k and 65k *Mycobacterium leprae* antigens defined by human T cell clones. *Eur. J. Immunol.*, **18**, 849–54
65. Gillis, T. P., Miller, R. A., Young, D. B., Khanolkar, S. R. and Buchanan, T. M. (1985). Immunochemical characterization of a protein associated with *Mycobacterium leprae* cell wall. *Infect. Immun.*, **49**, 371–7
66. De Bruyn, J., Bosmans, R., Turner, M., Weckx, M., Nyabenda, J., van Vooren, J.-P., Falmagne, P., Wiker, H. G. and Harboe, M. (1987). Purification, partial characterization, and identification of a skin-reactive protein antigen of *Mycobacterium bovis* BCG. *Infect. Immunol.*, **55**, 245–52
67. Young, D. B., Ivanyi, J., Cox, J. H. and Lamb, J. R. (1987). The 65kDa antigen of mycobacteria – a common bacterial protein? *Immunol. Today*, **8**, 215–19
68. Young, D., Lathigra, R., Hendrix, R., Sweetser, D. and Young, R.A. (1988). Stress proteins are immune targets in leprosy and tuberculosis. *Proc. Natl. Acad. Sci. USA*, **85**, 4267–70
69. Booth, R. J., Harris, D. P., Love, J. M. and Watson, J. D. (1988). Antigenic proteins of *Mycobacterium leprae*. Complete sequence of the gene for the 18kDa protein. *J. Immunol.*, **140**, 597–601
70. Engers, H. D., Bloom, B. R. and Godal, T. (1985). Monoclonal antibodies against mycobacterial antigens. *Immunol. Today*, **6**, 346-8
71. Hopwood, D. A., Kieser, T., Colston, M. J. and Lamb, F. I. (1988). Molecular biology of mycobacteria. *Br. Med. Bull.*, **44**, 528–46
72. Bloom, B. R. (1986). Learning from leprosy: a perspective on immunology and the third world. *J. Immunol.*, **137**, i–x
73. Snapper, S. B., Lugosi, L., Jekkel, A., Melton, R. E., Kieser, T., Bloom, B. R. and Jacobs, W. R. (1988). Lysogeny and transformation in mycobacteria. Stable expression of foreign genes. *Proc. Natl. Acad. Sci. USA*, **85**, 6987–91
74. Zainuddin, Z. F., Kunza, Z. M. and Dale, J. W. (1989). Transformation of *Mycobacterium smegmatis* with *E. coli* plasmids carrying a selectable resistance marker. *Molec. Microbiol.*, **3**, 29–34
75. Klatser, P. R., van Rens, M. M. and Eggelte, T. A. (1984). Immunochemical characterisation of *Mycobacterium leprae* antigens by the SDS-polyacrylamide gel electrophoresis immuno-peroxidase technique (SGIP) using patients' sera. *Clin. Exp. Immunol.*, **56**, 537–44
76. Vega-Lopez, F., Stoker, N. G., Locniskar, M. F., Dockrell, H. M., Grant, K. A. and McAdam, K. P. W. J. (1988). Recognition of mycobacterial antigens by sera from patients with leprosy. *J. Clin. Microbiol.*, **26**, 2474-9
77. Rook, G. A. W. (1980). The immunogenicity of killed mycobacteria. *Lepr. Rev.*, **51**, 295–301
78. Rook, G. A. W., Steele, J., Barnass, S., Mace, J. and Stanford, J. L. (1986). Responsiveness to live *M. tuberculosis*, and common antigens, of sonicate-stimulated T cell lines from normal donors. *Clin. Exp. Immunol.*, **63**, 105–10
79. Abou-Zeid, C., Smith, I., Grange, J., Steele, J. and Rook, G. (1986). Subdivision of daughter strains of Bacille Calmette-Guerin (BCG) according to secreted protein patterns. *J. Gen. Microbiol.*, **132**, 3047–53
80. Collins, F. M., Lamb, J. R. and Young, D. B. (1988). Biological activity of protein antigens isolated from *Mycobacterium tuberculosis* culture filtrate. *Infect. Immun.*, **56**, 1260–6

5
Pseudomonas aeruginosa immunization

J. E. PENNINGTON

BACKGROUND

Emerging pathogenic role

Pseudomonas aeruginosa, formerly known as *Bacillus pyocyaneus*, was described over 100 years ago by Gessard[1]. However, as recently as 1947 this ubiquitous environmental inhabitant was described as rarely pathogenic for man[2]. The advent of modern medical practices, however, including antimicrobial agents, immuno- and myelosuppressive chemotherapy and sophisticated life-support equipment, has produced a population of patients at increased risk for infection with opportunistic infectious agents. *P. aeruginosa* has emerged as one of the most common and most problematic among these modern opportunistic pathogens[3,4]. Perhaps of most concern has been the unusually high mortality associated with *P. aeruginosa* bacteraemia and pneumonia, often twice that observed with other Gram-negative bacillary infections[4–6].

A clear-cut pattern of *P. aeruginosa* infections has emerged in which certain high-risk target populations experience the bulk of *P. aeruginosa* infections (Table 1). Certain defects in the host-defence system thus appear more likely

Table 1 Clinical populations at highest risk for *Pseudomonas aeruginosa* infections

Burns
Cancer/neutropenia
Intensive-care unit
Respiratory assistance
Urinary catheters
Hypogammaglobulinaemia
Primary
Acquired (e.g. chronic lymphocytic leukaemia)
Cystic fibrosis

Table 2 Major pathogenic factors for *Pseudomonas aeruginosa* infections

Virulence factors	*Host-defence factors*
Endotoxin	Phagocytes
Exotoxin A	Opsonic antibodies
Exoenzyme S	Complement
Elastase	Mucocutaneous barriers
Alkaline protease	
Mucoid exopolysaccharide	
Pyocyanin	

to predispose to *P. aeruginosa* infection. Simply observing those groups at increased risk, one can predict that adequate numbers of phagocytes, intact natural epithelial barriers (e.g. skin, respiratory mucosa), and intact humoral immune systems are prime host-defence factors for *P. aeruginosa.* Indeed, numerous experimental studies on the pathogenesis of *P. aeruginosa* infection have verified these empirical observations.

Also appropriate to the emerging role of *P. aeruginosa* as an important human pathogen have been the large numbers of studies describing the major virulence factors of *P. aeruginosa*[7]. Table 2 presents a summary of the pathogenic factors involved in *P. aeruginosa* infection. Understanding these factors is basic to planning appropriate strategies for *P. aeruginosa* immunization. Importantly, the pioneering *in vitro* and *in vivo* work by Young[8], Reynolds *et al.*[9] and Bjornson *et al.*[10], clearly established the concept that serotype-specific humoral immunity against *P. aeruginosa* establishes a significant increase in host defence against this pathogen. These studies also suggest that the most protective type of *P. aeruginosa* antibodies are opsonic rather than bactericidal[8]. These studies thus provided the rationale for modern *Pseudomonas aeruginosa* immunization strategies which emphasize augmentation of humoral, rather than cell-mediated, immunity. Furthermore, most vaccines have utilized cell wall antigens designed to evoke opsonic antibody responses.

Immunization: older studies

Although *P. aeruginosa* is considered a modern pathogen, several older reports describe immunization strategies for *P. aeruginosa.* In general, those reports utilized autologous organisms in single-case situations[11,12], or else poorly described plasma or serum preparations[13,14].

The first *P. aeruginosa* vaccine developed with the intention of commercial availabiity was that described by Hanessian *et al.*[15] at Parke Davis and Company. This preparation (Pseudogen®) was a lipopolysaccharide (LPS) antigen vaccine, containing the seven immunotype antigens of the Fisher–Devlin–Gnabasik typing scheme[16]. These seven immunotypes represented about 94% of clinical strains studied at that time[15]. Numerous clinical studies were conducted with Pseudogen®, and some results suggested that type-specific immunization conferred a protective effect[17–19]. In other studies, immunogenicity for high-risk individuals was documented but clinical efficacy could not be demonstrated[20]. It should be noted that a prime motivation for the development of this vaccine was to immunize volunteer plasma donors and to produce a hyperimmune globulin for passive immune therapy. In fact, early trials suggested that this was feasible[18].

Despite some promising clinical observations, Pseudogen® was never licensed for clinical use, perhaps because the most promising clinical trials were uncontrolled. Furthermore, adverse effects with this LPS vaccine were common. Also, the time delay before achieving adequate immune reponse rendered active immunization less attractive in certain critical-care settings. Despite these setbacks, however, the early studies with Pseudogen® firmly established the rationale and clinical interest in *P. aeruginosa* immunization.

In addition to the development of Pseudogen® by the group at Parke Davis, the Wellcome Research Laboratories in England[21] were also developing a polyvalent cell-wall extract *P. aeruginosa* vaccine, called PEV-01. This vaccine contained 16 serotypes, based on a different serotyping scheme, and was claimed to be less toxic than Pseudogen®. Indeed, studies in volunteers suggested this to be true[22]. Subsequent trials in burned patients, however, disclosed both local and febrile reactions[23]. Recent work has identified LPS as the dominant antigen in this vaccine[24]. Clinical studies in India with PEV-01 have demonstrated decreased *P. aeruginosa* infections in burned patients[23]. However, these findings have not been reproduced in developed countries and the vaccine is currently unlicensed.

Other early efforts to develop *P. aeruginosa* vaccines represented attempts to side-step two important disadvantages of type-specific LPS vaccines, namely the adverse side-effects caused by LPS, and the need for polyvalent preparations due to LPS antigenic heterogeneity. A high-molecular weight polysaccharide vaccine was described by Pier *et al.* in 1978[25]. This vaccine contains the O-specific polysaccharide antigens of LPS, but lacks the toxic lipid A component. Recently this vaccine has been shown to be well tolerated and immunogenic in normal human volunteers[26].

In an attempt to offer cross-protection against LPS antigen diverse strains, vaccines based upon antigens other than O-specific LPS antigens were also developed. In 1968, Homma described a cell-wall protein antigen now known as original endotoxin protein (OEP)[27]. This protein was isolated from a single strain of *P. aeruginosa* but was found to be cross-protective for a wide range of O-serotype diverse isolates[28]. More recent work, however, has identified non-cross-reactive strains[29].

Yet another approach to reducing side-effects from immunization was to utilize non-cell wall antigens, such as the toxoid of endotoxin A. The majority of clinical *P. aeruginosa* isolates secrete exotoxin A[7], and this toxin is considered an important virulence factor in *P. aeruginosa* infection[7]. Furthermore, seroepidemiologic studies suggest that elevated natural antibody titres against exotoxin A confer protection against subsequent *P. aeruginosa* infection[30]. Several attempts to toxoid this potentially cross-reactive antigen have been described, and animal studies suggest at least partial protection[31]. Unfortunately, adjuvants may be necessary in order to elicit optimal immune response to exotoxin A toxoids[31]. Furthermore, several studies suggest that

Table 3 *Pseudomonas aeruginosa* vaccines under investigation

Lipopolysaccharide
Pseudogen
PEV-01
Polysaccharide
High molecular weight polysaccharide
Mucoid exopolysaccharide
Cell wall proteins
Original endotoxin protein
Outer membrane protein F (porin)
Pili
Flagella
Exoproducts
Exotoxin A
Elastase
Conjugate
O-specific polysaccharide plus exotoxin A

antibodies to exotoxin A are relatively weak compared to the protective effects of cell-wall directed antigens[32,33].

ACTIVE IMMUNIZATION: RECENT STUDIES

Based upon past observations, several facts regarding *P. aeruginosa* vaccines have become clear. These are: (1) native LPS-based vaccines are highly immunogenic but cause unacceptable side-effects in many vaccinees; (2) several candidate immunogens with reduced toxicity are available; and (3) O-serotype cross-protection might result from certain non-LPS antigen vaccines. Based upon these observations, recent vaccine development has emphasized less toxic and cross-reactive antigens (Table 3).

Pili and flagella

Most *P. aeruginosa* isolates are piliated. These pili appear to increase adherence to mucosal surfaces[34], and experimental evidence suggests that type-specific anti-pili antibodies might block mucosal adherence of *P. aeruginosa*[35]. Unfortunately, the antigenic heterogeneity of *P. aeruginosa* pili is extreme and only homologous antibodies offer protection against adherence[35].

Different protein-rich cell wall appendages, flagella, have also been implicated as a virulence factor for invasive *P. aeruginosa* infections[36]. Since most *P. aeruginosa* isolates are flagellated, and since only two major flagellar serotypes exist, efforts to develop a bivalent (type a and type b) flagellar vaccine have been described[37]. Early studies suggested that anti-flagellar antibodies act by reducing the motility and invasiveness of *P. aeruginosa*[37,38]. However, recent data suggest that flagellar antibodies also may act as opsonins[39]. Clinical data have not been reported.

Outer membrane proteins

The outer membrane of Gram-negative bacteria contains several proteins, some of which have been well characterized. Outer membrane protein (OMP) F (porin) is conserved in virtually all serotypes of *P. aeruginosa*[40], and elicits an antibody response in infected humans[41]. Thus, OMP-F is under investigation as a cross-protective immunogen against *P. aeruginosa*. Since it is difficult to purify OMP-F completely free of LPS, a recent study has evaluated OMP-F containing 7 μg LPS antigen per 10 μg protein[42]. Using a murine *P. aeruginosa* burn sepsis model, the OMP-F plus LPS vaccine conferred protection against six LPS heterologous *P. aeruginosa* challenge strains which was greater than the protection conferred by a control immunogen containing only the LPS constituent of the vaccine. It was concluded that the OMP vaccine constituent provided cross-protection. Unfortunately, controls receiving no vaccine were not included. In separate animal studies, monoclonal antibodies against OMP-F were compared to equivalent amounts of monoclonal antibodies directed to LPS antigens. For LPS homologous infecting strains the LPS antibodies were significantly more protective than the OMP antibodies[43,44]. Thus, while OMP-F vaccine or monoclonal antibodies appear to offer cross-protection for LPS heterologous strains, these antibodies appear less potent than LPS antibodies.

Conjugate vaccines

Attempts to reduce the toxicity of intact *P. aeruginosa* LPS vaccine by utilizing non-lipid A containing fragments of the LPS molecule clearly reduce vaccine immunogenicity[45]. Recent work suggests that immunogenicity can be increased by linking a protein molecule to the lipid A-free polysaccharide O-side chain molecules. The most extensively studied conjugate vaccine is that developed by Cryz and co-workers[46]. This vaccine contains O-polysaccharide derived from *P. aeruginosa* by extraction in phenol–water, and exotoxin A purified from culture supernates of an exotoxin A producing strain. The polysaccharide and exotoxin A moieties are linked covalently, and the final product contains about 30% polysaccharide and 70% toxin A[46]. To date, studies demonstrate that this conjugate vaccine is well tolerated and immunogenic in animals[46,47] and humans[47]. In humans, antibody levels reach peak at day 42 after vaccination and decline markedly by 15 months post-immunization[48]. Of interest is that a booster dose after 15 months elicited a rise only in toxin A antibodies[48]. To date, studies have utilized an LPS monovalent conjugate vaccine (immunotype 5). However, efforts are under way to produce an LPS polyvalent conjugate vaccine using this technology.

Mucoid exopolysaccharide

P. aeruginosa infection in cystic fibrosis (CF) patients is a unique problem. Rather than acute and fulminating episodes of sepsis, the CF patient experiences chronic bronchopulmonary infection which elicits a systemic immune response but is never eradicated from the lungs[20]. Also of interest is the peculiar and unique mucoid slime material produced by most *P. aeruginosa* strains isolated from CF patients' sputa. This mucoid exopolysaccharide (MEP) material has been characterized and is predominantly alginate[49]. Based upon *in vitro* studies it is hypothesized that MEP may act to inhibit opsonophagocytosis of *P. aeruginosa* by conventional antibodies, thereby allowing mucoid *P. aeruginosa* to persist in the CF lung[50].

Recently, MEP has been purified and shown in animal models to be immunogenic[49]. Furthermore, MEP antibodies have been shown to act as opsonins[51], and are associated with less *P. aeruginosa* colonization in older CF patients[52]. Consequently, work is under way to evaluate the safety, immunogenicity and efficacy of MEP vaccine in CF patients.

PASSIVE IMMUNIZATION

Why passive immunization?

Several drawbacks can be identified for active vaccination against *P. aeruginosa*. First, the onset of *P. aeruginosa* bacteraemia or pneumonia in the hospital setting (often in the intensive care unit) frequently occurs within the first week after admission. Active immunization, however, usually requires 10–14 days before an optimal immune response has developed. Second, *P. aeruginosa* infections account for only 10–15% of all nosocomial infections[53]. Finally, the more widely studied vaccines contain lipopolysaccharide (LPS), which has caused serious side-effects. Thus there has been reluctance to utilize potentially harmful LPS vaccines for a relatively small number of patients at risk. Passive immunotherapy offers the option of rapidly and safely administering type-specific antibodies by intravenous infusion to those with proven *P. aeruginosa* infections, or to those felt to be at the greatest danger of becoming infected.

Passive immunotherapy, however, also has potential drawbacks. For example, expensive immunological preparations may not be necessary for treatment of all patients, even those with proven *P. aeruginosa* infection. Which patients, then, should be treated with antibodies? This question unfortunately may remain moot, since it appears that the earlier antibody treatment is begun, the more likely it will offer therapeutic efficacy[54,55]. Thus, there may be little choice but to treat all patients recognized to have *P. aeruginosa* bacteraemia or pneumonia as soon as possible, rather than to wait for an evaluation of clinical response to antimicrobial therapy alone. The need to employ immunotherapy as early as possible also emphasizes the need for rapid and specific diagnosis.

Waiting for 48–72 h to fully identify a Gram-negative isolate as *P. aeruginosa* may preclude optimal use of antibody therapy. A fluorescent-labelled monoclonal antibody diagnostic kit is under development which may provide a more rapid and specific diagnostic method for *P. aeruginosa*[56]. Some of these diagnostic problems could be obviated if an effective broad-spectrum anti-Gram-negative bacteria antibody preparation were available. Unfortunately, the serotypic diversity of enteric and environmental Gram-negative bacillary pathogens makes preparation of an O-serotype-specific polyclonal antibody preparation a difficult task. Another strategy proposed for broad-spectrum immunotherapy is to employ antibodies directed at a 'common antigen' expressed in the core region of all Gram-negative bacterial cell walls[57]. However, several studies suggest that anti-LPS O-serotype-specific antibodies are more potent than anti-core-glycolipid antibodies in protection against Gram-negative bacterial infections, including *P. aeruginosa*[58–60]. Thus, development of serotype-specific anti-*P. aeruginosa* antibody preparations remains an objective with considerable clinical relevance.

A final consideration, prior to experimental and clinical studies of *P. aeruginosa* passive immunotherapy, is which antigen target is the most important for protective effect by antibodies. *P. aeruginosa* contains numerous candidate antigen targets (see above), and virulence properties have been identified for most of them[7]. However, when the relative protective potency of different antibodies has been studied, anti-LPS antibodies have uniformly exhibited the highest level of protection (Table 4). Thus the preparations currently under evaluation for *P. aeruginosa* passive immunization are based upon passive transfer of O-type specific antibodies.

Polyclonal antibodies

Passive immunotherapy is classically accomplished using animal or human serum, derived from hosts with pre-existing antibodies against the target pathogen. In recent years human plasma from normal or pre-immunized volunteers has been utilized to prepare immunoglobulin G fractions. These immunoglobulins contain antibodies which are concentrated four- to five-fold above their plasma concentration. Nevertheless, the level of natural *P. aeruginosa* antibodies in the final product is relatively low. Furthermore, while the maximum safe dosage of intravenous immunoglobulin G (IGIV) for humans is not known, concern about Fc receptor blockade in septic or high-risk humans limits peak recommended dosages of IGIV to about 500 mg protein per kg body weight. It may be noted that much higher doses of IGIV are used in non-septic individuals for non-anti-infective indications.

Thus, the goal of human plasma-derived IGIV preparations (polyclonal antibodies) is to prepare hyperimmune IGIV with enhanced antibodies

Table 4 Comparative studies demonstrating superior protection against *Pseudomonas* infection by lipopolysaccharide antibodies

Type of immunization	*Study (references)*	*Model*	*Antibody for Comparison*
Active	Pennington and Menkes, 1981[59]	Pneumonia	J5
Active	Cryz *et al.*, 1984[61]	Burn wound	Polysaccharide
Active	Pennington *et al.*, 1986[62]	Pneumonia	Detoxified LPS
Passive	Cryz *et al.*, 1983[32]	Burn wound	Elastase, exotoxin A
Passive	Cryz *et al.*, 1983[33]	Leukopenia, burn wound	Elastase, exotoxin A
Passive	Sawada *et al.*, 1984[43]	Peritonitis and burn wound	Outer membrane protein
Passive	Pennington *et al.*, 1986[44]	Pneumonia	Outer membrane protein

against the target organism. For *P. aeruginosa*, this may be done by pre-immunizing human volunteers with *P. aeruginosa* polyvalent vaccines or by screening donors for naturally high *P. aeruginosa* antibodies.

Several hyperimmune *P. aeruginosa* IGIV preparations have been made using plasma from humans immunized with polyvalent LPS vaccines. One preparation was studied in burned patients with *P. aeruginosa* sepsis, and shown to add an increment of protection to conventional therapy[18]. This preparation is no longer in production, however. Another such hyperimmune IGIV preparation has been evaluated only in animal models to date[63]. However, experimental results are promising.

A different approach was taken by Collins *et al.*, who used an enzyme-linked immunosorbent assay to screen normal human plasma donors for naturally elevated anti-LPS *P. aeruginosa* antibodies[64]. About one in 20 donors had elevated antibodies and these plasmas were combined to prepare a hyperimmune IGIV containing five-fold higher LPS antibody titres than conventional IGIV[64]. To date, animal studies employing this preparation have demonstrated promising results[44,64,65]. A pilot trial of this preparation as treatment for *P. aeruginosa* pneumonia in patients in an intensive care unit also gave favourable results[66]. Further clinical trials with this preparation are under way.

Monoclonal antibodies

The limited availability of human plasma-derived polyclonal *P. aeruginosa* hyperimmune antibody preparations, and the necessity to administer high doses of immunoglobulin G proteins in order to achieve protective antibody levels, have motivated development of *P. aeruginosa* monoclonal antibodies (MAbs). Simply developing a MAb with *P. aeruginosa* binding affinity does not guarantee anti-infective function. However, by screening candidate MAbs for opsonophagocytic activity or for protective activity in animal models, the most promising MAbs may be selected for clinical trials.

Early development of *P. aeruginosa* MAbs was focused on murine MAbs. Several murine anti-LPS MAb preparations have now demonstrated *in vivo* protection[43,44,67]. In two studies the protective capacity of anti-LPS MAb was compared to that of anti-OMP MAb, and in each study the anti-LPS MAb was superior[43,44]. In further studies a polyclonal hyperimmune IGIV preparation was compared to a MAb preparation for treatment of experimental *P. aeruginosa* pneumonia[44]. The MAb preparation provided protection at a protein dosage that was 100-fold less than that required for the polyclonal preparation. Thus, early studies with *P. aeruginosa* MAbs suggest that they function *in vivo* and that extremely low protein dosages can be used.

The desire to eliminate mouse protein from MAb preparations has led to recent development of human *P. aeruginosa* MAbs[68–71]. Again, these preparations are directed at O-specific LPS epitopes. Early studies in animals suggest that these preparations are functional *in vivo*. To date, clinical trials with MAb, murine or human in origin, have not been reported.

REFERENCES

1. Gessard, C. (1882). Sur les colorations bleue et verte des linges à pansements. *C.R. Sceances Acad. Sci. Serie D*, **94**, 536–8
2. Stanley, M. (1947). *Bacillus pyocyaneus* infections. A review, report of cases and discussion of newer therapy including streptomycin. *Am. J. Med.*, **2**, 253, 347–67
3. Reynolds, H. Y., Levine, A. S., Wood, R. E., Zierdt, C. H., Dale, D. C. and Pennington, J. E. (1975). *Pseudomnas aeruginosa* infections: persisting problems and current research to find new therapies. *Ann. Intern. Med.*, **82**, 819–31
4. Young, L. S., Wenzel, R. P., Sabath, L. D., Pollack, M., Pennington, J. E. and Platt, R. (1984). The outlook for prevention and treatment of infections due to *Pseudomonas aeruginosa. Rev. Infect. Dis.*, **6** (Suppl. 3), S769–74
5. Stevens, R. M., Teres, D., Skillman, J. J. and Feingold, D. S. (1974). Pneumonia in an intensive care unit. *Arch. Intern. Med.*, **134**, 106-11
6. Bryan, C. S. and Reynolds, K. L. (1984). Bacteremic nosocomial pneumonia. *Am. Rev. Resp. Dis.*, **129**, 668–71
7. Nicas, T. I. and Iglewski, B. H. (1985). The contribution of exoproducts to virulence of *Pseudomonas aeruginosa. Can. J. Microbiol.*, **31**, 387–92
8. Young, L. S. (1972). Human immunity to *Pseudomonas aeruginosa*. II. Relationship between heat-stable opsonins and type-specific lipopolysaccharides. *J. Infect. Dis.*, **126**, 277–87
9. Reynolds, H. Y., Kazmierowski, J. A. and Newball, H. H. (1975). Specificity of opsonic antibodies to enhance phagocytosis of *Pseudomonas aeruginosa* by human alveolar macrophages. *J. Clin. Invest.*, **56**, 376–85
10. Bjornson, A. B. and Michael, J. G. (1972). Contribution of humoral and cellular factors to the resistance to experimental infection by *Pseudomonas aeruginosa* in mice. II. Opsonic, agglutinative, and protective capacities of immunoglobulin G anti-*Pseudomonas* antibodies. *Infect. Immun.*, **5**, 775–82
11. Groves, E. H. (1909). Case of bacillus pyocyaneus pyaemia successfully treated by vaccine. *Br. Med. J.*, **1**, 1169-70
12. Feller, I. and Pierson, C. (1968). *Pseudomonas* vaccine and hyperimmune plasma for burned patients. *Arch. Surg.*, **97**, 225–9
13. Kefalides, N. A., Arana, J. A., Bazan, A., Boganegra, M., Stastny, P., Velarde, N. and Rosenthal, S. M. (1962). Role of infection in mortality from severe burns. *N. Engl. J. Med.*, **267**, 317–23
14. Bocanegra, M., Hinostroza, F., Bazan, A., Velarde, N., Yoza, V. and Rosenthal, S. M. (1966). Convalescent burn plasma therapy for severely burned children. *Ann. Surg.*, **163**, 461–9
15. Hanessian, S., Regan, W., Watson, D. and Haskel, T. H. (1971). Isolation and characterization of antigenic components of a new heptavalent *Pseudomonas* vaccine. *Nature*, **229**, 209–10
16. Fisher, M. W., Devlin, H. B. and Gnabasik, F. J. (1969). New immunotype schema for *Pseudomonas aeruginosa* based on protective antigens. *J. Bacteriol.*, **98**, 835–6
17. Young, L. S., Meyer, R. D. and Armstrong, D. (1973). *Pseudomonas aeruginosa* vaccine in cancer patients. *Ann. Intern. Med.*, **79**, 518–27
18. Alexander, J. W. and Fisher, M. W. (1974). Immunization against *Pseudomonas* in infection after thermal injury. *J. Infect. Dis.*, **130** (Suppl.), S152–8
19. Polk, H. C., Borden, S. and Aldret, J. A. (1973). Prevention of *pseudomonas* respiratory infection in a surgical intensive care unit. *Arch. Surg.*, **177**, 607–13
20. Pennington, J. E., Reynolds, H. Y., Wood, R. E., Robinson, R. A. and Levine, A. S. (1975). Use of *Pseudomonas aeruginosa* vaccine in patients with acute leukemia and cystic fibrosis. *Am. J. Med.*, **58**, 629-36
21. Miler, J. J., Spilsbury, J. F., Jones, R. J., Roe, E. A. and Lowbury, E. J. L. (1977). A new polyvalent *Pseudomonas* vaccine. *J. Med. Microbiol.*, **10**, 19–27
22. Jones, R. J., Roe, E. A., Lowbury, E. J. L., Miler, J. J. and Spilsbury, J. F. (1976). A new *Pseudomonas* vaccine: preliminary trial on human volunteers. *J. Hyg. Camb.*, **76**, 429–39
23. Roe, E. A. and Jones, R. J. (1983). Immunization of burned patients against *Pseudomonas aeruginosa* infection at Safdarjang Hospital, New Delhi. *Rev. Infect. Dis.*, **5** (Suppl.), 922–30
24. MacIntyre, S., McVeigh, T. and Owen, P. (1986). Immunochemical and biochemical analysis of the polyvalent *Pseudomonas aeruginosa* vaccine PEV. *Infect. Immun.*, **51**, 675–86

25. Pier, G. B., Sidberry, H. F., Zolyomi, S. F. and Sadoff, J. C. (1978). Isolation and characterization of high molecular weight polysaccharide from the slime of *Pseudomonas aeruginosa. Infect. Immun.*, **22**, 908–18
26. Pier, G. B. (1982). Safety and immunogenicity of high molecular weight polysaccharide vaccine from immunotype 1 *Pseudomonas aeruginosa. J. Clin. Invest.*, **69**, 303–8
27. Homma, J. Y. (1986). The protein moiety of the endotoxin of *Pseudomonas aeruginosa. Z. Allg. Microbiol.*, **8**, 227–48
28. Abe, C., Shionoya, H., Hirao, Y., Okada, K. and Homma, J. Y. (1975). Common protective antigen (OEP) of *Pseudomonas aeruginosa. Jpn. J. Exp. Med.*, **45**, 355–59
29. Okada, K., Kawaharajo, K., Kasai, K. and Homma, J. Y. (1980). Effects of somatic components of *Pseudomonas aeruginosa* on protective immunity in experimental mouse burn infection. *Jpn. J. Exp. Med.*, **50**, 53–61
30. Pollack, M. S. and Young, L. S. (1979). Protective activity of antibodies of exotoxin A and lipopolysaccharide at the onset of *Pseudomonas aeruginosa* septicemia in man. *J. Clin. Invest.*, **63**, 276-86
31. Pavlovskis, O. R., Edman, D. C., Leppla, S. H., Wretland, B., Lewis, L. R. and Martin, K. E. (1981). Protection against experimental *Pseudomonas aeruginosa* infection in mice by active immunization with exotoxin A toxoids. *Infect. Immun.*, **32**, 681–9
32. Cryz, S. J., Furer, E. and Germanier, R. (1983). Protection against *Pseudomonas aeruginosa* infection in a murine burn wound sepsis model by passive transfer of antitoxin A, antielastase, and antilipopolysaccharide. *Infect. Immun.*, **39**, 1072–9
33. Cryz, S. J., Furer, E. and Germanier, R. (1983). Passive protection against *Pseudomonas aeruginosa* infection in an experimental leukopenic mouse model. *Infect. Immun.*, **40**, 659–64
34. Woods, D. E., Bass, J. A., Johanson, W. G. Jr. and Straus, D. C. (1980). Role of adherence in the pathogenesis of *Pseudomonas aeruginosa* lung infection in cystic fibrosis patients. *Infect. Immun.*, **30**, 694–9
35. Woods, D. E., Straus, D. C., Johanson, W. G. Jr., Berry, V. K. and Bass, J. A. (1980). Role of pili in adherence of *Pseudomonas aeruginosa* to mammalian buccal epithelial cells. *Infect. Immun.*, **29**, 1146–51
36. Montie, T. C., Doyle-Huntzinger, D., Craven, R. C. and Holder, I. A. (1982). Loss of virulence associated with absence of flagellum in an isogenic mutant of *Pseudomonas aeruginosa* in the burned-mouse model. *Infect. Immun.*, **38**, 1296–8
37. Holder, I. A. and Naglich, J. G. (1986). Experimental studies of the pathogenesis of infections due to *Pseudomnas aeruginosa* immunization using divalent flagella preparations. *J. Trauma*, **26**, 118–22
38. Holder, I. A., Wheeler, R. and Montie T. C. (1982). Flagellar preparations from *Pseudomonas aeruginosa*: animal protection studies. *Infect. Immun.*, **35**, 276-80
39. Anderson, T. R. and Montie, T. C. (1987). Opsonophagocytosis of *Pseudomonas aeruginosa* treated with antiflagellar serum. *Infect. Immun.*, **55**, 3204–6
40. Mutharia, L. M., Nicas, T. I. and Hancock, R. E. W. (1982). Outer membrane proteins of *Pseudomonas aeruginosa* serotype strains. *J. Infect. Dis.*, **146**, 770–9
41. Lam, J. S., Mutharia, L. M., Hancock, R. E. W., Hoiby, N., Lam, K., Baek, L. and Costerton, J. W. (1983). Immunogenicity of *Pseudomonas aeruginosa* outer membrane antigens examined by crossed immunoelectrophoresis. *Infect. Immun.*, **42**, 88–98
42. Mathews-Greer, J. M. and Gilleland, Jr. H. E. (1987). Outer membrane protein F (porin) preparation of *Pseudomonas aeruginosa* as a protective vaccine against heterologous immunotype strains in a burned mouse model. *J. Infect. Dis.*, **155**, 1282–91
43. Sawada, S., Suzuki, M., Kawamura, T., Fujinaga, S., Masuho, Y. and Tomibe, K. (1984). Protection against infection with *Pseudomonas aeruginosa* by passive transfer of monoclonal antibodies to lipopolysaccharides and outer membrane proteins. *J. Infect. Dis.*, **150**, 570–6
44. Pennington, J. E., Small, G. J., Lostrom, M. E. and Pier, G. B. (1986). Polyclonal and monoclonal antibody therapy for experimental *Pseudomonas aeruginosa* pneumonia. *Infect. Immun.*, **54**, 239–44
45. Pennington, J. E. and Pier, G. B. (1983). Efficacy of cell wall *Pseudomonas aeruginosa* vaccines for protection against experimental pneumonia. *Rev. Infect. Dis.*, **5** (Suppl. 5), S852–7
46. Cryz, S. J., Jr, Fürer, E., Sadoff, J. C. and Germanier, R. (1986). *Pseudomonas aeruginosa* immunotype 5 polysaccharide-toxin A conjugate vaccine. *Infect. Immun.*, **52**, 161–5

47. Cryz, S. J. Jr, Fürer, E., Cross, A. S., Wegmann, A., Germanier, R. and Sadoff, J. C. (1987). Safety and immunogenicity of a *Pseudomonas aeruginosa* O-polysaccharide toxin A conjugate vaccine in humans. *J. Clin. Invest.*, **80**, 51–6
48. Cryz, S. J. Jr., Sadoff, J. C. and Fürer, E. (1988). Immunization with a *Pseudomonas aeruginosa* immunotype 5 O polysaccharide–toxin A conjugate vaccine: effect of a booster dose on antibody levels in humans. *Infect. Immun.*, **56**, 1829–30
49. Pier, G. B., Matthews, W. J., Jr and Eardley, D. D. (1983). Immunochemical characterization of the mucoid exopolysaccharide of *Pseudomnas aeruginosa. J. Infect. Dis.*, **147**, 494–503
50. Schwarzmann, D. and Boring, J. R. Jr (1971) Antiphagocytic effect of slime from a mucoid strain of *Pseudomonas aeruginosa. Infect. Immun.*, **3**, 762–7
51. Ames, P., DesJardins, D. and Pier, G. B. (1985). Opsonophagocytic killing activity of rabbit antibody to *Pseudomonas aeruginosa* mucoid exopolysaccharide. *Infect. Immun.*, **49**, 281–5
52. Pier, G. B., Saunders, J. M., Ames, P., Edwards, M. S., Auerbach, H., Goldfard, J., Speert, D. P. and Hurwitch, S. (1987) Opsonophagocytic killing antibody to *Pseudomonas aeruginosa* mucoid exopolysaccharide in older noncolonized patients with cystic fibrosis. *N. Engl. J. Med.*, **317**, 793–8
53. Nosocomial Infection Surveillance (1984). CDC morbidity and mortality weekly report **35**, 17ss–29ss
54. Finland, M. (1930). The serum treatment of lobar pneumonia. *N. Engl. J. Med.*, **202**, 1244–7
55. Pennington, J. E. and Pier, G. B. (1987). *Pseudomonas aeruginosa* immune globulin in experimental pneumonia. *Infection*, **15**, S47–9
56. Counts, G. W., Schwartz, R. W., Ulness, B. K., Hamilton, D. J., Rosok, M. J., Dunningham, M. D., Tam, M. R. and Darveau, R. P. (1988). Evaluation of an immunofluorescent-antibody test for rapid identification of *Pseudomonas aeruginosa* in blood cultures. *J. Clin. Microbiol.*, **26**, 1161–5
57. Ziegler, E. J., McCutchan, J. A., Fierer, J., Glauser, M. P., Sadoff, J. C., Douglas, H. and Braude, A. I. (1982). Treatment of gram-negative bacteremia and shock with human antiserum to a mutant *Escherichia coli. N. Engl. J. Med.*, **307**, 1225–30
58 Greisman, S. E., DuBuy, J. B. and Woodward, C. L. (1979). Experimental gram-negative bacterial sepsis: prevention mortality not preventable by antibiotics alone. *Infect. Immun.*, **25**, 538–57
59. Pennington, J. E. and Menkes, E. (1981). Type-specific versus cross-protective vaccination for gram-negative pneumonia. *J. Infect. Dis.*, **144**, 599–603
60. Sadoff, J. C., Futrovsky, S. L., Sidberry, H. F., Iglewski, B. H. and Seid, R. C. (1982). Detoxified lipopolysaccharide-protein conjugates. *Sem. Infect. Dis.*, **4**, 346–54
61. Cryz, S. J., Furer, E. and Germanier, R. (1984). Protection against fatal *Pseudomonas aeruginosa* burn wound sepsis by immunization with lipopolysaccharide and high-molecular-weight polysaccharide. *Infect. Immun.*, **43**, 795–9
62. Pennington, J. E., Pier, G. B., Sadoff, J. C. and Small, G. J. (1986). Active and passive immunization strategies for *Pseudomonas aeruginosa* pneumonia. *Rev. Infect. Dis.*, **8** (Suppl.), 426–33
63. Holder, I. A. and Neely, A. N. (1987). Experimental studies of the pathogenesis of infections due to *Pseudomonas aeruginosa*: passive intravenous immunotherapy using pseudomonas globulin. *Serodiagnosis Immunol.*, **1**, 153–62
64. Collins, M. S. and Roby, R. E. (1984). Protective activity of an intravenous immune globulin (human) enriched in antibody against lipopolysaccharide antigens of *Pseudomonas aeruginosa. Am. J. Med.*, **76**, 168–74
65. Pennington, J. E., Pier, G. B. and Small, G. J. (1986). Efficacy of intravenous immune globulin for treatment of experimental *Pseudomonas aeruginosa* pneumonia. *J. Crit. Care*, **1**, 4–10
66. Class, I., Junginger, W. and Klöss, Th. (1987). Einsatz von pseudomonas-immunglobulin bei beatmeten patienten einer interdisziplinären chirurgischen intensivstation. *Infection*, **15** (Suppl. 2), S67-70
67. Sadoff, J. C., Wright, D. C., Futrovsky, S., Sidberry, H., Collins, H. and Kaufmann, B. (1985). Characterization of mouse monoclonal antibodies directed against *Pseudomonas aeruginosa* lipopolysaccharides. *Antibiot. Chemother.*, **36**, 134–146
68. Sawada, S., Kawamura, T., Masuho, Y. and Tomibe, K. (1985). Characterization of a human

monoclonal antibody to lipopolysaccharides of *Pseudomonas aeruginosa* serotype 5: a possible candidate as an immunotherapeutic agent for infections with *P. aeruginosa*. *J. Infect. Dis.*, **5**, 965–70

69. Sawada, S., Kawamura, T. and Masuho, Y. (1987). Immunoprotective human monoclonal antibodies against five major serotypes of *Pseudomonas aeruginosa*. *J. Gen. Microbiol.*, **133**, 3581–90
70. Zweerink, H. J., Gammon, M. C., Hutchison, C. F., Jackson, J. J., Lombardo, D., Miner, K. M., Puckett, J. M., Sewell, T. J. and Sigal, N. H. (1988). Human monoclonal antibodies that protect mice against challenge with *Pseudomonas aeruginosa*. *Infect. Immun.*, **56**, 1873–9
71. Hector, R. F., Trawinski, J., Besemer, D., Collins, M. S. and Pennington, J. E. (1987). *In vitro* and *in vivo* evaluation of a human immunoglobulin M monoclonal antibody to *Pseudomonas aeruginosa* immunotype 3. Presented at the 27th Interscience Conference on Antimicrobial Agents and Chemotherapy, New York, No. 547

6
Varicella vaccines

R. B. HEATH

INTRODUCTION

Primary infection with varicella zoster virus (VZV) results in the common childhood illness varicella or chickenpox. However, in common with other members of the herpesvirus family, VZV is not completely eliminated from the body following recovery from the primary infection, and enters into a latent state. After a period of time, which is usually decades, the virus reactivates and produces the recurrent illness herpes zoster (or shingles).

PATHOGENESIS

A knowledge of the pathogenesis of the disease is essential when contemplating means of its prevention, but unfortunately there are few detailed studies on the pathogenesis of VZV infections. It is, for example, uncertain how the virus spreads. The lesions of both varicella and herpes zoster are teeming with virus particles, and so it is possible that these lesions are the source of the virus. However, as varicella most commonly occurs in the winter months, many have presumed that, in common with most respiratory viral infections, it is spread by aerosols from infection of the upper respiratory tract. This must, however, remain a presumption as it is virtually impossible to isolate VZV from respiratory secretions either in the incubation period or during the course of the disease. It is generally presumed that the respiratory tract is the portal of entry for the virus[1]. It should be noted at this stage that prevention of upper respiratory viral infections has proved to be one of the least successful aspects of the otherwise outstanding success of viral prophylaxis by means of vaccination.

What is certain about the pathogenesis of varicella is that the virus spreads from the portal of entry to reach virtually every organ of the body. This involves viraemic spread, and it is at this stage that the infection can be most easily aborted by vaccines in a manner similar to what has been so successfully achieved with smallpox and poliomyelitis. Following viraemia, the virus replicates in many of the organs which it has reached. However, apart from the skin it is unusual for viral replication to cause sufficient damage that will manifest clinically. There are exceptions to this generalization, and in particular replication in the lungs[2] and central nervous system[3] can on occasions cause serious complications of the disease. These and other major complications of varicella are listed in Table 1.

The damage caused to tissues such as the skin and lungs is due to a direct lytic effect of viral replication since the pathological changes, which include giant-cell formation, are similar to the cytopathic changes seen in infected culture systems. In this respect it should be noted that the pathogenesis of the varicella rash is very different from that of measles, which is certainly immune-mediated.

As with varicella, we have no precise information on the pathogenesis of herpes zoster. It is presumed that the virus establishes a latent state in posterior root ganglia and in the ganglia of cranial nerves. However, unlike herpes simplex virus (HSV), VZV has never been recovered from ganglia. The possibility that virus remains latent elsewhere in the body and, at a late stage, migrates to the ganglia cannot be excluded, although this is very unlikely. What is certain is that recurrent lytic infection occurs in these ganglia since histology reveals that they are extensively damaged as a result[4]. The virus then proceeds down the sensory nerve of the affected ganglia and infects the dermatome supplied by that nerve, producing the classical lesions of shingles. Apart from distribution, the lesions of zoster are identical to those of varicella. With recurrent HSV infection there is frequently a history of an event such as a common cold, pyrexia, exposure to ultraviolet light, etc., which is thought to have triggered the recurrence. It is very unusual to obtain a history of any event which might have induced herpes zoster.

Since this disease usually appears several decades after the primary infection, it is thought that it is mainly due to the weakening of the immune response, induced by the primary infection, with time. Strong support for this hypothesis comes from the finding that herpes zoster occurs at a younger age and is more severe in those who are immunocompromised.

When considering the pathogenesis of VZV infection it is important to note that whilst chickenpox can be 'caught' from individuals with either chickenpox or herpes zoster, the latter, as explained above, can only be 'caught' from oneself.

A knowledge of the pathogenesis of VZV infection, and particularly the fact that the recurrent infection is at least partly due to diminished effectiveness of the immune response, prompts the intriguing question – can vaccination

Table 1 The complications of varicella

Secondary bacterial infection	Reye syndrome
Pneumonitis	Purpura
Cerebellar ataxia	Hepatitis
Encephalomyelitis	Glomerulonephritis
Transverse myelitis	Uveitis
Optic neuritis	Arthritis
Guillian-Barré syndrome	Appendicitis

be used to prevent a recurrent infection? This possibility cannot be dismissed and is worthy of further consideration.

CLINICAL MANIFESTATIONS

The clinical presentations of both varicella and herpes zoster are so well known that it will be unnecessary to describe them here. Instead, consideration will be given to the morbidity and mortality of these infections as this is, of course, particularly relevant to consideration of the introduction of varicella vaccines.

It is unquestionably true that varicella is one of the mildest diseases of childhood. It is unusual for it to be of any concern to either parent or medical practitioner. Isolation of infected individuals is rarely practised, and indeed it is sensibly considered preferable for the disease to be contracted in childhood because it is frequently more serious in adults. The complications which have been listed in Table 1 are more frequently seen in adults than in young children. Although some of these are serious, particularly when the lungs and brain are involved, it has to be recognized that these complications are rare. It is also true that the complications of varicella occur less frequently and are generally less severe than those of measles. This is the reason that, to date, no serious consideration has been given to prevention by means of mass vaccination. In contrast to measles, however, varicella can be a problem to pregnant women. If the infection occurs early in pregnancy the virus may cross the placenta and infect the fetus. The child will be born severely damaged with what is now known as the congenital varicella syndrome[5], the distinct features of which are listed in Table 2. If the infection occurs late in pregnancy, then VZV, in common with other viruses, can cross the placenta, and this can result in neonatal varicella. The '5-day rule' is important in this context. This, in essence, states that if the onset of symptoms in the mother occurs more than 5 days before delivery, then the child is likely to be born protected by passively transferred maternal antibodies and, if the child is infected, the illness is unlikely to be severe. In contrast, if the onset of symptoms in the mother was 5 or less days before delivery then the child will be born without the benefit of maternal antibodies, and it is in these instances that the severe neonatal forms of varicella are seen. It is fortunate that the congenital varicella syndrome, although very serious, is extremely rare. Further, the serious effects of neonatal varicella can be obviated to a large extent by the prophylactic administration of zoster immune globulin, and if necessary by the therapeutic administration of acyclovir. In view of this it is not easy to justify the introduction of mass vaccination to prevent the problems caused by varicella in pregnancy.

Table 2 The congenital varicella syndrome

Scarring of skin	Corneal atrophy
Hypoplasia of the limbs	Mental retardation
Muscular atrophy	Choreoretinitis
Rudimentary digits	Cataracts

Whilst it is unquestionably true that varicella is one of the mildest of infections, an important exception to this generalization is when it occurs in the immunocompromised. It is important to appreciate that patients of this kind are comprising an ever-increasing proportion of, at least, hospital patient populations. This is mainly the result of the increasing success in both the treatment of malignant diseases, particularly of the blood and reticuloendothelial system, and of organ and tissue transplantation. Varicella in the immunocompromised is essentially similar to that seen in normal individuals, but complications occur with much greater frequency and severity. It is in these patients that the so-called 'disseminated' forms of varicella occur, in which organs other than the skin are seriously affected. The lungs are the most important of these and VZV pneumonitis is a common cause of death.

Feldman and his colleagues, in 1975[6], reported on the outcome of varicella in 77 children with cancer. They observed that the serious effects occurred more frequently in those who were on therapy than in those who were in remission. In particular, a white cell count of less than $500/mm^3$ was found to increase the chances of visceral dissemination. In this study, varicella was found to have a mortality of 7%, but even this is appreciably lower than the 30% mortality reported by Japanese workers[7].

An analysis of the epidemiology of chickenpox in England and Wales has recently been published[8]. This report is worthy of detailed study by all concerned with the prevention of varicella, but only one aspect of the paper will be considered here. From mortality statistics, and from data on annual consultation rates for varicella provided by the Royal College of General Practitioners, the authors have estimated an overal fatality rate of 7.7 per 100 000 cases, and that immunosuppression was a contributory cause of nearly 30% of the deaths. It was of interest that although varicella is a rare disease in the elderly, the overal fatality rate per 100 000 cases in 45-year-olds was estimated to be 213 compared with a rate of 3.1 in those aged 5-14 years. Immunosuppression was a contributory cause of death in nearly half of these older patients.

Herpes zoster is an extremely unpleasant and painful condition, and post-herpetic neuralgia can be extremely disabling. Nevertheless the disease has a low mortality. As with varicella, recurrent VZV infection in the immunocompromised is frequently more severe. With these patients the infection may disseminate, second attacks can occur and the disease may appear in childhood.

Although varicella is generally a very mild disease, mortality rates are sufficiently high to warrant serious consideration of prevention by vaccination, particularly for those who are immunocompromised. Such a strategy would, however, require a safe vaccine capable of inducing long-lasting immunity. Experience with currently available live varicella vaccines will now be described.

THE VACCINES

The development of a live varicella vaccine was first described by Japanese workers in 1974[9]. The source virus for the vaccine was a clinical isolate obtained from a young 3-year-old boy – called Oka – with typical varicella. Attenuation was attempted by 10 serial passages in human embryo lung (HEL) cells followed by 12 serial passages in guinea-pig embryonic fibroblasts. A final passage was made in WI38 cells to produce a master seed for the initiation of vaccine production. Further passages have been carried out by manufacturers in WI38 and MRC5 human diploid cells, sometimes including cloning passages before production of vaccine lots. Others have attempted, and perhaps are still attempting, to produce attenuated varicella vaccines, but currently only vaccines using the Oka strain virus are available.

Evaluation of live attenuated varicella vaccines

A series of studies of the newly developed vaccine was carried out in healthy individuals, which showed that it produced good seroconversion rates without serious reactions. It was shown that immediate inoculation prevented the spread of varicella in hospital wards[10] and in family contacts[11]. In a study of 181 seronegative children it was shown that the seroconversion rate was 97.8% and that in a 2-year follow-up of 51 of these children it was found that 98% had retained induced antibodies over a 2-year period, but there was a decline in the levels of these antibodies during this period[12]. In a collaborative study with American workers it was shown that the levels of antibody induced by the vaccine were 4–8-fold lower than those observed after natural infection[13].

The results of these initial studies carried out by Japanese workers on mainly healthy children have in essence been confirmed by investigators in other countries[14–16]. One of the most impressive of these was a large placebo-controlled trial carried out in the USA involving nearly 1000 children aged 1–14 years without a history of varicella[17]. Ninety-four per cent of those who were vaccinated were shown to have seroconverted within 8 weeks. The protective efficacy of the vaccine during a 9-month surveillance period was shown to be 100%. None of the 468 vaccinees developed varicella compared with 38 cases amongst 436 placebo recipients. However, in other studies with healthy children, an occasional vaccinee has developed mild varicella following exposure[18].

In all these studies the vaccine has in general been well tolerated. A few children have had either local pain and tenderness at the injection site or mild pyrexia. Some vaccinees have developed a mild papulovesicular rash, but in most studies there has been no convincing evidence of spread of the virus from these cases; but this cannot be excluded[17].

In the early studies carried out by the Japanese and other workers virtually all of the vaccinees were immunocompetent. However, some of these children were suffering from underlying conditions, including the nephrotic syndrome, or were receiving steroids which may have impaired their immunity to some extent. Severe varicella, as discussed above, is most likely to be seen in immunocompromised children, particularly those with leukaemia and other childhood malignancies. With this in mind the Japanese workers then proceeded with the next obvious, but potentially dangerous, step of vaccinating susceptible children immunocompromised because of malignant disease.

In an early study[7], 11 children in remission from leukaemia and six with solid tumours (neuroblastoma 3, retinoblastoma 3) were vaccinated. Cytotoxic therapy for the children with solid tumours was suspended for 1 week before and 1 week after vaccination. All of the children seroconverted and the only reactions were mild rashes with incomplete vesicles which appeared in two children 2–4 weeks after vaccination. Three of the children were subsequently exposed to varicella, but none developed symptoms of this disease. Encouraged by these early results the live attenuated varicella vaccine has been evaluated in immunocompromised patients by several investigators in many parts of the world. Further experience in Japan on the use of the vaccine in 326 leukaemic children has been reported by Takahashi *et al.*[19]. A large multicentre trial of the vaccine in leukaemic children has been carried out in the USA[20] and the vaccine has been evaluated in children with solid tumours in the UK[21]. The worlwide experience with live varicella vaccines up to 1985 involving more than 10000 subjects, of which over 1000 were immunocompromised, has been reviewed[18]. The essential findings in all these studies can be briefly summarized as follows:

Reactogenicity

It is encouraging that immunocompromised patients have, in general, tolerated the vaccine well. A mild reaction at the injection site has ocurred with some of these patients, but this has always been short-lived. There is a single report[21] of a child who developed a 5 cm indurated area at the injection site, the centre of which became necrotic. This lesion rapidly healed and was not associated with general symptoms.

The commonest reaction to the vaccine is the development of a generalized maculopapular, or more commonly, a vesicular, rash which is indistinguishable from mild varicella, and from which the vaccine strain can be isolated. The incidence of these rashes is usually less than 10% but can be as high as 42% in those currently on, or who have just been taken off, cytotoxic chemotherapy[19]. These rashes are of short duration and are rarely accompanied by systemic symptoms. Few investigators have felt the need to administer acyclovir, although it has been shown that the vaccine is sensitive to this drug[22]. Reactions are much less frequent after a second dose of vaccine even if therapy has not been suspended[20].

As mentioned above, in the studies involving vaccination of healthy children no evidence was obtained of transmission of virus from vaccinees to seronegative close contacts. However, in comparable studies with immunocompromised children it has been shown that those who develop rashes may transmit the virus to susceptible siblings[20]. Transmission to the contacts has most frequently been demonstrated by seroconversion, but some of these have developed mild vesicular rashes similar to that seen in vaccinees.

It is perhaps unfortunate that zoster has been shown to develop in vaccinees, and that it has in some instances been shown to be due to reactivation of the vaccine strain[23]. Comparative studies have consistently shown that the vaccine-related risk of zoster is less than that seen in those who were infected naturally, but the difference may not be statistically different[24]. The severe disseminated form of the disease due to the vaccine strain has not been observed. It has been shown that vaccination, with suspension of therapy, has no adverse effect on underlying disease such as leukaemia[19].

Immunogenicity

It has been shown that there is considerable variation in the seroconversion rates of immunocompromised vaccinees which have varied from 63 to 100%[18]. Such variation could be expected, because of the differing degrees of immunosuppression of the vaccinees. It has also been found that the longevity of the vaccine-induced immune response is shorter than that seen in healthy subjects. It is because of this that it is now the usual practice to administer a second dose of the vaccine either at about 3 months after the primary vaccination[20] or when follow-up testing has shown that seroconversion has not occurred, or that antibody induced by the vaccine has either disappeared or has fallen to very low levels[21].

Some investigators have used skin testing[19] and lymphocyte transformation[15] assays to assess the induction of immunity by the vaccine. In general there is good agreement between the results of these assessments of cell-mediated immunity and the humoral immune response. It is of interest that cell-mediated immunity can be detected within 4 days after vaccination, which has enabled its use for post-exposure prophylaxis[11].

Protection

In general it has been found that vaccination of immunocompromised patients affords good protection, but this is not complete. In one study[21] none of nine vaccinees who subsequently came into close contact with varicella developed any symptoms of the disease. However, in a larger study[20] involving 307 children with leukaemia, 38 of the vaccinees had household contact with varicella and seven (18%) developed the disease. This attack rate should be compared with an expected rate of 80-90% for household contact[25]. In this same study a further 94 vaccinees were exposed outside their households and 10 contracted varicella.

Although live attenuated varicella vaccines afford appreciable protection to at-risk patient this is far from ideal. In the future it will be important to consider new vaccination schedules aimed at providing better protection.

Current indications for vaccinations

High-risk patients

The vaccine is primarily indicated for high-risk patients who are most likely to experience the severe effects of varicella, and for susceptible children and adults who are in close contact with such patients. The categories of patients that can be considered as high risk have been listed in Table 3. These patients will usually, but not exclusively, be children, because children are less likely to have previously been exposed to infection. Although it is certainly true that these patients will be more seriously affected by natural infection than

Table 3 Patients at risk of contracting the severe forms of varicella

Leukaemias, Hodgkin's disease and other neoplasms of the lymphoreticular system, whether or not treatment is being given.
Other cancers which are being treated with cytotoxic drugs or other regimens which are immunosuppressive.
Primary immunodeficiency syndromes.
Bone marrow transplant recipients, irrespective of their own or the donors' VZV status.
Diseases requiring systemic steroids at a dosage equivalent to at least 2 mg prednisone/kg per day.
Children of women who contracted varicella during pregnancy.
Premature infants whose mothers have no history of varicella or any infant whose birth weight was <1000 g.

by vaccination, it has to be appreciated that it is theoretically possible that the vaccine might produce severe reactions in those who are highly immunosuppressed. Consideraton should therefore be given to the following:

1. The vaccine should not as a general rule be administered to patients receiving intense immunosuppressive therapy or during a course of radiation.
2. If possible the vaccine should be administered when patients are in full remission and off cytotoxic therapy, or in the intervals between courses of treatment. The intervals should be at least 1 week before vaccination and 1 week before treatment is resumed.
3. The lymphocyte count should be at least 1×10^9/l.
4. There should be other evidence of cellular immune competence such as positive responses in delayed skin hypersensitivity tests or *in vitro* lymphocyte proliferative assays.
5. Serum IgG levels should be greater than 1000 mg/l.

Future indications

Mass vaccination

The successful large-scale trial of a varicella vaccine involving 1000 children, referred to above, has provided sufficient evidence for serious consideration of mass vaccination to prevent varicella. Indeed, it has been estimated, at least in the USA, that a mass vaccination programme would be cost-effective[26]. This calculation has been based on a number of assumptions. For example, that there would be no deleterious effect on the occurrence and complications of zoster, which is most unlikely. Further, the vaccine would have to be given as a single dose in combination with measles, mumps and rubella vaccine strains, and that there would be no increase in the number of varicella cases in older persons who are at increased risk of complications. It has already been shown that a combined measles, mumps, rubella and varicella vaccine is feasible[27], but there must be serious doubts about the longevity of protection afforded by current varicella vaccines.

Vaccination of health-care workers

It is known that about 10% of nurses are susceptible to varicella, and that outbreaks of varicella in nurses' homes are not infrequent. Infected nurses can be a potential risk to seronegative immunocompromised patients, particularly since it is well known that infection can be transmitted before the development of the rash. Vaccination of this category, and indeed other categories, of staff, closely associated with high-risk patients is worthy of future investigation.

Prevention of zoster
Since it has been shown that the administration of live varicella vaccine can enhance both cell-mediated and humoral immunity in previously seropositive adults[28], there is clearly the possibility that it could be used for the prevention of zoster. This could be a fruitful area for future research.

Administration

Current vaccines
These are supplied in lyophilized form and should be reconstituted, in the sterile saline solution provided, before injection. Unfortunately the vaccine virus is unstable even when lyophilized, and consequently has to be stored at -20°C. This can cause problems for some pharmacies, and difficult logistic distribution problems. There is clearly a need to discover effective stabilizers which, if added to the vaccine, would permit it to be more conveniently stored at temperatures above freezing point. The standard inoculum of reconstituted vaccine should be 0.5 ml, containing not less than 2000 plaque-forming units. This should be inoculated subcutaneously but never intravenously or intradermally. For reasons given above, two doses of vaccine should be administered to at-risk patients with an interval of about 3 months between doses. If follow-up serological assessment indicates that induced levels of antibodies have disappeared, or fallen to very low levels, then further inoculations may be required to ensure continuous protection. At the present time there is insufficient information available to say whether just one dose of vaccine will be sufficient to give long-term protection to healthy subjects.

Contraindications
For reasons that have been stated above it is currently considered unwise to vaccinate severely immunosuppressed patients except in those circumstances where there has been close contact with an infected individual, when on balance the risks of reaction to the vaccine strain are outweighed by the risks of natural infection. It is perhaps of interest that to date there are no reports on the vaccination of patients with Hodgkin's disease or those infected with the human immunodeficiency virus, undoubtedly because of the high degree of defective cellular immunity in these patients. The only other contraindications are systemic hypersensitivity to neomycin and, for theoretical reasons, pregnancy.

CONCLUSION

Professor Takahashi and his colleagues in Japan are to be congratulated for their courage and determination in developing and initiating evaluation of a live varicella virus vaccine. This pioneering work has aroused considerable worldwide interest, which in turn has led to fruitful extension of the initial investigative work.

The vaccine has clearly been shown to have an important role in preventing the serious effects of varicella in high-risk patients. For the future, consideration needs to be given to first preventing infection in healthy individuals by mass vaccination, and then perhaps to the prevention of zoster. Although the initial studies of live varicella vaccines are encouraging it is apparent that they are far from ideal. It is unquestionably true that they are not as effective as the live virus vaccines curently in use for the prevention of measles, mumps and rubella. The major defect of current vaccines is their comparatively poor immunogenicity and, in particular, the short duration of the induced immunity. The fact that varicella vaccines can be reactogenic in immunocompromised patients, although undesirable, cannot be regarded as a serious criticism because the reactions are mild compared with the effects of the natural infection in this category of patient. For the immediate future there is a need to expand the use of current varicella vaccines in high-risk children, and to explore the use of alternative vaccination regimens with the aim of prolonging the duration of induced immunity. It is important, therefore, that current vaccines should be licensed for use with this category of patient in those countries which have not yet done this. This will enable those who have responsibility for children with, for example, malignant disease and renal failure, to have easier access to the vaccine.

REFERENCES

1. Grose, C. (1981). Variation on a theme by Fenner: the pathogenesis of chickenpox. *Pediatrics*, **68**, 735–7
2. Triebwasser, J. H., Harris, R. E. and Rhoades, E. R. (1967). Varicella pneumonia in adults: Report of seven cases and a review of the literature. *Medicine*, **46**, 409–23
3. Johnson, R. and Milbourn, P. E. (1970). Central nervous system manifestations of chickenpox. *Can. Med. Assoc. J.*, **102**, 831–4
4. Heath, R. B. (1987). Varicella-zoster. In Zuckerman, A. J. *et al.* (eds), *Principles and Practice of Clinical Virology*, p. 58. (Chichester: John Wiley & Sons)
5. Hanshaw, J. B. and Dudgeon, J. A. (1978). Varicella-zoster infections. In *Viral Diseases of the Fetus and Newborn*, pp. 192–208. (Philadelphia: W. B. Saunders)
6. Feldman, S., Hughes, W. T. and Daniel, C. B. (1975). Varicella in children with cancer: seventy-seven cases. *Pediatrics*, **56**, 388-97
7. Izawa, T., Ihara, T., Hattori, A., Iwaza, T., Kamiya, H., Sakurai, M. and Takahashi, M. (1977). Application of a live varicella vaccine in children with acute leukaemia or other malignant diseases. *Pediatrics*, **60**, 805–9
8. Joseph, C. A. and Noah, N. D. (1988). Epidemiology of chickenpox in England and Wales, 1967–85. *Br. Med. J.*, **296**, 673–6
9. Takahashi, M., Otsuka, T., Okuna, Y., Yazaki, T. and Isomura, S. (1974). Live vaccine to prevent the spread of varicella in children in hospital. *Lancet*, **2**, 1288–90
10. Asano, Y., Nakayama, H., Yazaki, T., Ito, S., Isomura, S. and Takahashi, M. (1977). Protective efficacy of vaccination in children in four episodes of natural varicella and zoster in the ward. *Pediatrics*, **59**, 8–12
11. Asano, Y., Nakayama, H., Yazaki, T., Kato, R., Hirose, S., Tsuzuki, K., Ito, S., Isomura, S. and Takahashi, M. (1977). Protection against varicella in family contacts by immediate inoculation with live varicella vaccine. *Pediatrics*, **59**, 3–7

12. Asano, Y. and Takahashi, M. (1977). Clinical and serological testing of a live varicella vaccine and two-year follow-up for immunity of the vaccinated children. *Pediatrics*, **60**, 810–14
13. Bogger-Goren, S., Baba, K., Hurley, P., Yabuuchi, M., Takahashi, M. and Ogra, P. L. (1982). Antibody response to varicella-zoster virus after natural or vaccine-induced infection. *J. Infect. Dis.*, **146**, 260–5
14. Arbeter, A. M., Star, S. E., Weibel, R. E. and Plotkin, S. A. (1986). Varicella vaccine studies in healthy children and adults. *Pediatrics*, **78**, 748–56
15. Ndumbe, P. M., Cradock-Watson, J. E., Heath, R. B. and Levinsky, R. J. (1985). Live varicella immunization in healthy non-immune nurses. *Postgrad. Med. J.*, **61**, 133–5
16. Gershon, A. A., Steinberg, S. P., LaRussa, P., Ferrara, A., Hammerschlag, M., Gelb, L. and the NIAID Varicella Vaccine Collaborative Study Group. (1988). Immunization of healthy adults with live attenuated varicella vaccine. *J. Infect. Dis.*, **158**, 132-7
17. Weibel, R. E., Neff, B. J., Kuter, B. J., Guess, H. A., Rothenberger, C. A., Fitzgerald, A. J., Connor, K. A., McLean, A. A., Hilleman, M. R., Buynak, E. B. and Scolnick, E. M. (1984). Live attenuated varicella virus vaccine. *N. Engl. J. Med.*, **310**, 1409–15
18. Andre, F. E. (1985). Worldwide experience with the Oka-strain live varicella vaccine. *Postgrad. Med. J.*, **61**, 113–20
19. Takahashi, M., Kamiya, H., Baba, K., Asano, Y., Ozaki, T. and Horiuchi, K. (1985). Clinical experience with Oka live varicella vaccine in Japan. *Postgrad. Med. J.*, **61**, 61–7
20. Gershon, A. A., Steinberg, S. P., Gelb, L. and the National Institute of Allergy and Infectious Diseases Varicella Vaccine Collaborative Study Group (1986). Live attenuated varicella vaccine use in immunocompromised children and adults. *Pediatrics*, **78**, 757–62
21. Heath, R. B., Malpas, J. S., Kangro, H. O., Ward, A., McEniery, J. M. and Kingston, J. E. (1987). Efficacy of varicella vaccine in patients with solid tumours. *Arch. Dis. Child*, **62**, 569–72
22. Shiraki, K., Yamanishi, K. and Takahashi, M. (1984). Susceptibility to acyclovir of oka-strain varicella vaccine and vaccine-derived viruses isolated from immunocompromised patients. *J. Infect. Dis.*, **150**, 306–7
23. Hayakawa, Y., Torigoe, S., Shiraki, K., Yamanishi, K. and Takahashi, M. (1984). Biologic and biophysical markers of live varicella vaccine strain (Oka): identification of clinial isolates from vaccine recipients. *J. Infect. Dis.*, **149**, 956–63
24. Lawrence, R., Gershon, A. A., Holzman, R., Steinberg, S. P. and the NIAID Varicella Vaccine Collaborative Study Group (1988). The risk of zoster after varicella vaccination in children with leukaemia. *N. Engl. J. Med.*, **318**, 543–8
25. Ross, A. H., Lencher, E. and Reitman, G. (1962). Modification of chickenpox in family contacts by administration of gamma globulin. *N. Engl. J. Med.*, **267**, 369–76
26. Preblud, S. R. (1986). Varicella: complications and costs. *Pediatrics*, **78**, 728–35
27. Brunell, P. A., Novelli, V. M., Lipton, S. V. and Pollock, B. (1988). Combined vaccine against measles, mumps, rubella and varicella. *Pediatrics*, **81**, 779–84
28. Berger, R., Luescher, D. and Just, M. (1984). Enhancement of varicella-zoster-specific immune responses in the elderly by boosting with varicella vaccine. *J. Infect. Dis.*, **149**, 647

7
The application of molecular biology to the development of new vaccines against poliomyelitis

J. W. ALMOND

INTRODUCTION

Over the past decade the poliovirus has become one of the best understood of all viruses which affects humans. The application of increasingly sophisticated molecular biological and immunological techniques to the study of this virus has provided detailed insights into its molecular and genetic structure, its mode of replication and the molecular basis of its pathogenicity (for reviews see refs 1–3). Poliomyelitis, the disease caused by the poliovirus, has been successfully controlled in many countries of the world through the use of two very good vaccines, the inactivated 'Salk' vaccine and the live attenuated 'Sabin' vaccine. Although both of these vaccines have considerable merits, they also have some relative disadvantages when compared with each other and with other viral vaccines. For example, the killed vaccine is more expensive than the live attenuated, and has seldom found widespread use in developing countries. Its use has also been occasionally linked to problems; for example an outbreak of poliomyelitis in Finland in 1984 suggested that the immunogenicity of at least the type 3 component of the killed vaccine may have been inadequately antigenic[4]. It has also been suggested that the immune response to the killed vaccine may not provide herd immunity due to the lack of induction of secretory antibodies[5]. For these reasons, and because of its advantages of lower cost and ease of administration, most countries prefer the live attenuated 'Sabin' vaccine. However, here too there are some drawbacks. Seroconversion rates following vaccination in many developed countries are sometimes rather poor[6], and because of the instability of the vaccine a comprehensive cold chain needs to be maintained from supplier to site of use. In developed countries there is also a low but detectable paralysis associated with the use of the live attenuated vaccine[7].

In light of the recent advances made in our understanding of the molecular biology and pathogenicity of polioviruses, and the fact that the existing vaccines are based on technologies of more than a quarter of a century ago, researchers have begun to propose that it should now be possible to develop improved vaccines which overcome some of the above difficulties[8]. Encouragement to this view was given at the Forty-third Assembly of the World Health Organization, which in 1988 accepted a motion calling for the global eradication of poliomyelitis by the year 2000. This now forms one of the aims of the WHO's Expanded Programme of Immunization (EPI) which has recommended the development of improved vaccines with better thermostability, better take-rates, and which would be absolutely free of side-effects in vaccinees. The stage is therefore set to exploit the knowledge of polioviruses that we have gained during the 1970s and 1980s, to develop new candidate strains which could be used as new vaccines in the 1990s. This chapter summarizes recent important research in this area, and discusses the possible new routes to improved poliovirus vaccines. Although it is possible that recombinant DNA technology may provide a way of producing new killed or subunit vaccines, e.g. through yeast or baculovirus expression vectors, this chapter will concentrate on possible new developments in the field of live attenuated poliovirus vaccines.

THE MOLECULAR STRUCTURE OF POLIOVIRUSES

Polioviruses are members of the *Enterovirus* genus of the family Picornaviridae, a large group of human pathogens associated with a wide array of disease syndromes. On the basis of serum neutralization tests polioviruses can be divided into three serotypes – P1, P2 and P3 – each of which is capable of causing paralytic poliomyelitis in humans. The viruses of all three serotypes have identical morphology. In each case the particle is composed of 6 copies each of the structural proteins VP-1, VP-2, VP-3, and VP-4. These proteins form a shell which surrounds a single strand of messenger sense RNA of approximately 7450 bases in length[3]. The RNA has a 22 amino acid protein (VPg) covalently linked to its 5′ terminus and a poly-A tract at its 3′ terminus. The genome, whose organization is shown in Figure 1, contains a 5′ non-coding region of about 750 nucleotides, the detailed functions of which remain largely unknown but include the control of protein translation[9] and probably the control of messenger RNA synthesis[10] and RNA encapsidation. This sequence is followed by a single large open reading frame, which encodes the polyprotein precursor of the structural and non-structural polypeptides[11]. At the end of the open reading frame is a short untranslated region of about 70 bases before the polyadenylate tract. The virus-encoded polyprotein has a molecular weight of around 200 kd and is processed during its synthesis by at least two virus-coded proteases. Comparison of amino and carboxy terminal sequences of individual virus proteins with the polyprotein sequence predicted from the sequence of the cDNA sequence has allowed the comprehensive genetic map of poliovirus type 1 to be deduced (Figure 1)[3]. Although the corresponding data have not been obtained for poliovirus types 2 and 3, there is sufficient homology in the

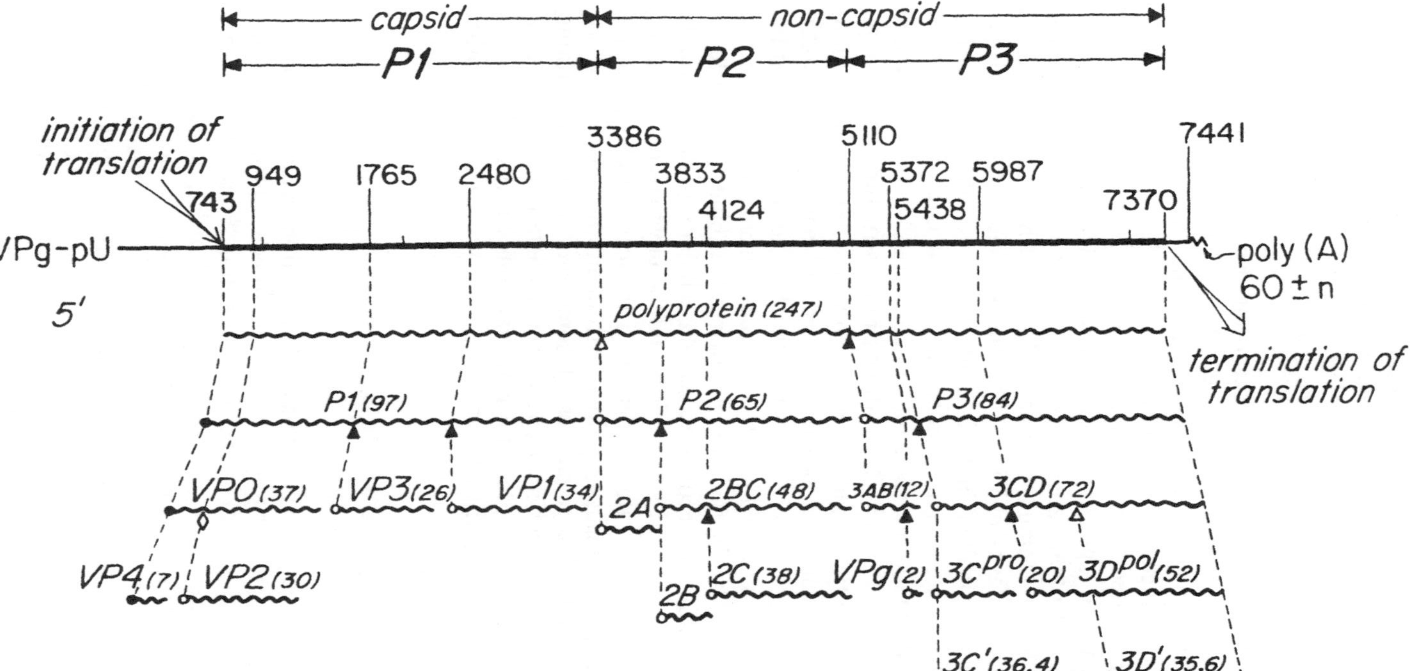

Figure 1 Gene organization of poliovirus RNA. Virion RNA, terminated at the 5′ end with the genome-linked protein VPg and at the 3′ end with poly(A), is shown as a solid line, the translated region being more pronounced than the non-coding regions. The numbers above the virion RNA refer to the first nucleotide of the codon specifying the N-terminal amino acid for the virus-specific proteins. The coding region has been divided into three regions (P1, P2, P3), corresponding to rapid cleavages of the polyprotein. Numbers in parentheses are calculated molecular weights. Open circles indicate that the terminal amino acid has been experimentally determined. The N-termini are glycine in all cases except for VP2 where it is serine. The C-terminal amino acid of protein 3D is phenylalanine. Closed circles indicate that the N-termini are known to be blocked. Closed trianlges correspond to Gln-Gly pairs that are cleaved during proteolytic processing of a polypeptide by the virus-coded proteinase 3C. Open triangles correspond to Tyr–Gly pairs cleaved by viral proteinase 2A[3]. The open diamond corresponds to an Asn-Ser pair cleaved only during morphogenesis. Polypeptides 3C′ and 3D′ are products of an alternative cleavage, the biological significance of which is unknown. (Reproduced with permission from Nomoto and Wimmer[2].)

polyprotein to allow a fairly precise alignment and the identification of likely cleavage sites for these two serotypes also. The non-structural P2 and P3 regions of the polyprotein contain the RNA-dependent RNA polymerase, the genome-linked protein VPg, the two proteases and other non-structural proteins whose functions are not known.

The protein structures of poliovirus types 1 and 3 have been determined to near atomic resolution by X-ray crystallography[12,13]. Three of the proteins, VP-1, VP-2, and VP-3 – molecular weights 33.5, 30 and 26.5 kd respectively – have a similar three-dimensional structure: a core made up of eight anti-parallel srands of β-pleated sheet forming a β-barrel type structure, plus two α-helical regions lying at right angles to each other. The major differences between these three proteins are in the size and conformations of their termini, and of the loops joining the domains that contribute to the common core structures. The similarity of VP-1, VP-2 and VP-3 is such that they can be considered quasi-equivalent in their contribution to the $T = 3$ virion architecture. VP-4 is a somewhat smaller protein (7.4 kd) and occupies a position on the interior of the shell that is analogous to the N-terminal domains of VP-1 and VP-3. The three-dimensional structure reveals high points or projections on the surface of the virion which have been shown to be important in antigenicity (see below). It has also been suggested that a cleft or canyon 25 Å deep and 12–30 Å wide, which separates a peak on the five-fold axis of the virion formed by VP-1 molecules, from a plateau formed by VP-2 and VP-3, may be the region of poliovirus that binds to the cellular receptor[14]. Since the ability to recognize a specific cellular receptor is thought to be crucial to the poliovirus's tissue tropism, and thereby to its pathogenesis, it is likely that the shape and the properties of this canyon constitute the essential feature that distinguishes a polovirus from another enterovirus. To date the complete nucleotide sequences of some nine poliovirus strains, including representatives of each serotype, have been determined[15]. This has provided information on the degree of genetic variability between strains as compared with the level of divergence between polioviruses and other enterovirus types.

ANTIGENIC STRUCTURE

Humoral immunity is thought to be the basis of protection against poliomyelitis in humans. The antigenic structures giving rise to neutralizing antibodies have therefore been the subject of intensive investigation. Several approaches have been taken to the study of poliovirus antigenicity, including the comparison of amino acid sequences of different serotypes[15], the analysis of antigenicity of synthetic peptides[16], and the expression of virus proteins in *E. coli*[17]. Perhaps the most informative approach, however, has been the characterization and sequence analysis of monoclonal antibody-resistant variants of the virus[18]. Such studies have suggested that there are at least four antigenic sites on the poliovirus particle, although the relative immunodominance of these sites may differ between serotypes. Although most antigenic studies were carried out without reference to the three-dimensional structure, it was reassuring to note that the sites identified could be assigned to high spots on the surface of the virus particle once the model became available. This detailed knowledge of antigenic structures of the poliovirus has suggested new ways for the development of alternative vaccines (see below).

An interesting and potentially important embellishment of the antigenic character of polioviruses concerns the trypsin cleavability of site 1 in poliovirus type 3[19]. This site is immunodominant in mice, and probably also in humans. However, it contains an arginine at position 99 and is therefore susceptible to cleavage by trypsin and trypsin-like enzymes in the gut of the human host. It has been noticed that virus excreted from the gut of healthy vaccinees is in a cleaved form, and is thus not neutralizable by antibodies directed against this site. Antibodies against the site, however, are present in the blood of vaccinees, indicating that at some stage during the infection virus with an intact site 1 is presented to the immune system[19]. These observations may provide the reason for the persistence of the type 3 virus in the gut following vaccination, and suggest also that the protective immune response may be qualitatively different in the gut and the blood.

ATTENUATION OF POLIOVIRUS NEUROVIRULENCE

As discussed above, most countries use Sabin's live attenuated vaccines as their major means of controlling poliomyelitis. These avirulent strains infect and induce immunity in humans without causing disease. Although the Sabin vaccines are arguably the safest and most effective live virus vaccines currently in use, it has been shown that in a small number of cases (estimated at 0.84 cases per million recipients) poliomyelitis may develop as a consequence of vaccination. Such disease is mainly associated with type 2 and type 3 vaccine strains and much less frequently with type 1[7]. An understanding of the molecular basis of attenuation of the Sabin vaccines is important because it could lead to improved methods of production and quality control, as well as to the development of modified type 2 and 3 vaccines which might be of comparable safety to the excellent type 1 strain.

All three of the vaccine strains were developed empirically by passage of wild-type virus in monkey tissue *in vivo* and *in vitro*[20]. Over the past few years much has been learnt about the genetic basis of attenuation in these strains. The work has been based primarily on the comparison of sequences of neurovirulent and attenuated strains, together with the construction of defined recombinants from infectious cDNAs of vaccine strains and their wild-type progenitors[1,2].

Our previous work has concentrated on poliovirus type 3, the serotype most commonly implicated in vaccine-associated disease, and that which has presented most problems in vaccine manufacture. Comparison of the nucleotide sequences of the genomes of the Sabin type 3 vaccine strain P3/Leon/12a$_1$b and its neurovirulent progenitor P3/Leon/37, indicated that they differ by just 10 point mutations in their 7432 base genome (Figure 2). These mutations must therefore account for the attenuated phenotype of the

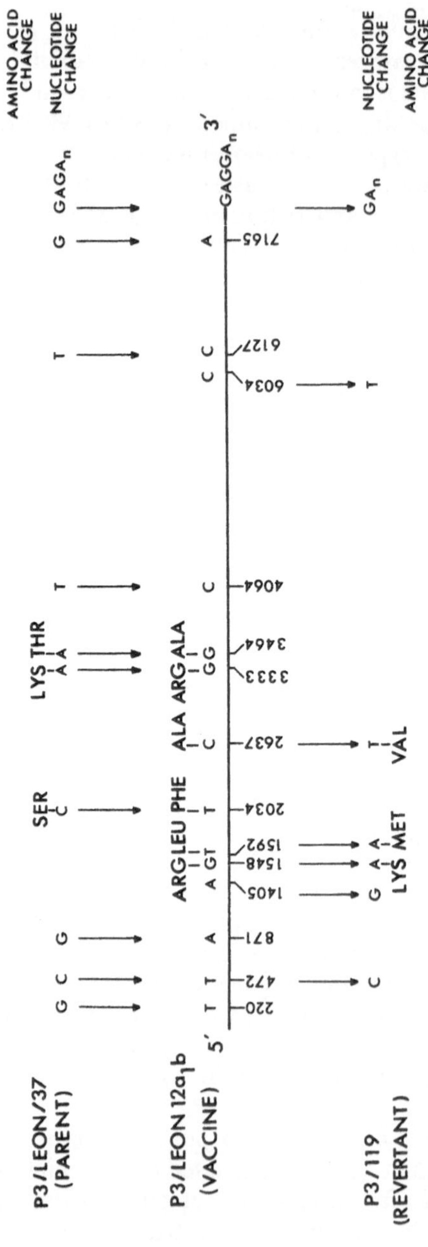

Figure 2 Nucleotide and predicted amino acid sequence differences between poliovirus type 3 strains P3/Leon/37 (parent), P3/Leon $12a_1b$ (vaccine), and P3/119 (revertant)

vaccine. Information on which of these might be responsible for the attenuation phenotype was obtained from the genome sequence of P3/119, the neurovirulent revertant of the vaccine isolated from a fatal case of vaccine-associated paralysis. P3/119 showed seven changes from the vaccine but significantly was vaccine-like at eight of the 10 positions where the vaccine differed from its progenitor. This showed that the P3/119 strain was a direct descendant of the vaccine and was therefore a *bona-fide* revertant. The mutations in P3/119 are also indicated in Figure 2. From these results it was concluded that attenuation is likely to be effected by one of three genetic changes: the base change at 472 which directly back-mutated in P3/119, the changes which give rise to structural protein changes or the mutation just prior to the poly-A tract[21]. The most direct information bearing on which of these mutations are responsible for the attenuation phenotype of poliovirus type 3, however, has come from studies of recombinant viruses prepared from infectious cDNA[22]. A series of recombinants was prepared to examine the effects of each mutation either singly or in combination with others. Viruses recovered from recombinant cDNAs were tested for neurovirulence by a modified version of the WHO neurovirulence test for vaccine safety. The results are indicated in Figure 3, and are interpreted as follows. Virulent viruses rapidly paralyse all animals and usually give a high lesion score of <2.2. In contrast attenuated viruses comparable to the vaccine cause clinical signs in only about 2% of animals, and show histological lesion scores in a range between 0.2 and 0.9, indicating a low degree of invasion and neurological damage. It can be seen from Figure 3 that virus recovered from the P3/Leon/37 cDNA, like the virus from which it was derived, was highly virulent, with an average lesion score of 2.7 and all animals showing clinical disease. Similarly the virus recovered from the Sabin vaccine cDNA was also of the phenotype expected, giving an average lesion score of 0.41 with no animals showing signs of disease. Thus the process of cloning the virus genome and recovery of transfection did not have a significant effect on the virulence phenotype of these viruses. Recombinant viruses containing the 5′ portion of their genome from the vaccine strain and the 3′ portion from the progenitor strain were significantly less virulent than P3/Leon/37, giving fewer animals with clinical signs and a lower lesion score. Similarly recombinant viruses containing the VP-3 of the Sabin vaccine (residue 2034) in a genome otherwise derived from P3/Leon/37, were of an intermediate character. While few of these animals showed clinical signs, their lesion scores were significantly higher than for the Sabin vaccine strain. These findings are consistent with the view that mutations in the 5′ portion of the genome and in VP-3 both contribute to the attenuated phenotype, and that neither of these fully attenuates the virus on its own. Recombinant viruses which contained the VP-1 or the P2A mutation of Sabin in a genome which was otherwise P3/Leon/37 were virulent, suggesting that these two mutations had no effect on the level of neurovirulence of the virus. A similar conclusion was reached concerning the 3′ portion of the vaccine genome. It was concluded from these studies that the Sabin vaccine strain is attenuated by just two point mutations, a C-U mutation at 472 and a C-U mutation at 2034 which causes a serine to

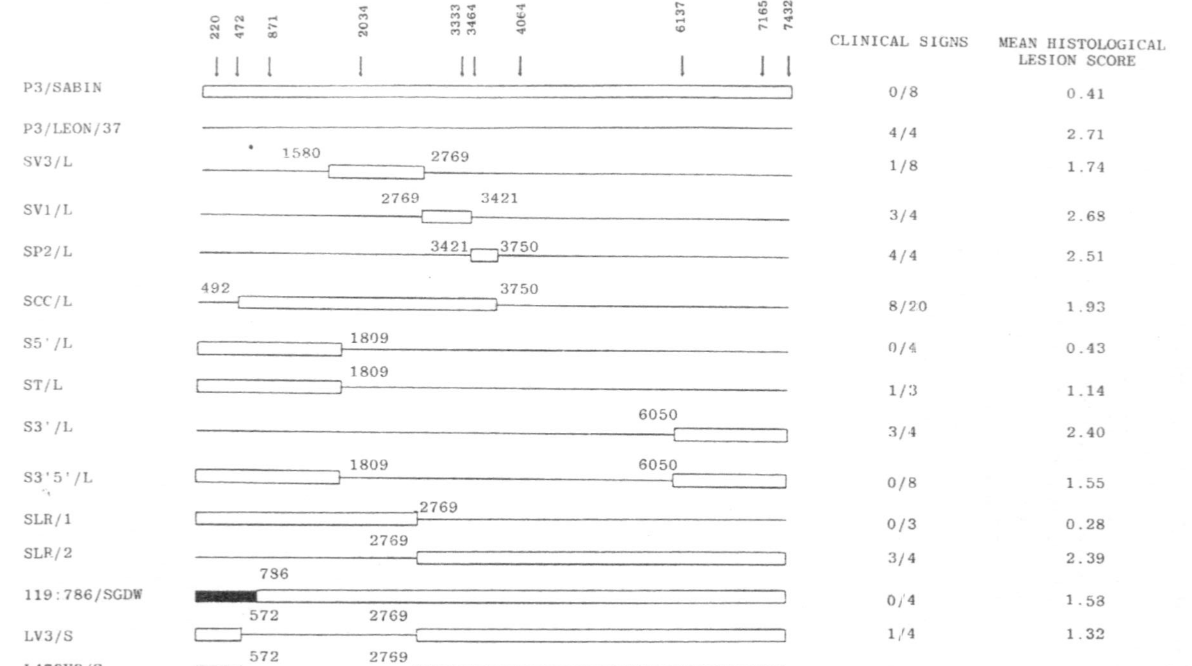

Figure 3 Structure of recombinant viruses between the progenitor strain P3/Leon/37 and the vaccine strain P3/Leon/$12a_1b$ constructed from infectious cDNAs. Recombinants were constructed using convenient restriction endonuclease cleavage sites falling between the mutations considered to be important to the attenuation phenotype[21]. After recovery of recombinant viruses by transfection of Hep2C cells in culture at 35°C the identity of the recombinants was verified using the primer extension sequencing on purified virus RNA covering sites of sequence difference at both side of each cross-over point. Recovered viruses were tested for neurovirulence in animals[1]. Clinical signs refer to the development of obvious weakness or paralysis in one or more limbs. Single lines correspond to genome regions derived from P3/Leon/37, open bars to P3/Leon $12a_1b$ and filled bars

phenylalanine substitution in virus coat protein VP-3[22]. This latter mutation also confers a temperature-sensitive phenotype to the vaccine, and this is therefore linked to the rct 40 marker (reproductive capacity at supraoptimal temperature). Based on an analysis of the likely effect of this mutation on the three-dimensional structure of the virus, and on consideration of suppressor mutations which lead to a reversion of the ts phenotype without direct back-mutation at 2034, we suggest that the temperature-sensitive phenotype is caused by the weakening of interactions between protomers along the five-fold axis of the virus (unpublished). Suppressor mutations probably cause reversion to ts^+ by strengthening these protomer–protomer interactions.

Our conclusion that the C-U mutation at position 472 in the non-coding region of the poliovirus type 3 genome plays a role in attenuation comes not only from the studies described above, but also from the analysis of viruses excreted from healthy vaccinees[23] and from the sequence analysis of other viruses isolated from cases of vaccine-associated disease[24]. In all virulent viruses examined to date the 472 U of the Sabin strain has directly back-mutaed to a C. Moreover in healthy vaccinees this back-mutation occurs rapidly following vaccination. Thus it was reported by Evans *et al.*[23] that virus excreted just 2 days following vaccination had reverted to C at position 472. Although such viruses have usually retained the attenuation mutation at 2034 they are significantly more neurovirulent than the vaccine strain, suggesting that the reversion at 472 does cause an increase in neurovirulence. Further evidence for the role of the C–U mutation at 472 in attenuation comes from studies using the mouse model for polio virulence developed by Racaniello and colleagues[25]. This system uses the mouse-adapted P2/Lansing strain of virus which is virulent for mice when injected intracranially. By construction of intertypic recombinants between P2/Lansing and either P3/Leon/37 or the type 3 vaccine P3/Leon/12a_1b, such that the recombinants derive their 5′ terminal non-coding region from the type 3 strains, but otherwise are entirely P2/Lansing, it was possible to show that the C–U at 472 had a significant attenuating effect on the P2/Lansing virus for mice. A similar recombinant deriving its 5′ non-coding region from P3/119 derivative was neurovirulent, as expected. The replication of the three recombinant viruses in HeLa cell cultures was very similar but the virus containing U at position 472 showed very little, if any, replication in the mouse brain. The importance of this mutation was underscored by the isolation of virus from the brain and spinal cord of diseased animals which had received a large dose ($>10^7$ p.f.u.) of the vaccine recombinant. Sequencing of these isolates reveals that position 472 had back-mutated to wild-type C. These isolates showed a level of neurovirulence comparable to that of P2/Lansing when injected into further mice.

It seems, then, that a single nucleotide change of C–U at position 472 renders the virus incapable of replicating and of causing pathological damage in mouse brain. This suggests that the mouse model accurately reflects the results obtained in primates[25]. Thus the mouse model may provide a useful animal model in which to study the poliovirus pathogenesis and in which to develop alternative safer vaccines (see below).

Similar studies to those described above have been carried out with poliovirus type 1 by Nomoto and colleaues[2,26]. Comparison of the sequences between the neurovirulent progenitor of the type 1 vaccine, P1/Mahoney, and the vaccine strain, P1/LS-c,2ab, reveals that these two viruses differ by 57 nucleotide point mutations in the 7441 base genome[27]. Twenty-one of these give rise to amino acid changes. Analysis of recombinants between these two strains constructed via infectious cDNAs has been used to map attenuating mutations. Although the results of this analysis prove to be rather complicated, Nomoto and colleagues were able to draw several conclusions[26]. First, mutations scattered over the first 5601 bases of the genome seem to contribute to attenuation of the Sabin type 1 strain. Second, a strong attenuating mutation was observed in the first 1122 bases. Subsequent work by Nomoto and colleagues identified the mutation at 481 in the genome as having a major attenuation effect[28]. The greater number of attenuating mutations in this strain than in type 3 probably accounts for its better safety record. Complications due to vaccine with type 1 appear to be at least an order of magnitude lower in frequency than those associated with types 2 or 3.

Recently studies have been initiated attempting to identify mutations in the type 2 vaccine strain responsible for its attenuation, and to determine how this virus reverts to neurovirulence. Although this work is incomplete, it appears that the type 2 vaccine strain, like the type 1 and type 3 described above, has an attenuating mutation in the non-coding region of its genome at position 481 (Pollard, unpublished). Thus the structure of the region of the genome around bases 460–540 seems to be important for the neurovirulence phenotype. All three vaccine strains seem to possess a major attenuating mutation in this region.

EVOLUTION OF POLIOVIRUSES IN THE HUMAN GUT

Minor and colleagues have shown that the attenuating mutations in the 5′ non-coding region of the genome described above for poliovirus types 1, 2 and 3 are rapidly selected against upon replication of the virus in the human gut[29]. In types 2 and 3 most, if not all, vaccinees begin to shed virus which has reverted to the wild-type sequence within a few days following vaccination. The case of type 1 is less clear-cut where approximately 50% of vaccinees shed reverted virus, whereas the remainder shed virus which is vaccine-like at position 480 throughout their period of shedding. These observations suggest that vaccine virus is not well adapted for growth in the human gut, and that the mutations in the 5′ non-coding region cause some disadvantage to the virus for replication at this site. This relative disadvantage compared with wild-type viruses may be the basis of the attenuation of the vaccine strains.

Studies on viruses shed from the gut of vaccinees following vaccination with the trivalent oral polio vaccine have also revealed that recombination between the three types occurs with high frequency[29]. Moreover, it has been observed that recombination between strains characteristically takes place in regions of the genome encoding proteins believed to be involved in RNA synthesis. In several individuals examined, the timing of the appearance of various recombinants showed a similar pattern, suggesting that recombination may play a role in adaptation to grow in the human gut. In particular, it was observed that some feature of the region of the genome encoding non-structural proteins of the type 3 virus seems relatively poorly adapted to replication in the gut. The molecular basis of the selection of these recombinants is unknown, but these observations are possibly of some practical interest in that it may be possible to produce optimal genomic arrangements of the type 1, type 2 and type 3 viruses which are suited for growth in the human gut. Such viruses, providing they carry appropriate attenuating mutations, may well provide a means of producing vaccinees with improved take rates.

POSSIBLE APPROACHES TO NEW LIVE ATTENUATED POLIOVIRUS VACCINES

As discussed above, the live attenuated vaccines have several attractions such as cost, ease of administration and efficacy, and have been the vaccines of choice for most countries for the past 25 years or so. New approaches to the development of alternative live attenuated strains are based on our recent improvement in knowledge of the genetic basis of attenuation, and of the determinants of antigenicity. Underscoring the conviction that it should be possible to produce safer and more effective type 2 and type 3 vaccine strains than those presently available is the observation that in the case of the type 1 we have a vaccine strain of outstanding safety and efficacy[7]. The new approaches therefore have addressed one or more of the following questions:

1. Can the existing type 3 and type 2 vaccine strains be further attenuated using site-direted mutagenesis techniques to the point where they are comparable in safety to the present excellent type 1 strain?
2. Can the existing type 1 strain be modified antigenically using protein engineering so that it resembles the type 2 and/or type 3 viruses, and therefore potentially be used as a vaccine against these two serotypes?
3. Is it possible, based on our knowledge of evolution of polioviruses in the human gut and on observations relating to virus stability, to improve the rate of seroconverson in vaccinees and the stability of vaccine batches in the field?

MODIFICATION OF THE 5′ NON-CODING REGION

Evans *et al.*[23] suggested that the mutation at base 472 of poliovirus type 3 involved in attenuation might act through its effect on the secondary structure of the RNA molecule, and these authors proposed a secondary structure for the 5′ non-coding region based on computer-predicted minimum energy folding. We have recently further investigated the secondary structure of the

5′ non-coding region using a combination of computer and biochemical techniques. Our results suggest[30] that the model proposed by Evans *et al.* is incorrect, and that the region around 472 involves substantial base pairing with the region from 520 to 540 in the RNA. This refined secondary structural model for poliovirus type 3 RNA is conserved in a number of different entero- and rhinoviruses. We have employed the technique of site-directed mutagenesis to assess the effect of further mutations in this area. Of 10 mutations introduced into this region four gave rise to viable virus. These four mutants have been tested for neurovirulence in mice and the results are shown in Table 1. Mutations 7 and 13 clearly attenuate the virus in terms of LD_{50} as compared with the wild-type virus, whereas mutation 14 has little or no effect. Thus we have been able to introduce new attenuating mutations into this region of the genome of poliovirus type 3, suggesting that the region is capable of being further manipulated to develop new vaccines. We were therefore interested to construct a double-mutant containing two independently attenuating mutations. Mutant 8 contains the mutation found in the vaccine strain of type 3, that is U472, plus the A at 482 present in mutant 7. This double-mutant has been tested in mice, and our results suggest that it is more attenuated than either of the single-mutant strains. By inoculating high doses of this virus into mice it has been possible to isolate revertants of the double-mutant. These have either an intermediate level of neurovirulence or have reverted fully to the wild-type level of virulence. One isolate, SFP8/FC10/0, was intermediate and had reverted at 482 but not at 472. Another isolate, SFP8/ST10, was fully neurovirulent and had reverted at both 472 and 482. The third isolate, SFP8/FC10/1, was also neurovirulent but had only reverted at 472 and not 482. However, this isolate had a second mutation at 529 and in the new secondary structure model this base pairs with 482. Moreover the mutation at 529 restores the base pairing between 529 and 482. Thus it appears that the stability of the helix and the secondary structure of this region is important to the neurovirulence of the virus. The analysis of further site-directed mutants and revertants thereof is consistent with the idea that viruses require extensive base pairing in this region in order to retain a neurovirulent phenotype. Disruption of base pairing in this region seems to attenuate. We are presently unaware of the precise function of this region, although it is interesting to note that it is included in the region identified by Sonnenberg and colleagues as being

Table 1 LD_{50} values in mice (25) for parental mouse adapted strain P2/Lansing, the type 3 vaccine and progenitor recombinants (PRV7.3 and PRV6.1) and various site-directed mutants of PRV6.1 (SFPs)

Virus		LD_{50} (p.f.u.)
P2/Lansing		1.6×10^3–1×10^5
PRV 6.1 (Leon)	472 C	$<6 \times 10^2$
7.3 (Sabin)	472 U	$>2 \times 10^7$
SFP 7	482 A	7.5×10^6
8	472 U, 482 A	1.6×10^8
13	479 C	9.1×10^6
14	480 C	$<7 \times 10^4$

necessary for the internal initiation of protein synthesis in the poliovirus genome[9]. The observation that the structure of this region is important for neurovirulence raises the prospect of disrupting it further to produce strains of even greater attenuation. We are therefore experimenting with several mutants including deletion mutants in this region. Viruses which are observed to have a sufficient level of attenuation in the mouse system (in which the protein coding region of the virus is provided by P2/Lansing) will be built into the existing Sabin type 3 vaccine strain. These modified vaccine viruses will be fed to monkeys to assess their ability to immunize via the oral route, and their ability to revert to wild-type upon replication in the monkey gut. The introduction of mutations in this region which are highly unlikely to back-mutate to wild-type may be very important in the development of vaccines which are incapable of reverting to neurovirulence in humans.

PROTEIN ENGINEERING OF THE SABIN TYPE 1 VACCINE STRAIN

As stated above, the Sabin type 1 vaccine strain is rarely associated with paralysis in vaccinees, and is at least an order of magnitude safer than the type 2 and type 3 vaccines[7]. Indeed, this virus is probably the safest live virus ever used in humans. The knowledge of the three-dimensional crystal structure of type 1, plus the availability of infectious Sabin type 1 cDNA, has raised the possibility of the redesign of the poliovirus particle for vaccine purposes. In particular we have been interested in the possibility of modifying the antigenic sites of Sabin type 1 so that they resemble those of the more problematical type 2 and type 3 viruses[31]. The antigenic sites involved in neutralization of poliovirus type 3 have been identified (Table 2). We have extensively modified the counterparts of these sites in Sabin type 1 so that they resemble those of type 3. In our first experiments on this theme site-directed mutagenesis was employed on a 1174 base pair restriction endonuclease fragment of poliovirus Sabin type 1 cDNA. This mutagenesis resulted in the coding region for eight amino acids from site 1 of the type 1 vaccine strain (SASTKNKD) being replaced by the corresponding amino acids from a poliovirus type 3 strain 3.370 (EQPTTRVQ). Mutant or 'chimaeric' virus was recovered from a full-length cDNA incorporating the modified restriction fragment. The new virus, designated S1/3.10, was shown to contain an altered RNA genome by direct nucleotide sequence analysis

Table 2 Location (amino acid numbers) of antigenic sites in poliovirus type 3

Site	*Location*
1	VP1; 89–100
2a	VP1; 220–222
2b	VP2; 164–172
3a	VP1; 286-290
3b	VP3; 58-60, 70, 71, 77, 79

through the region covering 2762–2785. Characterization of S1/3.10 indicated that it had antigenic properties of type 3 poliovirus as well as those of type 1. In a standard typing assay an unknown poliovirus is incubated with pairs of specific antisera (i.e. type 1 + type 2; type 2 + type 3; type 1 + type 3) to neutralize all but one serotype of virus in each test. The chimaera S1/3.10 was neutralized by all three combinations of antisera, by the type 1 and type 3 antisera alone, but not by the type 2 antisera. This demonstrates that the virus chimaera has antigenic characteristics of both type 1 and type 3, but is not a mixture of these two viruses. The antigenicity of S1.310 was also examined using panels of Sabin 1- and Sabin 3-specific monoclonal antibodies in both antigen blocking and neutralization tests. These results confirmed that the particle had composite antigenicity. All type 3 antibodies against site 1 which reacted with the parental 3.37 host strain, also reacted with the chimaeric virus, whereas type 3 antibodies against other sites failed to react. As expected, antibodies against site 1 of type 1 also failed to react (since this site had been replaced), whereas monoclonal antibodies against sites 2 and 3 of type 1 reacted as well with the chimaeric virus as they did with the Sabin 1 vaccine strain.

The immunogenicity of chimaera S1/3.10 was tested in mice, rabbits and monkeys, following a single inoculation of the virus. As can be seen from Table 3, animals inoculated with this virus showed a good immune response

Table 3 Antibody titres against intact and trypsin-cleaved virus in antigen blocking tests

Animal	*Immunized with*	*Antibody titre to virus*					
		S1/3.10	*s1/3.10 TRP*	*Sabin type* 1	*Sabin type* 1 *TRP*	3.370	3.370 *TRP*
Mouse							
1	Sabin type 1	160	160	320	160	<10	<10
2		160	160	160	160	<10	<10
3		640	640	640	640	<10	<10
4		640	640	640	320	<10	<10
5		160	160	160	160	<10	<10
6	S1/3.10	160	160	160	160	10	<10
7		2560	2560	2560	2560	1280	<10
8		80	80	80	80	<10	<10
9		80	80	80	80	20	<10
10		160	160	160	160	20	<10
Rabbit							
1	S1/3.10	80	80	80	80	10	<10
2		320	320	80	80	80	<10
3		160	160	40	40	160	<10
Monkey							
1	S1/3.10	160	160	160	160	20	<10

Animals were immunized with 0.1 ml of sucrose purified poliovirus of titre approximately 10^8 $TCID_{50}$ per ml. Mice were inoculated twice by the intraperitoneal route, and rabbits twice by the intramuscular route. A cynomolgus monkey was fed 1 ml of virus tissue culture fluid, and blood samples and faecal specimens taken twice a week for 4 weeks. Antibody titres were measured in the antigen blocking test and are expressed as the end-point dilution which inhibits the diffusion of virus. Viruses were treated with trypsin[31]. TRP = trypsin-treated virus.

against type 3 poliovirus 3.370 as well as against type 1. In contrast mice immunized with the Sabin 1 strain produced antibody against the chimaera and the homologous virus but failed to produce antibody against virus 3.370. Because of the sensitivity of antigenic site 1 to trypsin digestion it was possible to analyse further the type 3 antibody induced by the chimaera. All antisera raised against this virus, and showing neutralization of intact type 3 virus, failed to react with trypsin-cleaved type 3 virus, indicating that the type 3 response in these sera was against intact site 1 in the configuration found in normal infectious virus. It was also of interest to note that the monkey used in these experiments developed an anti-type 3 antibody response following infection via feeding. It has been shown previously (discussed above) that antigenic site 1 of excreted viruses of type 3 is in a cleaved form, presumably as a result of the action of intestinal proteases. This implies that the virus in the gut differs antigenically from that grown in tissue culture in respect of the presence of site 1. The fact that anti-site 1 antibodies were observed in the serum of the monkey suggests that at least some of the virus presented to the immune system in this animal must have been in an uncleaved form, and therefore was likely to have undergone replication in body sites other than the gut. These results indicate that after exchange of one of its antigenic sites the very safe poliovirus type 1 vaccine can induce neutralizing antibodies against polio type 3[31]. This modification was introduced into a region of the genome of the type 1 strain which is highly unlikely to contain attenuating mutations[2]. It is therefore reasonable to expect that the chimaera should retain the stable attenuation phenotype of the type 1 vaccine strain. To date we have constructed 13 viable poliovirus type 1/3 and 1/2 chimaeras, some of which may constitute serious alternatives to the existing type 3 and type 2 vaccine strains. Further careful characterization of antigenic domains is probably necessary, however, as some of the viruses which have extensive modifications at sites 2 and 3 do not show precisely the antigenic properties predicted. This suggests that the antigenic sites may encompass more amino acids than have so far been recognized through the analysis of monoclonal antibody escape mutants. Type 1 chimaeras incorporating more extensive areas of antigenic sites 2 and 3 are now under construction.

CONCLUSIONS

The past decade has seen considerable advances in our knowledge of the genetic and molecular basis of poliovirus pathogenesis, and of the antigenic structures important in stimulating immunity. We have now reached the point from which the design of improved vaccines against poliomyelitis is a realistic objective. In order to be serious rivals to the existing Sabin strains the new vaccines would need to show improved thermostability, better take-rates among vaccinees, and hold the promise of being completely safe from side-effects. A well-understood molecular basis of their attenuation might also provide a means by which quality and efficacy could be controlled and monitored *in vitro*, rather than through the use of the present expensive and cumbersome monkey neurovirulence test.

The most likely routes to new vaccines presently seem to be through:

1. The introduction of further attenuating mutations into the genomes of polioviruses types 2 and 3 – particularly in the region 460–490, the secondary structure of which is believed to be important to the neurovirulent phenotype.
2. The construction of intertypic antigen chimaeras based on the very stable poliovirus type 1 strain.

It has been suggested that replacement of the existing Sabin vaccine strains would be extremely unlikely because of the difficulty of establishing that new strains were of comparable or improved safety in humans. However, the proposals described above are all based on modifications to the existing vaccines, and have a sound scientific rationale. After cautious initial trials in immune individuals it should be possible to proceed to larger trials, and even to widespread use, with a far greater degree of confidence than would be the case for the introduction of completely new vaccine strains.

REFERENCES

1. Almond, J. W. (1987). The attenuation of poliovirus neurovirulence. *Ann. Rev. Microbiol.*, **41**, 153–80
2. Nomoto, A. and Wimmer, E. (1986). Genetic studies of the antigenicity and the attenuation phenotype of poliovirus. In Russell, W. C. and Almond, J. W. (eds), *Molecular Basis of Virus Disease*, Vol. 40, pp. 107–34. SGM Symposium
3. Kuhn, R. J. and Wimmer, E. (1987). The replication of picornaviruses. In Rowlands, D. J., Mahy, B. W. J. and Mayo, M. (eds), *The Molecular Biology of Positive Strand RNA Viruses*, pp. 17-51. (New York: Academic Press)
4. Hovi, T., Huovilainen, A., Kuronent, T., Poyry, T., Salama, N., Cantell, K., Kinnunen, E., Lapinleimu, K., Roivainen, M. and Stenvik, M. (1986). Outbreak of paralytic poliomyelitis in Finland: widespread circulation of antigenically altered poliovirus type 3 in a vaccinated population. *Lancet*, **1**, 1427–42
5. Melnick, J. L. (1978). Advantages and disadvantages of killed and live poliomyelitis vaccines. *Bull. WHO*, **56**, 21-38
6. Montefiore, D. Q., Jamieson, M. F., Collard, P. and Jolly, H. (1963). Trial of type 1 oral poliomyelitis vaccine (Sabin) in Nigerian children. *Br. Med. J.*, **1**, 1569-72
7. Assaad, F. and Cockburn, W. C. (1982). The relationship between acute persisting spinal paralysis and poliomyelitis vaccine – results of a ten-year enquiry. *Bull. WHO*, **60**, 231–42
8. Almond, J. W., Stanway, G., Cann, A. J., Westrop, G. D., Evans, D. M. A., Ferguson, M., Minor, P. D., Spitz, M. and Schild, G. C. (1984). New poliovirus vaccines: a molecular approach. *Vaccine*, **2**, 177–84
9. Pelletier, J. and Sonnenberg, N. (1988). Internal initiation of translation of eukaryotic mRNA directed by a sequence derived from poliovirus RNA. *Nature*, **334**, 320–5
10. Lubinski, J. M., Kaplan, G., Racaniello, V. R. and Dasgupta, A. (1986). Mechanism of *in vitro* synthesis of covalently linked dimeric RNA molecules by the poliovirus replicase. *J. Virol.*, **58**, 459–67
11. Kitamura, N., Semler, B., Rothberg, P. G., Larsen, G. R., Adler, C. J., Dorner, A. J., Emini, E. A., Hanecak, R., Lee, J. J., van der Werf, S., Anderson, C. W. and Wimmer, E. (1981). Primary structure, gene organisation and polypeptide expression of poliovirus RNA. *Nature*, **291**, 547-53
12. Hogle, J. M., Chów, M. and Filman, D. J. (1985). The three-dimensional structure of poliovirus at 2.9Å resolution. *Science*, **229**, 1358-65
13. Filman, D. J., Syred, R., Chow, M., Minor, P. D., Neadham, A. J. and Hogle, J. M. (1989).

Structural factors that control conformational transitions of serotype specificity in type 3 poliovirus. *EMBO J.* (Submitted)

14. Rossmann, M. G., Arnold, E., Erickson, J. W., Frankenberger, E. A., Griffith, J. P., Hecht, H-J., Johnson, J. E., Kamer, G., Luo, M., Mosser, A. G., Rueckert, R. R., Sherry, B. and Vriend, G. (1985). Structure of a human cold virus and functional relationship to other picornaviruses. *Nature*, **317**, 145–53
15. Toyoda, H., Kohara, M., Kataoka, Y., Siganuma, T., Omata, T., Ionura, N. and Nomoto, A. (1984). Complete nucleotide sequences of all three poliovirus serotype genomes. Implications for genetic relationship, gene function and antigenic determinants. *J. Mol. Biol.*, **174**, 561–85
16. Emini, E. A., Jameson, B. A. and Wimmer, E. (1983). Priming for and induction of anti-poliovirus neutralizing antibodies by synthetic peptides. *Nature*, **304**, 699–703
17. Van der Werf, S., Wynchowski, C., Bruneau, P., Blondel, B., Crainic, R., Horodniceanu, F. and Girard, M. (1983). Localization of a poliovirus type 1 neutralization epitope in viral capsid polypeptide VP1. *Proc. Natl. Acad. Sci. USA*, **80**, 5080–4
18. Minor, P. D., Ferguson, M., Evans, D. M. A, Almond, J. W. and Icenogle, J. P. (1986). Antigenic structure of polioviruses of serotypes 1, 2 and 3. *J. Gen. Virol.*, **67**, 1283-91
19. Icenogle, J. P., Minor, P. D., Ferguson, M. and Hogle, J. M. (1986). Modulation of humoral response to a 12-amino-acid site on the poliovirus virion. *J. Virol.*, **60**, 297–301
20. Sabin, A. B. and Boulger, L. R. (1973). History of Sabin attenuated poliovirus oral live vaccine strains. *J. Biol. Stand.*, **1**, 115–18
21. Cann, A. J., Stanway, G., Hughes, P. J., Minor, P. D., Evans, D. M. A., Schild, G. C. and Almond, J. W. (1984). Reversion to neurovirulence of the live-attenuated Sabin type 3 oral poliovirus vaccine. *Nucl. Acids Res.*, **12**, 7787–92
22. Westrop, G. D., Wareham, K. A., Evans, D. M. A., Dunn, G., Minor, P. D., Magrath, D. I., Taffs, F., Marsden, S., Skinner, M. A., Schild, G. C. and Almond, J. W. (1989). Genetic basis of attenuation of the Sabin type 3 oral polio vaccine. *J. Virol.* (In press)
23. Evans, D. M. A., Dunn, G., Minor, P. D., Schild, G. C., Cann, A. J., Stanway, G., Almond, J. W., Currey, K. and Maizel, J. V. Jr. (1985). Increased neurovirulence associated with a single nucelotide change in a non-coding region of the Sabin type 3 poliovaccine genome. *Nature*, **314**, 548–50
24. Almond, J. W., Westrop. G. D., Cann, A. J., Stanway, G., Evans, D. M. A., Minor, P. D. and Schild, G. C. (1985). Attenuation and reversion to neurovirulence of the Sabin poliovirus type 3 vaccine. In Lerner, R. A., Chanock, R. M. and Brown, F. (eds), *Vaccines* 85, pp. 271–83. (Cold Spring Harbor Laboratory)
25. La Monica, N., Almond, J. W. and Racaniello, V. R. (1987). A mouse model for poliovirus neurovirulence identifies mutations that attenuate the virus for man. *J. Virol.*, **61**, 2917–20
26. Omata, T., Kohara, M., Kuge, S., Komatsu, T., Abe, S., Semler, B. L., Kameda, A., Itoh, H., Arita, M., Wimmer, E. and Nomoto, A. (1986). Genetic analysis of the attenuation phenotype of poliovirus type 1. *J. Virol.*, **58**, 348–58
27. Nomoto, A., Omata, T., Toyoda, H., Kuge, S., Horie, H., Kataoka, Y., Genba, Y., Nakano, Y. and Imura, N. (1982). Complete nucleotide sequence of the attenuated poliovirus Sabin 1 strain genome. *Proc. Natl. Acad. Sci. USA*, **79**, 5793–7
28. Nomoto, A., Kohara, M., Kuge, S., Abe, S., Semler, B. L., Komatsu, T., Arita, M. and Itoh, H. (1988). The development of new poliovirus vaccines based on molecular cloning. In Kurstak, E., Marusyk, R. G., Murphy, F. A. and Van Regenmortel, M. H. V. (eds), *Applied Virology Research*, Vol. I: *New Vaccines and Chemotherapy*, pp. 43–62. (New York, London: Plenum)
29. Minor, P. D. and Dunn, G. (1988). The effect of sequences in the 5′ non-coding region on the replication of polioviruses in the human gut. *J. Gen. Virol.*, **69**, 1091–6
30. Skinner, M. A., Racaniello, V. R., Dunn, G., Cooper, J., Minor, P. D. and Almond, J. W. (1989). A new model for the secondary structure of the 5′ non-coding RNA of poliovirus is supported by biochemical and genetical data which also show that RNA secondary structure is important in neurovirulence. *J. Mol. Biol.* (In press)
31. Burke, K. L., Dunn, G., Ferguson, M., Minor, P. D. and Almond, J. W. (1988). Antigen chimaeras of poliovirus as potential new vaccines. *Nature*, **332**, 81–2

8
Rabies vaccines

K. G. NICHOLSON

INTRODUCTION

Rabies is an acute infectious encephalomyelitis caused by a *Lyssavirus*, a bullet-shaped virus belonging to the *Rhabdovirus* family. The disease is uniformly fatal in man once symptoms and signs develop. Nevertheless its 'disease burden value' is low in comparison with other infectious diseases, so rabies is not generally considered a priority for vaccine development or delivery. The true extent of human rabies is unknown but as many as 100 000 deaths are believed to occur annually. Rabies is prevalent throughout most of the world and many millions of doses of vaccine are given each year following genuine or possible exposures to the virus. Comparatively little is given for pre-exposure prophylaxis.

RABIES – TRANSMISSION TO MAN

By far the most common mode of infection in man is by the bite of a rabid animal or the contamination of scratch wounds by virus-laden saliva. Intact skin appears impenetrable to the virus, but infection across undamaged mucous membranes of the mouth, conjunctiva, anus and genitalia, either directly from rabid animals[1–4], or indirectly through licking contaminated cord or material[1] are feasible. Infection by aerosol transmission has also been amply demonstrated in laboratory animals[5–8] and has been implicated in human infection acquired in bat-infested caverns in Texas and in several laboratory accidents[9–12]. Human-to-human transmission by transplantation of infected corneas has been reported in five instances with the diagnosis in the donors only being made retrospectively[13–16]. Occasional cases of human-to-human transmission are described in the older literature, and in a large Indian survey 1 of 11 134 contacts of human cases developed the disease[17]. Judging by the absence of reports of cases in nursing and medical staff, however, human-to-human transmission seems to be an extremely rare event. Nonetheless, close medical attendants are at genuine risk of being bitten or contaminated by saliva[18–22], especially when it is in aerosol form, e.g. in patients undergoing respiratory care, and should be considered for post-exposure therapy.

Initiation of treatment in severely exposed persons should never await the results of laboratory diagnosis. Specific guidelines for the treatment of persons following bites by suspect or confirmed rabid domestic or wild animals, or animals unavailable for observation, or laboratory testing, follow in a later section.

EPIDEMIOLOGY OF RABIES IN ANIMALS

Apart from the nature of the exposure, the decision to initiate rabies post-exposure treatment should take into account the distribution of the disease and the known species involvement. Rabies is distributed in all continents except Australasia and Antarctica among a variety of warm-blooded animals, primarily the Canidae and Chiroptera. Most other disease-free areas are islands or less commonly peninsular land masses where stringent quarantine regulations can be rigidly enforced. All warm-blooded animals are susceptible to the virus, including birds, though these are rarely if ever infected in nature. The disease exists in two epidemiological forms; urban rabies which is propagated chiefly in feral and domestic dogs and is prevalent in many developing countries of the world; and sylvatic rabies which occurs in a wide range of species, principally small carnivores and Mustelids.

According to the 1981 WHO survey[23] and figures from the United States[24] rabies is most prevalent among wild canids (foxes, wolves, and jackals; 35.5% of 38 089 cases), followed by dogs (33.8%), skunks (11.8%), farm animals (7%), cats (3.8%), bats (2.3%), mongooses (0.3%), and other species (5.5%). Extensive surveys show rodent rabies to be extremely uncommon[25-31]. Rabies is unusual among lagomorphs (i.e. rabbits and hares) and insectivores (i.e. shrews, moles, and hedgehogs), though Mustelids (i.e. skunks, weasels, badgers and martens) and the Viverridae (i.e. mongoose, suricate, ferret, genet, civet cat and polecat) are regularly found infected[23,26,27,29,32].

Non-human primates are occasionally infected, and isolated cases have been reported throughout Africa, South America, and parts of Asia[33,34]. Among the wild felidae, sporadic cases have been identified in lions, hyaenas, leopards, cheetahs, lynxes, tigers, and ocelots[33]. Rabies among wild ungulates is regularly identified in central European deer[27,31,34,35], and is recorded in camels in North Africa and the Near and Middle East[33,36]; kudu and eland antelopes in South-West Africa[37]; and occasionally in buffalo and moose in North America[32].

The Chiroptera are of major importance as reservoirs and transmitters of infection in the Americas. In Latin America bites by haematophagous vampire bats cause losses of more than 100 000 cattle each year[38], and in the United States bats represent the most most widely distributed vector. In Europe and Asia, bat rabies has been reported but generally seems rare[39-42].

EPIDEMIOLOGY OF HUMAN RABIES; AND RABIES POST-EXPOSURE TREATMENT

Official reporting of rabies in man is grossly deficient in many lesser-developed countries and the true extent of the disease in man is largely unknown. In India, a survey of teaching hospitals showed an incidence of one case of human rabies per 2000 admissions, and in certain areas the incidence was four times higher[43]. Thus from estimates of the total population and the numbers hospitalized, it is suggested that at least 17 000 deaths occur in India each year. Still higher figures might be expected, since many cases never reach hospital. In addition, many cases undoubtedly go unnoticed, either through lack of appropriate diagnostic facilities or because cases are not suspected to occur. Sanmartin *et al.*[44] discovered that 27 of the 1596 people (1.7%) on whom post-mortems were carried out in Cali, Colombia, in 1962 had died of rabies, although only one or two cases had been diagnosed annually in years past. Similary, 21% of all cases in the United States between 1960 and 1979 were not diagnosed until after death, and may have gone undiagnosed if post-mortem pathological or virological studies had not been undertaken.[45].

Apart form the Indian subcontinent and South-east Asia, hydrophobia is prevalent throughout much of Africa, South and Central America, and Mexico[34,46–50]. Few tropical countries have rabies under control, and the risk of exposure in most developing countries is still formidable. Indeed, a study of missionaries and foreign aid personnel working in the Third World showed that the overall risk, based on a mean stay of 4–5 years, was 16% per household[51]. More extensive analyses in 30 tropical countries show the incidence of rabies to be 0.1–28.8 cases per million population (mean, 3.7), and the number of treatments to be 2.7–4570 (mean, 867) per million population[52]. Dog bites are responsible for the majority of human cases and for virtually all post-exposure rabies vaccinations.

RABIES VIRUS STRUCTURE

Members of the *Lyssavirus* genus contain a common cross-reacting N protein[53] which can be detected by standard fluorescent antibody, complement fixation, and precipitation techniques[54]. They are distinguished by virus-neutralization and cross-protection tests, indicating that their surface glycoproteins are different[55]. The application of monoclonal antibody technology to the study of antigenic relationships among rhabdoviruses[56] has confirmed the distinction between rabies and rabies-related viruses, and has revealed extensive antigenic variation in both glycoprotein and nucleocapsid proteins of a number of laboratory and street strains[57–60]. Analysis of several hundred isolates from animals and man in different parts of the world has revealed both geographic and species patterns of reactivity[59–61]. Similarly, live virus strains used for the immunization of animals can be distinguished from wild-type viruses. When the antigenic make-up of a large number of field isolates was compared with that of the PM-HDCS vaccine strain, the proportion of common antigenic determinants ranged from 44 to 100%[62]. The relevance of these observations to recommendations concerning vaccine strains for vaccine and antiserum production has yet to be established, although preliminary investigations provide no indication that antigenic differences account for vaccination failures.

ASSESSING IMMUNITY TO RABIES

For more than 40 years the mouse neutralization test (MNT) devised by Webster and Dawson[63], has been invaluable in assessing humoral response to rabies vaccines and in establishing optimum regimens for pre- and post-exposure prophylaxis. The test has provided a useful diagnostic tool and remains an important method of assessing vaccines, although it suffers from a number of disadvantages, primarily the requirement for large numbers of young adult mice and the facilities necessary to contain them. The test also suffers with an inherent variability which makes it difficult to correlate results between laboratories, even when standard antiserum is included in each test[64,65].

To overcome these problems a number of attempts have been made in recent years to develop an *in vitro* assay for virus neutralizing antibody. A cytopathic effect with rabies virus, although reported by some authors[66–73] has not been sufficiently reliable to permit routine tissue culture neutralization tests such as inhibition of cytopathic effect or plaque-inhibition. However, the introduction of immunofluorescent staining techniques led to the rapid fluorescent focus inhibition test (RFFIT) which requires only 24 h for completion[74] and correlates well with the MNT[74–76].

More recently the enzyme-linked immunosorbent assay (ELISA) has been introduced as a possible alternative to neutralization tests for rabies[77–79]. Investigations reported by Wiktor *et al.*[80] indicate that antibodies specific for the virus surface glycoprotein are responsible for neutralisation. The whole-virus particles with intact glycoprotein used in most ELISAs should measure neutralizing antibody mostly, and indeed the close agreement found initially between the MNT and ELISA supported this supposition. However, recent unpublished data indicate that the ELISA measures antibodies other than those directed against the glycoprotein, and that such antibodies are present at high titre following the successful post-exposure use of neurotissue vaccine (NTV). Interestingly, there is recent evidence that an immune response to the ribonucleoprotein is important in protection[81], hence the ELISA may be a better guide of protection than has hitherto been considered. This view is strengthened by the ability of ELISA to detect antibodies of the IgG class. It is well known that IgM antibody is the initial humoral response to infection or immunization, and that in infections with viraemia IgM is especially important. However, neither passively transferred nor actively induced IgM neutralizing antibody protects mice infected experimentally[82]. Thus IgG antirabies antibody detected by ELISA may be of greater importance than the early antibody response to infection or immunization measured by neutralization tests.

Historically virus neutralizing antibody has been considered to be the key to successful rabies prophylaxis, both before and after virus exposure[83-87], and inadequate antibody responses to neurovaccine and duck embryo vaccine have generally been held responsible for occasional treatment failures.

Nilsson *et al.*[88] challenged immunized mice, selected genetically for 'high' and 'low' antibody responses, and found that 'high' responders were the more resistant to rabies. The possible involvement of other immune systems was not excluded and intracerebral challenge with a fixed strain of rabies virus hardly simulates natural infection. However, review of the older literature, in which pre-exposure immunization of various animal species was followed by peripheral challenge with street rabies virus, reveals a 96% reduction in mortality when antibody was present at the time of challenge. In the absence of antibody, survival was 57.5% if a humoral response had been demonstrated previously and 23.6% if it had not. Hence the presence of actively induced antibody seemed definitely to be associated with protection to vaccine given before infection. Inspection of the antibody titres of the 14 animals that died revealed a range of 1 in 2 to 1 in 1750 (GMT 1 in 18), implying that even substantial titres of antibody cannot always guarantee protection. Recent studies in pre-immunized dogs and cats show a relation between the titre of neutralizing antibody and protection against rabies virus challenge: a neutralizing antibody titre of approximately 0.5 IU/ml at the time of challenge is necessary for uniform protection[89,90].

The association between antibody and protection is much less clear for treatment given post-exposure. In several studies in monkeys in which challenge with street virus was followed by a single injection of potent rabies vaccine of tissue culture origin, animals succumbing to infection showed high titred antibody responses comparable in height and time of appearance to those of survivors[89,91-93]. Habel and Koprowski[85] and Chowdhuri *et al.*[94] also showed that the antibody profiles of patients dying after NTV treatment were equivalent to those of survivors. In addition, many workers have found that passively administered antibody may prolong survival but has little influence on mortality[91,95-97]. It must be assumed that interferon induction and cellular immunity have key roles in post-exposure protection.

PASTEUR AND ANTIRABIES VACCINATION

The prolonged incubation period of rabies, the terrifying course of the disease in man and its unavoidable fatal outcome must have been foremost in Pasteur's mind when he selected rabies for vaccine development. In 1881 Pasteur declared: 'the central nervous system and especially the bulb joining the spinal cord to the brain are particularly concerned and active in the development of the disease'[98]. He then announced that his group had successfully transmitted rabies by inoculating brain with infected nervous tissue, and that the incubation period was shortened accordingly. In 1885, after promising attempts at virus attenuation by intracerebral passage in monkeys[99], Pasteur described a new method of attenuation and its application to the first human post-exposure treatment[100].

By repeatedly passaging a bovine isolate through rabbits by intracerebral inoculation, Pasteur obtained a virus characterized by a shortened incubation period of 6–7 days and stereotyped clinical illness. He called this 'fixed' virus, in contrast to natural infection caused by 'street' virus. His method of attenuation consisted of desiccating infected rabbit cords for periods of up to 2 weeks. Dogs that were inoculated with extensively desiccated cord followed by injections of progressively less desiccated material resisted intracerebral challenge with virulent virus. More importantly, experiments made on dogs treated after rabid animal bites gave promising results[100].

Accordingly Pasteur felt justified in treating Josef Meister, a 9-year-old boy from Alsace, who was bitten at 14 sites on the hands, legs and thighs by a rabid dog. The worst of the wounds were cauterized and on the evening of 6 July, after the attack, the boy was inoculated with material desiccated for 15 days. Over the next 10 days he received a further 12 injections of increasingly less desiccated cord, ending with fully virulent virus. The boy survived without ill-effects and in October 1885 a second patient was treated. Pasteur's vaccine became widely available in Paris, and by November 1886, 2490 people had been treated. Sadly more than a century later the vast majority of antirabies post-exposure treatments are still with vaccines that differ little from Pasteur's original product.

NEUROTISSUE VACCINE PREPARED FROM ADULT BRAIN

With the increasing demand for Pasteur's treatment it soon became evident that difficulties in maintaining large numbers of freshly infected cords would restrict its application. The problem was resolved by the introduction of glycerol as a vaccine preservative[101,102]. Other modifications were soon advocated. Höyges[103] reduced virulence by diluting infected rabbit cords 1 in 10 to 1 in 5000 in NaCl; heat inactivation was introduced by Puscariu and Vesesco[104] (at temperatures of 30–80 °C for 10 min) and Babes[105] (exposure at 50 °C for different times) to overcome the vagaries of desiccation; and Fermi[106] first used a chemical method, 1% phenol, to attenuate the virus. Fermi's method differed from those previously used in so far as there was no gradation of virulence of successive doses; this greatly simplified the manufacturing process and the method became widely accepted. Concern about the danger of inoculating residual live virus led Semple[107] to modify the phenol treatment so as to render the vaccine completely non-infectious but still to retain its immunizing capacity. Semple's method became well established, and although other methods of inactivation were introduced; namely – ether[108,109], chloroform[110], ether and phenol[111], formalin[112], and ultraviolet light[113], they never became so universally accepted.

Today the infected brain tissue of adult rabbits, sheep and goats remains the principal source of virus for vaccine production in many parts of the world, and Semple vaccine is the most widely used. There have been several minor modifications in its preparation; complete inactivation of the virus is usually achieved with phenol at a concentration of 0.5–1%, at temperatures between 20 and 30 °C for 48–72 h[114]. Due to poor antigenicity, courses consist of up to 24 5-ml injections of a 5 or 10% brain suspension, equivalent to 6–12 g of brain tissue.

NTV usage has long been associated with an unacceptably high incidence of post-vaccine reactions including inflammation, malaise, and paralysis[115]. Localized redness, swelling and pruritus commonly occur[116]; they often appear within several hours of vaccination, reach their maximum within 6–8 h, and are usually gone by the following day. Delayed tuberculin-type reactions are less common; they are often associated with malaise, headache, low-grade fever, lymphadenopathy, urticaria and nausea, and may herald the development of paralysis[117,118]. At first the neurological reactions were considered to be due to the street virus, or to its modification during the course of treatment[117]. This view was challenged by Tonin in 1902, who reported a case of post-vaccine paralysis with the animal suspected of being rabid remaining healthy[117]. Subsequently a number of cases of 'rage de laboratoire' were described in which fixed rabies virus could be recovered from the brains of vaccinees[118–120]. In 1908, Marinesco[121] first suggested that the brain tissue component of the vaccine might itself exert a toxic effect, but only when immune adjuvants became available and brain tissue was tested did animal experiments establish the encephalitogenic nature of uninfected brain[122–125].

Remlinger, at the first international conference on rabies in Paris in 1927, reported 329 neurological reactions among 1 164 264 persons treated (1 per 3539 treatments), but considered this to be an underestimate and suggested a figure of 1 episode per 500–1000 treatments[118]. Greenwood[17] reported 222 cases among 1 290 758 treatments (1 per 5814 treatments). Analysis of 22 smaller series indicates the overall incidence of neurological reactions to be 1 in 1180 treatments, a quarter of which terminate fatally. The risk of developing neural complications is notably higher for persons with a history of allergy[117] or previous rabies treatment[126]. Other factors affecting the incidence include the type of vaccine used[17], its neural tissue content[127], the total number of injections given[128], and the presence of phenol-killed bacterial contamination, which behaves as an adjuvant[129]. Also children and teenagers are a lower risk than older persons[118,130,131].

Five forms of neurological complication are described, namely: peripheral neuritis, transverse myelitis, acute ascending paralysis, encephalitis, and 'rage de laboratoire'[117,118,132,133]. Of these dorsolumbar myelitis is the most common[118]. They usually develop 8–21 days after the first injection[117,118,126–128,134–136], but may appear several weeks after the last[118,137]. About 15% of vaccinees develop EEG abnormalities during treatment[138], and more than 50% produce antibodies against brain[139,140].

The animal model for post-vaccine encephalomyelitis provided a method of characterizing the encephalitogenic factor and of studying its pathogenesis. Skin testing of animals with post-vaccine encephalomyelitis suggested that a cell-mediated response might be important[141,142]. This view was supported by passively transferring lymphoid cells from sensitized animals, which reproduced the condition[143,144]. By contrast there was no correlation between the disease process and antibody to brain[144]. The sensitizing factor appeared to be associated with myelin, since it was absent from the unmyelinated neural tissue of newborn mammals, frog, or fish brain[124]. This led to the treatment of vaccine preparations with aromatic hydrocarbons[145], low-speed centrifugation[146,147], ECTEOLA-cellulose chromatography[148], and fluorocarbon[149] in attempts to remove the factor. All were claimed to be successful, but none has been used routinely in vaccine manufacture.

Contrary to expectation, the literature contains only meagre evidence that NTVs actually protect laboratory animals. In 1939, Webster[150] published a critical review of all published work performed under relatively controlled conditions. He concluded, on the basis of the small number of animals employed per test, that Pasteur's data on post-exposure immunization of dogs were unsuitable for analysis. Only one set of data showed significant post-exposure protection, but this was only achieved providing at least 25% of the animals' body weight in vaccine was given in divided doses[106]. The results of later experimental work were similarly considered unimpressive[151].

The influence of prophylactic treatment in preventing rabies has been estimated by comparing the mortality in treated and untreated groups of persons bitten by animals causing the death from hydrophobia of one or more subjects or animals. Semple[152] quotes the outcome following bites by two infective dogs. Of 18 persons bitten, nine received treatment and remained well, whereas seven of the nine who were untreated died from rabies. According to Veeraraghavan and Subrahmanyan[153], the mortality from rabies among the completely treated is 6.5% rising to 20% among the incompletely treated, and 42.1% among the untreated. Thus Semple vaccine apparently saves approximately 84% of those who would otherwise develop rabies and die. Kitamoto *et al.*[154] followed up 460 people who had been bitten by proven rabid animals and treated with ultraviolet ray-inactivated vaccine. Altogether 4.4% died, but the mortality rose to 10.8% following bites to the head.

Another method of assessment is to take instances in which a *presumably rabid animal* has bitten several persons of whom some accept treatment and others refuse. Cornwall[155] estimated the mortality among the treated and untreated to be 2.9% and 6.2%, respectively. Yu[156] similarly reports mortalities of 4.5% and 10.0%, suggesting that only one out of every two persons is spared by brain tissue vaccine. A number of reports stress, however, that the mortality after severe bites by 'infective' or rabid wild animals is virtually as high as in individuals who receive no treatment[157-161]. It may be concluded that although adult NTV is of value in protecting against minor exposures, it is less effective following head bites, and there is no evidence that it is effective following particularly severe exposures.

NEUROTISSUE VACCINES PREPARED FROM IMMATURE BRAIN

The rapid multiplication of fixed rabies virus to high titres in the brains of immature animals, and the relative absence of myelin from their neural tissue, have been exploited in the preparation of potent vaccines from suckling mouse[162] suckling rat[129] and suckling rabbit brains[163]. All three vaccines had successful preliminary clinical trials[129,164,165]. No cases of post-vaccine encephalitis were recorded among 16943 persons treated with suckling mouse brain (SMB) vaccine in Chile[166] or among 9500 subjects given suckling rat brain vaccine in Russia[129], and no-one died from rabies. SMB vaccine inactivated by ultraviolet light, β-propiolactone, or phenol is now the most extensively used treatment in Latin America.

Although originally considered to be free from the encephalitogenic factor, there have been a number of reports of paralytic reactions associated with its use[137,167–169,384], even after a reduced schedule of immunization[170]. In contrast to the neurological disease developing after the use of other types of NTV, the majority of cases develop the Guillain–Barré syndrome. Held and Adaros[167] collected details of 32 cases from eight countries, and estimated the complication rate to be 1 case per 7865 persons treated. A further 21 cases were reported by Toro *et al.*[168], who estimated the complication rate to be 1 in 4615 treatments with a 52% mortality. Thus, from the available data, suckling mouse brain vaccine appears to be only marginally safer than vaccines derived from adult neural tissue. Moreover, the extremely large number of animals required for its manufacture increases both the problem of harvesting the brains aseptically and the risk of contamination by endogenous viruses[114]. Attempts were made to purify SMB vaccine by centrifugation and chromatography[171,172], but events in the field of tissue culture vaccine have overshadowed these developments.

AVAIN TISSUE VACCINES

Avian tissue vaccines evolved from attempts to avoid neural tissue substrates completely. Two, the Flury low egg passage (LEP) and Flury high egg passage (HEP) vaccines, were prepared in chick embryos and used as live virus vaccines. The Flury strain of rabies virus was originally isolated from a girl of that name[4,173]. It was 'fixed' by serial passage in day-old chicks and then adapted to the developing chick embryo[174]. At the low egg passage level (40–50 passages) the virus was innocuous for most mammals when injected parenterally[96,173,175]. At high egg passage level (~180 passages), it became apathogenic for adult mice, rabbits and dogs when given intracerebrally, but remained lethal for suckling mice and rhesus monkeys[176]. Flury HEP vaccine was given extensive trials in man[177–184], but with disappointing results. Many grams of infected embryo material were necessary to elicit a humoral response, and anaphylaxis and suppuration at the injection site were unacceptable complications[177,178,180]. The use of this material was based upon the belief that it underwent limited replication in non-neural tissue in the recipient. Schwab *et al.*[177] and Sharpless *et al.*[180] found no evidence to support this hypothesis, so the vaccine had no advantage over inactivated material containing the same quantity of antigen. Moreover the attenuated state was lost upon further passage[176], making this live vaccine potentially far more dangerous. Accordingly, the WHO Expert Committee on Rabies, in its 5th Report, recommended that the use of Flury vaccines be restricted to animals[185].

The successful adaptation to growth of fixed strains of rabies virus in embryonated duck eggs[186] permitted the development of an attenuated vaccine for human use[187] from tissue possessing little or no encephalitogenic activity[188]. The vaccine was subsequently inactivated with β-propiolactone which had been found to yield vaccine of greater antigenicity than formalin or phenol[189,190]. According to Greenberg and Childress[191], duck embryo vaccine (DEV) evoked humoral responses in humans more rapidly than Semple vaccine; seroconversion occurred in about 90% of subjects with either vaccine, but the titres were subsequently greater with Semple vaccine. In contrast to Semple vaccine, DEV produced no EEG abnormalities in humans[138].

DEV became commercially available during the late 1950s and early 1960s, and until recently it was used to treat approximately 30 000 people annually in the USA, although its efficacy has never been established by clinical trial. Some data suggest that it conferred no greater immunity than NTVs – between 1957 and 1967, when both DEV and NTV were available in the USA, there were 6 deaths among 117 700 treated with NTV, and 7 deaths among 172 000 treated with DEV[192]. There have been conflicting reports on the ability of DEV to evoke antibody responses, some investigators noting good seroconversion[193,194], others finding the vaccine to be poorly antigenic, particularly when given with passive immunization[195–197,385]. Multiple inoculations were necessary to ensure adequate responses, but in other animals and humans receiving repeated daily injections, transition to IgG synthesis is delayed and the IgM response prolonged[82,198,199]. In rabies, where neural rather than viraemic spread is important, IgM is of questionable value since it is largely restricted to the intact cirulation[200,201]. By contrast IgG antibodies enter the tissues and, unlike IgM, they afford protection to laboratory animals infected with rabies[82].

Because of DEV's apparent freedom from serious adverse effects it has been widely recommended for pre-exposure use. The results have generally been disappointing. Even after three of four doses seroconversion was rarely found in more than 80% of vaccinees and the titres are generally low[182,184,202–208]. Comparison of the potency of DEV and NTV consistently showed the avian vaccine to be inferior despite having an equivalent protein content[209]. The concentration of DEV was subsequently increased by 40%[68], but this had no appreciable effect[171] except on adverse local and systemic reactions which occurred in 67% of subjects during pre-exposure prophylaxis and in up to 100% during post-exposure treatment[210]. The spectrum of reactions included anaphylaxis, occuring in 0.5–0.9% of vaccinees, and neurological accidents occurring with an estimated incidence of 1 in 32 600 and fatality rate of 1 in 210 000[210–216] Schlenska[217] reported two cases of neuroparalytic reactions among an estimated 6000–8000 vaccinees. According to Schell *et al.*[218], there have been only six neurological reactions among the persons who received the more than 6.5 million doses of DEV produced in Switzerland. Nonetheless, concern regarding both the antigenicity and safety of DEV prompted the same authors to purify and concentrate their product.

The new purified duck embryo vaccine (PDEV) consists of a suspension of β-propiolactone-inactivated rabies virus prepared by density gradient ultra-centrifugation. It is of high potency and purity, containing only about 1% of the protein of previous DEV, and is comparable to the new tissue culture vaccines[219]. Potency testing of consecutive batches has consistently shown antigenic values in excess of 5 IU/ml, and in a preliminary clinical study PDEV and human diploid cell strain rabies vaccine (HDCSV) were equally antigenic in man. Mild local reactions occur only slightly more frequently than with HDCSV. Subsequent studies[220] have confirmed the early findings and have established the immunogenicity and safety of PDEV.

TISSUE CULTURE VACCINES

Until recently licensing authorities would consider only primary cultures of embryonic tissue or strains of diploid cells of human origin as being suitable for the preparation of tissue culture vaccines for use in man.

Primary cell culture vaccines

The adaptation to growth of rabies virus to hamster kidney cells[221] permitted the development of experimental rabies vaccines prepared using primary hamster kidney cells as the substrate[68,222–224]; most batches were of adequate potency and several that were studied contained 20- to 25-fold less protein than NTV or DEV. Nonetheless, low virus yields, slow growth, and the risk of anaphylaxis to serum present in the culture medium made this approach to vaccination seem impracticable. Fenje and Pinteric[225] overcame these difficulties by using a chemically defined medium, by concentrating the virus by ultracentrifugation, and using aluminium adjuvants. Their vaccine was given clinical trials in 1966 and was licensed in Canada in 1968 for pre-exposure prophylaxis[226]. There are few published reports concerning its use. According to Cho *et al.*[227] and Fenje[226], approximately 15 000 doses were distributed annually with most subjects responding to a three-dose schedule of immunization. However, doubts were expressed about this vaccine when low or absent titres were found in almost 70% of veterinarians vaccinated during the previous 6 years[228].

In Russia an ultraviolet light-inactivated vaccine was prepared from primary hamster kidney cells infected with the Vnukovo-32 strain of rabies virus[229]. By 1978 almost 60 000 persons had received up to 125 ml of the vaccine for post-exposure prophylaxis. No neuroparalytic reactions were observed, and only two cases of rabies developed among those treated[230,231]. The Russian vaccine is now used widely in Eastern bloc countries and by spring 1988, 17 human cases of rabies were believed to have developed after post-exposure treatment with the Soviet vaccine. Details of these 17 cases are unavailable, but it is understood that most, if not all, of these cases were associated with delayed or inadequate therapy, and should not be regarded as true treatment failures.

In China, Semple NTV was partially substituted by a primary hamster kidney cell rabies vaccine (PHKCRV) in 1980 and was replaced completely in 1981[232]. Post-exposure use of PHKCRV was evaluated in 301 individuals, 97 of whom had been bitten by proven rabid animals. None of the patients contracted rabies in 7 months to 3 years after exposure[233]. However, four deaths were described in later report following wounds by a rabid wolf to the head (three cases) and the forearm (one case); none received antirabies serum and treated with PHKCRV was either delayed or incomplete[232].

Primary chick embryo cells have been used to prepare live adjuvant HEP Flury virus vaccine[183] and HEP[234] and LEP[235] vaccines inactivated with β-propiolactone. All three products are immunogenic and the inactivated vaccines have been given post-exposure trials in man[236,237]. The purified chick embryo cell rabies vaccine (PCECV) developed in Germany by Behringwerke has been shown to be clinically acceptable and to generate high titred antibody responses comparable to those evoked by human diploid cell strain rabies vaccine[235,238,239]. More importantly, results of preliminary studies of post-exposure use in 115 patients[240,241] have shown the vaccine to be highly immunogenic. It is now licensed for post-exposure use, and is used extensively in Europe, the Indian subcontinent, and Thailand.

Vaccines have similarly been prepared on primary cultures of duck embryo cells[242,243] fetal bovine kidney cells[244,245], canine kidney cells[246], and quail embryo cells[247]. Primary bovine kidney cell rabies vaccine (FBKCV), produced by Institut Pasteur Production, Paris, using the PV/RV-31 Pasteur strain of rabies virus, is licensed for post-exposure treatment in France, and by 1984 a total of 3000 doses had been administered for both pre- and post-exposure use[248]. A number of reports attest FBKCV and HDCSV to be comparable with regard to tolerance and antigenicity, and FBKCV has been used successfully for the post-exposure treatment of 153 rabies-exposed persons[249].

Continuous cell culture vaccines

Vaccines derived from human cell substrates

From the early 1970s to the mid-1980s most attention focused on the vaccine developed at the Wistar Institute in WI-38 human diploid cells[70,250]. The cells, which were isolated from human embryonic lung[251], have been extensively tested and used for vaccines against polio[252], rubella[252], cytomegalovirus[253], and varicella[254]. The virus used was the Pitman Moore 1503-3M strain of fixed rabies virus derived from a strain originally isolated by Pasteur and maintained by the National Institute of Health, Bethesda, Md, USA[255]. In 1962–63 the virus was adapted to growth in WI-38 cells and was propagated in WI-38 cells for 52 passages. Subsequently a master seed pool was prepared in 1965, and the seed virus was transferred to l'Institut Merieux, a vaccine-producing laboratory, in 1966. The seed strain was distributed to two further vaccine manufacturers, Behringwerke and Wyeth, in 1969 and 1971, respectively. The Wyeth product was a subunit vaccine inactivated with tri(*n*-butyl)-phosphate. In contrast the vaccines produced by l'Institut Merieux and Behringwerke are both whole-virion preparations grown in MRC-5 human diploid lung fibroblasts and inactivated with β-propiolactone. The early batches of the Merieux vaccine, however, were prepared on WI-38 cells. The current European products differ only in so far as the Behringwerke vaccine is concentrated and purified by rate zonal untracentrifugation[269], whereas the Merieux product is concentrated by ultrafiltration. The American (Wyeth) vaccine was never produced commercially due to manufacturing and potency problems.

Early experimental batches of β-propiolactone-inactivated[189] HDCSV were immunogenic in mice[70] and monkeys[91,250], but because the virus yields from WI-38 cells are relatively poor[256] it was necessary to concentrate the cell supernatants to obtain vaccine of high potency. Using either ultrafiltration through nitrocellulose membrane; continuous zonal centrifugation; or zinc acetate precipitation, desalting on a Sephadex column, and concentration by high-speed centrifugation, it was possible to concentrate the virions present in the tissue culture fluids 100–200-fold and to increase purity to a considerable degree[257–260]. The Wistar group, in collaboration with CDC, Atlanta, then gave a single dose of concentrated HDCSV to monkeys that had previously been inoculated with street rabies virus[91,92]. These investigators found that the new vaccine gave greater protection than 14 daily doses of DEV or a massive dose of homologous antirabies serum, and soon afterwards the first human trials were performed on members of the Wistar Institute[261].

The first human trial of HDCSV was reported in Lyon in 1972[262,263]. Eight subjects who had received a rabies vaccination previously developed an anamnestic response after a single dose of the Wyeth split-product HDCSV; the new vaccine was given intradermally to seven and intramuscularly to one subject. Intramuscular vaccination of eight other individuals who had not previously received rabies vaccine evoked an antibody response in five persons after the first dose, and substantial antibody titres in seven after the second.

During the next few years the clinical trials with HDCSV were directed towards establishing optimal regimens for pre- and post-exposure immunization and freedom from troublesome reactions. When volunteers were immunized with a 1 ml dose of whole virion HDCSV (HDCSV-WV) produced by l'Institut Merieux, Bahmanyar[264] found that antibodies were not detectable on day 7, but on days 21 and 35 the titres were similar to those of persons given seven or twelve daily doses of phenolized brain tissue vaccine. The highest levels were seen in groups given four doses of vaccine on days 0, 1, 2, 3, or 0, 3, 7 and 21, the latter schedule, however, produced the highest levels and a more prolonged response. Nonetheless, administration of 50 IU/kg of mule antirabies serum on day 0 markedly suppressed the antibody response of subjects receiving HDCSV-WV on days 0, 3, 7 and 21.

In 1976, trials in Germany and Iran showed HDCSV, together with serum or HRIG, to afford complete protection to persons bitten by known rabid animals[265,266]. The vaccination schedule consisted of six doses of 1 ml given on days 0, 3, 7, 14, 28 and 90; this regimen is now officially recommended by WHO, though in some countries, notably in the USA, the day 90 dose has been dropped.

Reactions to HDCSV

In contrast to the high incidence of neuroparalytic reactions to NTVs the rate of neurological side-effects with HDCSV is extremely low. In a large study of reaction rates conducted in Britain between 1976 and 1983, and covering more than 40000 doses for both pre- and post-exposure immunization[267], two neurological reactions were observed: one was transient in a person who experienced paresthesiae and weakness of the right arm after the fourth dose of a post-exposure course; the second had pain and weakness of the right arm with muscle wasting after a routine booster dose. Two other cases have been reported. Boe and Nyland[268] describe one case of Guillain–Barré syndrome (GBS) in a 15-year-old boy who received two i.d. doses of Merieux vaccine 30 days apart and who developed GBS 50 days after the first injection. Bernard *et al.*[269] reported an 11-year-old boy with transient muscular leg weakness. Even if all four cases are accepted as being due to vaccination by HDCSV, the neuro-complication rate would be only $\leq 1:250000$, similar to the values of most safe vaccines such as oral poliomyelitis, yellow fever, and tetanus toxoid.

In general HDCSV is extremely well tolerated. In the MRC studies local erythema and induration were noted after approximately 50% and 20%, respectively, of intradermal injections, and were transient and clinically insignificant[270–272]. Erythema and induration were recorded after less than 5% of i.m. injections, but local pain was noted after 16% compared with only 3% for i.d. injections. Generalized reactions such as malaise, headache, fever, and lymphadenopathy were reported infrequently after either route of injection, and with the exception of headache, which occurred in 6% of subjects after i.m. and s.c. injections, there was no consistent relationship between generalized symptoms and vaccination, and the reaction rates were not statistically different in those receiving vaccine i.d. or i.m.

The only hypersensitivity reaction seen in the MRC studies, involving many hundreds of injections, was in a known atopic individual following primary and booster doses of vaccine. In contrast, Cox and Schneider[273] observed local reactions in seven of 14 subjects after i.d. primary and booster inoculations with Merieux HDCSV. More worrisome, two of the seven individuals complained of generalized pruritus, urticaria, and oedema of the face, legs, arms, and hips 9–10 days after the booster. By May 1984, over a period of 48 months, 108 allergic reactions, mostly in association with booster, had been reported in the USA, with reactions ranging from urticaria to anaphylaxis (a rate of 11 per 10000 vaccinees)[274]. Preliminary analysis of epidemiological features of the illness revealed a male/female relative risk of 2.3. However, no significant associations were demonstrated between persons who reported presumed type III hypersensitivity reactions and age, route of primary or booster immunization (i.m. or i.d.), timing of booster after primary immunization, history of other allergies, or history of previous immunization with rabies vaccines other than HDCSV. These reports of systemic allergic reactions included nine cases of presumed type I hypersensitivity (1:10000), 87 cases of presumed type III delayed hypersensitivity (9:10000), and 12 cases of indeterminate type allergic reactions[275]. Skin testing of five persons experiencing the reaction showed that all five reacted strongly to the Merieux HDCSV, but only one showed any reactivity to the more purified Behringwerke HDCSV, and the reaction was very weak[276]. Radio-allergosorbent testing (RAST) on sera from four patients who had also experienced allergic reactions showed that they all reacted positively to the Merieux HDCSV and to β-propiolactone treated human serum albumin, but not to an HDLV not activated by β-propiolactone, to DEV inactivated by β-propiolactone, or to human serum albumin[277]. It was concluded that the β-propiolactone-treated human serum albumin component of the vaccine induced the allergic reactions seen clinically[276]. Few patients required hospitalization and there were no fatalities. Subsequent experiments showed that β-propiolactone-treated homologous serum albumin caused anaphylaxis in 70% of guinea-pigs[277a].

Notwithstanding the above incidents, numerous studies involving thousands of subjects testify to the virtual freedom of troublesome reactions to HDCSV.

Post-exposure experience with HDCSV

No other vaccine has been so rigorously assessed as HDCSV in persons bitten by proven rabid animals. A study conducted during 1980–82 in the USA showed that of 511 patients who had been bitten by proven rabid animals and treated with five doses of vaccine plus RIG, none died of rabies[275]. These cases, together with more than 300 successful treatments reported in the literature, leave little doubt concerning the efficacy of combined sero-vaccine therapy with HDCSV.

By October 1983 a total of 2 million doses had been used to treat an estimated 533 000 patients worldwide, but the number who had been genuinely exposed to rabies is unknown. By June 1988, 17 people had developed rabies after treatment with HDCSV, purified chick embryo cell culture vaccine, and Vero cell vaccine; 11 had been treated with HDCSV. Review of all 17 fatalities at an informal WHO Meeting revealed that 13 had severe or category III exposures, i.e. had licks of mucosal surfaces or 'major' bites, namely multiple bites, or bites to the face, head, fingers or neck. At least 11 of these 13 patients did not receive passive immunization as recommended by WHO. Only one definitely received immune globulin around the wound as recommended by WHO. A total of four patients had category II exposures, i,e, licks on the skin, scratches or abrasions, or minor bites on covered areas of arms, trunk and legs. After careful analysis of the 17 cases, it was agreed that only one – a South African case – could definitely be considered a treatment failure. In all other cases (with the possible exception of an Iranian case in whom the site of passive immunization is unknown, and in whom the extent and severity of the facial wounds would have posed considerable difficulties with respect to effective wound infiltration), treatment flaws were noted, mostly the lack of antiserum, the failure to infiltrate antiserum locally, and delays in treatment. In the South African case the vaccine was applied in the buttocks, a route now known to be inferior to the injection of vaccine in the deltoid region. The overall 'failure' rate (i.e. including cases with less than optimal therapy) has been evaluated as $< 1:80\,000$ treatments in the USA, Canada, and Europe, 1 in 12 000–20 000 in Thailand, and 1 in 30 000 in the remaining tropical countries.

It must be stated that the proportion who were genuinely exposed to rabies is unknown, and that the true treatment failure rate remains uncertain.

Although the expense of HDCSV has severely limited its use in underprivileged countries there is convincing evidence that as little as 1.4 ml of HDCSV given in multiple intradermal sites affords equally good protection. The rationale for the use of multiple intradermal sites is that it evokes high titres of antibody rapidly. After several volunteer studies[278,279,281–283] and a post-exposure protection trial using street rabies virus infection in rabbits[281], a post-exposure study was carried out in 78 patients who were bitten by a dog or cat whose brain was positive for rabies antigen by immunofluorescence[284]. Thirty-six patients with 'severe' exposures and 42 with mild exposure were recruited to the study. All were treated with a regimen of 0.1 ml i.d. at eight sites (on both sides of the deltoid, lateral thigh, suprascapular and lower abdominal regions) on day 0, 0.1 ml i.d. at four sites on day 7 (the deltoids and lateral thighs only), and 0.1 ml on days 28 and 91 at one i.d. site; severe exposures were treated with 40 IU/kg of equine ARS in addition. All patients were alive and well 1 year after their bite, though one patient was lost to follow-up after 6 weeks to 6 months of starting vaccination. The investigators recommended the multi-site regimen as the treatment of choice when finance is limited, and where passive immunization is not available. Multi-site intradermal vaccination is currently used in Africa, India and Thailand, and in Bangkok a variation of the regimen[285–287] has been applied in more than 10 000 treatments.

The approach adopted by other investigators has been to marginally reduce the overall cost of immunization by reducing the total number of doses to four, but to evoke high titres of antibody more rapidly than the current WHO regimen by giving two doses of the vaccine on day 0, with subsequent single doses on days 7 and 21 – the so-called 2–1–1 regimen[288,289].

Pre-exposure experience with HDCSV

Recommendations for pre-exposure immunization against rabies advise that a minimum antibody level of 0.5 IU/ml should be attained 4 weeks after the last inoculation[290]. In the British MRC studies, 96% of subjects given a single dose of 0.1 ml of vaccine i.d., and 94% given 1.0 ml i.m., had titres equal to, or in excess of, this arbitrary level[272]. However, the titres rapidly declined, and by 6 months 28% of vaccinees had titres less than 0.5 IU/ml and 19% had no detectable antibody (< 0.1 IU/ml), clearly indicating that more than one dose is necessary.

Twenty-eight days after a second injection on day 28 by either the i.m. or i.d. routes, 100% of vaccinees had titres in excess of 0.5 IU/ml. These results are in accord with those of many similar studies in Europe where two doses of the Merieux HDCSV were given 28 days apart. After several injections the titres were several times greater by the i.m. (1.0 ml) route compared with the i.d. (0.1 ml) route, but the proportion of vaccinees who were without antibody 6–24 months after immunization were similar whether the i.d. or i.m. routes were used, and it is questionable whether the significantly higher titres which develop after i.m. vaccination are clinically important. A third injection administered on day 56 provided a further increase in antibody titre and reinforced the humoral response, so that antibody was still present in 100% of vaccinees at 2 years, and 86% at 3 years. The antibody response to boosters administered at 6, 12 or 24 months by either the i.d. or s.c. routes was rapid, with an upward trend in mean titre being apparent at 48 h, well within the incubation period for rabies.

Thus for pre-exposure prophylaxis where the risk of exposure is low, the MRC group suggested that two doses of vaccine, by either the i.d. or i.m. route, should be adequate, and that with vaccine of adequate potency (antigenic potency > 2.5) there is little justification in monitoring the antibody response. The necessity for frequent booster injections seemed doubtful, and the American reports of allergic reactions to the Merieux product reinforced this view. For those at high risk of exposure to rabies virus, i.e. those working with rabies virus in research, diagnostic laboratories, and in vaccine production facilities where the risks of accidental exposure may be higher, the MRC group considered that it was necessary to monitor antibody titres at 6-monthly intervals and give boosters when required. The US Immunization Practices Advisory Commitee has identical recommendations[291].

The economic benefits of using the i.d. route are quite considerable, and in July 1982 the public health authorities in the USA tentatively endorsed the use of a 0.1 ml i.d. HDCSV dose as an alternative to the 1.0 ml i.m. dose then approved for pre-exposure immunization[24]. This decision was based on a review of data from 11 carefully conducted trials in Europe and the USA involving over 1500 persons; satisfactory responses were observed in all subjects given a three-dose regimen, each i.d. dose containing only 10% of the standard i.m. formulation. Reassuringly, data from four studies indicate that all persons should seroconvert in the unlikely event of all three 0.1 ml injections going percutaneously[292,294296]. However, the neutralizing antibody response to HDCSV given i.d. is superior to the same amounts given i.m.[296].

In August 1983 the rabies death of a Peace Corps volunteer in Kenya who had been pre-immunized with HDCSV by the intradermal route raised questions concerning the efficacy of the i.d. regimen and the recommendation for i.d. vaccination was temporarily suspended. It should be noted that this individual did not receive booster doses of vaccine recommended for immunized persons who are subsequently exposed. Intensive review of i.d. vaccination revealed that, in the USA, persons receiving the i.d. vaccine responded adequately as had been demonstrated in the earlier trials. In contrast, people who had been immunized overseas, whether by the i.d. or i.m. routes, often had lower antibody responses than expected[297,298]. There was no obvious explanation for the discrepancies. A defect in the cold-chain was considered a possiblity, but none was found, and from a field trial in Pakistan we know that lyophilized HDCSV can withstand prolonged exposure to high ambient temperature[299]. Indeed, stability testing of Merieux rabies Vero cell vaccine shows that lyophilized rabies vaccine is stable at 20 °C, 37 °C, and 45 °C for more than 1 year, and that at 4 °C it is stable for more than 5 years (Roumiantzeff, personal communication). It has also been established[300] that the immunogenicity of HDCSV is not lost by reconstitution and storage at 4 °C for 18 h. Faulty i.d. technique would not explain the extent of the discrepancies; moreover, on observation, administration of vaccine was satisfactory. Taylor *et al.*[301] compared the 12 week rabies antibody titres of Peace Corps volunteers (PCVs) in Thailand who were taking or not taking antimalarials at the time of vaccination. PCVs who took chloroquine for more than 7 weeks had a significantly lower geometric mean titre than those who did not take the antimalarial. Pappaioanou *et al.*[302] then reported the results of a randomized controlled trial to evaluate the antibody response of veterinary students to i.d. HDCSV administered concurrently with chloroquine. Chloroquine was administered weekly starting 9 days before the first dose of vaccine (administered on days 0, 7, and 28) and continuing until day 48. Since the mean rabies neutralizing antibody titre for the chloroquine group was significantly lower than that for the control group on each day of testing an explanation for the lower than anticipated results had been confirmed.

For hepatitis B vaccine vaccination into the gluteal region results in a lower antibody response compared to injections into the deltoid region. In 1987, Shill *et al.*[303] reported a case of rabies in a 19-year-old South African man who was bitten on the finger by a rabid mongoose and promptly received both local wound treatment and the recommended doses of human rabies immune globulin and HDCSV. The authors speculated that administration of the vaccine in the gluteal area may have led to a failure of the vaccine. Subsequently Fishbein *et al.*[304] undertook a limited survey of rabies post-exposure treatment in the USA and found not only that administration of HDCSV into the gluteal area was common practice, but also that the titres were lower in the subjects who had received at least one dose in the buttock. It is recommended that, in adults, the vaccine should always be administered into the deltoid area; in children the anterolateral aspect of the thigh is considered acceptable.

It is well known that antibody responsiveness to certain vaccines decreases with age. In the British MRC HDCSV studies, although the height of antibody response to the first injection decreased with age, the proportion of people aged 50 and above who failed to develop titres of ≧ 0.5 IU/ml was no different from those who were younger; moreover the titres were indistinguishable from those of younger people following a second dose. Hefti *et al.*[305] similarly found that the antibody response of persons 50 years of age and over is less than in persons aged under 25, and that antibody levels of < 0.5 IU/ml are no more frequent in the elderly than in the young.

CONTINUOUS CELL CULTURE VACCINES DERIVED FROM NON-HUMAN CELL SUBSTRATES

Institut Merieux has prepared a new vaccine using Vero cells grown on a micro-carrier system and infected with the same virus strain used for HDCSV production[306]. The use of such a heteroploid cell substrate for producing human vaccines was excluded until recently because it was thought that potentially oncogenic DNA might be released from the cells during viral replication. Provided that appropriate tumorigenicity tests are carried out, and the product is free from cellular DNA, continuous cell lines are generally considered acceptable for human vaccine production. Vero cell vaccine satisfied the stringent safety requirements and has shown excellent antigenicity and protective efficacy in humans, again with antibody responses comparable to those of HDCSV[289]. Use of the micro-carrier technique and greater yield of virus from Vero cells compared to HDSCV have resulted in a considerable reduction in price. The vaccine is purified by zonal centrifugation and chromatography and is well tolerated. Study of 328 injections given to 174 healthy adult volunteers[307] showed erythema to occur in 4%, induration in 3%, local pain in 7%, and fever of $> 38\,°C$ in 1%. Vero cell vaccine is produced commercially and is used extensively for rabies post-exposure treatment.

INTERFERON RESPONSE TO RABIES VACCINES IN HUMANS

Studies in experimental animals have shown that rabies can often be prevented if interferon is administered or induced before or after the time of infection[308–320]. Inactivated Kern Canyon virus, influenza B virus and some tissue culture rabies vaccines are capable of inducing interferon and protecting animals against challenge with rabies virus, and in these studies the rabies vaccines gave no protection if interferon could not be detected[309,320]. In contrast, Pille and Matevoysan[322] compared the protective effects of two rabies vaccines, only one of which induced interferon, and found no association between interferon induction and protection in mice. A post-exposure study in non-human primates at the US Center for Disease Control showed that HDCSV induced low titres of interferon in a proportion of monkeys but the outcome of infection could not be related to the interferon response[323]. Studies in man show interferon induction by rabies vaccines to occur inconsistently. Low titres are sometimes found after primary vaccination with 1.0 ml doses of HDCSV, but not after revaccination[279]. These observations are in agreement with those found in rabbits[320]. The interferon response to HDCSV and PCECV is related to vaccine dosage[280,324], and peak titres of 20–100 U/ml are observed in man 17–25 h after vaccination with HDCSV[280]. It may be concluded that interferon is a valuable adjunct to rabies post-exposure therapy, but the ability of vaccines to induce interferon does not appear to be essential for protection.

PASSIVE IMMUNIZATION

Studies in animals

As early as 1889, Babes and Lepp[105] demonstrated experimentally the efficacy of antirabies serum. Since then many workers have examined the value of passive immunization. The results, which ranged from complete protection[325] to none at all[326], are difficult to interpret since they were often based on a small number of experimental animals, control animals were often few or not included, and the titration of rabies antibody with any degree of reproducibility could not be assured at the time[327]. Following improvements in study design, a few workers showed no benefit of serum[328-331], but others obtained consistently good results in various animals, ranging from mice to monkeys, if large doses were given shortly before, during, or after infection[83,84,95,332-335].

Experiments on combined active and passive immunization were also undertaken. Hoyt *et al.*[336] reported that a single injection of antiserum, given at the beginning of active immunization, largely nullified the effects of 12 daily doses of vaccine. However, other workers[83,84,96,337] presented experimental evidence in mice, hamsters, guinea pigs, dogs and monkeys that post-exposure treatment with vaccine and subcutaneous or intramuscular antiserum would prevent street rabies virus infection following peripheral virus inoculation. Moreover, the protection attained was generally better than that observed after serum or vaccine treatment alone. The difference between these results and those of Hoyt *et al.*[336] no doubt reflects that the dosage of antiserum is critical, particularly when given with a poor immunogen – too small a dose may fail to give adequate antibody levels, and too large a dose may suppress active immunity. Habel's observation[338] that street rabies virus could be demonstrated up to 72 h afterwards in the muscle at the site of peripheral inoculation seems at first to have been overlooked, since more than 15 years were to elapse before experimental evidence stressed the importance of prompt infiltration of wounds with antiserum[339-343]. However, a number of earlier studies had suggested the usefulness of local infiltration[337] and in 1957 the World Health Organization Expert Committee on Rabies recommended its use[344].

The high incidence of serum sickness that accompanies use of heterologous antitetanus serum[345] and antirabies serum[196,346,347] in man prompted further studies in animals. Some experimental data provide evidence that homologous antibody preparations may provide superior protection when compared with heterologous antibody[86,348,348a]. In contrast, other workers found homologous antiserum to give greater immunosuppression than a heterologous product[349]. Although the adjunctive effect of antiserum is generally not in doubt, there is abundant evidence that passively administered antibody often prolongs the incubation period but gives little, or no, protection by itself[91,92,95-97,326,331].

Passive immunization – studies in man

Babes and Cerchez[350] first reported the use of antirabies serum in the treatment of man in 1891; 12 person who were severely bitten by a rabid wolf received, in addition to Pasteur's treatment, four to six injections of hyperimmune whole blood from dogs or man. All 12 survived, but an untreated person who was bitten by the same wolf died, indicating that they had all been exposed to an infective animal[351]. Marie[326] reported most encouraging results from mixtures of antiserum and virus for the treatment of more than 300 persons. Semple[351] treated 202 exposures to rabies with equine antiserum and vaccine and reported three deaths. These early studies and a succession of others[329,330,352–354,354a] claiming a beneficial effect of sero-vaccine therapy over vaccine treatment alone were flawed by the failure to include vaccine-only controls, and/or by neglecting to establish the diagnosis of rabies in the biting animals by laboratory methods.

One of the most rigorous tests of antirabies therapy is the post-exposure treatment of persons bitten by proven rabid wolves. The bites are often multiple and deep, and in Iran, despite a course of treatment with NTV, they carry a 25% risk of mortality overall and a 42% mortality among individuals wounded on the head or face[159]. It was in this setting that a convincing demonstration of the value of antirabies serum in man was first made. In August 1954 a rabid wolf entered village in Iran and bit 29 persons, some very severely. Five individuals with head wounds and treated with a course of NTV alone showed no demonstrable antibodies in their sera until the nineteenth day following the start of treatment; three of these five persons died from rabies. In contrast, 11 of 12 survivors among 13 individuals similarly exposed, who received antirabies serum plus a course of vaccine, had demonstrable antibodies early and throughout an 8-week period of observation[85,355]. Selimov *et al.*[356] and Fathi et al.[161] have provided further evidence for the beneficial effect of antiserum following bites by rabid animals, mostly wolves. Aggregated data from Balatazard and Bahmanyar[355], Selimov *et al.*[356] and Fathi *et al.*[161] show that antiserum saves the lives of approximately 85% of persons who would otherwise develop rabies and die, despite treatment with NTV.

From a series of studies coordinated by WHO it was concluded that antibody was demonstrable no sooner than 7–10 days following the start of treatment with NTV, HEP Flury vaccine, or DEV[357–360]. By contrast passively administered antirabies serum given at the start of treatment produced circulating antibody within 24 h and persisted until the active antibody response became measurable. However, it was also noted that immune serum suppressed the antibody response to vaccination[179,357–360] and that this interference could be overcome by booster injections 10 and 20 days after a 14-day course of inoculations[360]. Despite the extra protection afforded by passive immunization treatment failures were still reported following combined sero-vaccine therapy[94,160,161,355,361–364,364a]. It remains unclear whether these failures were caused by delay in giving the serum, inadequacy of the antibody preparation, low potency of the vaccine, refractoriness of the subject to the antigenic stimulus, or the interfering effect of the serum on vaccine.

Immune globulin preparations of human origin were developed during the late 1950s to overcome the problems of anaphylaxis and serum sickness that were commonly associated with the use of crude equine preparations[196,346,347]. Hosty *et al.*[365] used the methods of Cohn[366] and Oncley[367] to fractionate a serum pool prepared from volunteers hyperimmunized with DEV and HEP Flury vaccine. Although the final product was low-titred in comparison with equine antiserum, satisfactory blood levels were obtained after doses of 0.5 ml/kg and the decrease in titre was more gradual than with the heterologous product[365]. This was consistent with the findings of others that homologous tetanus antibody in humans is far superior to equine antibody on a unit basis[368]. The subsequent production of human rabies immune globulin (HRIG) of similar or greater potency[86,193,348,369] was followed by trials to establish the dosage to be used with DEV[193,210,370,371,385]; administration of 15–40 IU/kg of HRIG generally resulted in early appearance of antibody but inhibited the development of active antibody. Based on these data, the regimen recommended for prophylaxis of severe exposure consisted of 20 IU/kg HRIG combined with 21 doses of DEV given over 21 days and two booster injections given 10 and 20 days after completion of the primary series[197].

Many investigators have studied the effect of passive immunization on the active antibody response to 1.0 ml quantites of HDSCV. Hafkin *et al.*[372] and Kuwert *et al.*[372a] showed that passive immunization had no immunosuppressive effect; Mertz *et al.*[373] similarly obtained no evidence of immunosuppression, but the groups were not strictly comparable. Keller *et al.*[374], Nicholson and Turner[374a], Steck *et al.*[375], and Hefti *et al.*[305] showed that the titres were consistently lower, but not significantly so, after passive immunization. Méan *et al.*[376] compared day 30 antibody titres of 151 Swiss subjects undergoing post-exposure treatment with and without antibody, and observed significantly lower titres in the sero-vaccine group. They attributed this to vaccine of low potency (antigenic value 1.6), but in a subsequent study, Méan[377] again found consistently lower titres in sero-vaccine groups, even when batches of adequate potency were used. Moreover, it appeared that there was indeed a relationship between vaccine potency and the suppressive effect of passive immunization. Overall, it is evident that 20 IU/kg of HRIG has only a modest immunosuppressive effect on the stimulus provided by 1.0 ml quantities of vaccine.

In the MRC study[374a] detectable antibody was present in only 47–80% of subjects 24–48 h after the administration of Lister HRIG. Low or absent antibody titres, similar to those reported by the MRC group, have been noted by other workers in subjects passively immunized with 20 IU/kg HRIG[372a,373,374,378], and if detectable antibody within the first 48 h is a criterion of protection, then it seems that 20 IU/kg HRIG may be inadequate, and that 30–40 IU/kg would be more valuable, particularly in the presence of potent vaccines such as HDCSV.

POST-EXPOSURE PROPHYLAXIS

The essential components of post-exposure prophylaxis are active and passive immunization (see Table 1).

Wound treatment

Experimentally the incidence of rabies can be reduced markedly with local therapy alone. It is of maximal value when applied immediately after exposure but should not be neglected even if several hours or days have elapsed. It is imperative that the wounds are thoroughly cleansed and flushed with soap

Table 1 Specific systemic treatment

Nature of exposure	*Status of biting animal (irrespective of any earlier vaccination)* — *At time of exposure*	*During next 10 days*[a]	*Recommended treatment*
I. Contact, but no lesion; indirect contact; no contact	Healthy	Healthy	None
	Suspected as rabid[b]	Rabid	
II. Licks on the skin; scratches or abrasions; minor bites (on covered areas of arms, trunk, and legs)	Healthy	Healthy	None
		Rabid[c]	Start vaccination schedule.[c]
	Suspected as rabid[b]	Healthy	Start vaccination schedule; stop treatment if animal remains healthy for 5 days.[a,d]
		Rabid	Start vaccination schedule; upon postive diagnosis, complete the course of vaccine.
	Rabid; wild animal[e] or animal unavailable for observation		Give complete course of vaccine.
III. Licks of mucosa; major bites (multiple, or on face, head, finger, or neck)	Suspect[b] or confirmed rabid domestic or wild[e] animal, or animal unavailable for observation		Serum + vaccine. Stop treatment only in the case of domestic animal under observation[a] which remains healthy for 5 days.

[a]This observation period applies only to dogs and cats. Other domestic and wild animals suspected as rabid should be killed and examined using the fluorescent antibody technique.

[b]All unprovoked bites in endemic areas should be considered suspect unless proved negative by laboratory examination of the animal's brain.

[c]During the usual period of 10 days, begin treatment with vaccine at first sign of rabies in a dog or cat that has bitten someone. The symptomatic animal should be killed immediately and examined using the fluorescent antibody technique.

[d]Or if the animal's brain is found to be negative by fluorescent antibody examination.

[e]In general, exposure to rodents, rabbits and hares seldom, if ever, requires specific antirabies treatment.

and water, detergent, or water alone. This procedure is recommended by the World Health Organization (WHO) for all bite wounds, including those unrelated to possible exposure to rabies. Then apply either 40–70% alcohol, tincture or aqueous solutions of iodine, or quaternary ammonium compounds (QAC), e.g. 1–2% benzalkonium chloride, 0.1% cetrimonium bromide

(Cetavlon). QAC may be neutralized by tapwater in 'hardwater' areas, as well as by soap; wounds cleaned with a soap solution therefore should be rinsed throughly with water before application of a QAC. Extensive deep lacerations may require surgical debridement. The WHO recommends that suturing of the wounds should be delayed whenever possible. If suturing is considered essential for haemostasis or cosmetic reasons, use antiserum or immune globulin locally, as directed in the following section. Antibiotics and specifc tetanus prophylaxis should be given where indicated to control infections other than rabies.

Human rabies immune globulin (HRIG), equine rabies immune globulin (ERIG), or antirabies serum (ARS)

When employed, HRIG, ERIG, or ARS is administered only once, at the beginning of antirabies prophylaxis at the same time as the vaccine, to provide antibodies until the patient responds to active immunization. The dose of HRIG recommended by WHO is 20 IU/kg of body weight and 40 IU/kg for ERIG and ARS. To facilitate administration it may be necessary to further dilute particularly viscous or concentrated solutions in normal saline. This can usually be accomplished using a 10 ml or 20 ml syringe. At least half should be applied to the wounds by careful instillation in the depth of the wounds (i.e. avoiding further puncture wounds to the bite site) and by infiltration around the wound. The rest is administered intramuscularly, but at a different site to the vaccine.

There is evidence that administration of passive immunization prior to vaccination reduces the overall efficacy of treatment. Thus only in exceptional circumstances, i.e. when vaccine is temporarily unavailable, should antirabies immune globulin be administered before active immunization. Should this occur, it was suggested at an informal WHO meeting that double the normal dose of vaccine should be given in two sites at the first available opportunity.

Vaccine treatment

Currently six 1 ml doses of potent tissue culture vaccine given i.m. on days 0, 3, 7, 14, 30 and 90 are recommended by the WHO; five 1 ml doses given on days 0, 3, 7, 14 and 28 are recommended by the US Immunization Practices Advisory Committee of the Centers for Disease Control, Atlanta.

Recent work suggests that abbreviated 'multi-site' schedules evoke more rapid antibody responses than the current recommended regimens. One schedule, the 2–1–1 regimen, may ultimately supplement or replace the current five- or six-dose schedules. Unfortunately the cost of the 2–1–1 schedule is still too high for most tropical countries. Rabies antibody is evoked more rapidly in response to eight 0.1 ml intradermal (i.d.) injections on day 0 (in both deltoid regions, thighs, suprascapular area, and lower abdominal wall), four 0.1 ml injections on day 7 (to thighs and deltoid region), and a single 0.1 ml injection on days 28 and 90, than to the five- or six-dose regimens currently recommended. This regimen is envisaged to be of particular value in developing countries where cost considerations are of paramount importance. It should be stressed that the response to single

0.1 ml i.d. injections on days 0, 3, 7, 14, 30 and 90 is inferior to 1.0 ml volumes administered by the same schedule, and is definitely not recommended.

Post-exposure treatment in previously vaccinated persons

Previously vaccinated persons with *proven* seroconversion should receive at least two doses of tissue-culture vaccine, one immediately and one 3–7 days later. Passive immunization may interefere with the anamnestic response, and should not be given. If the immune status of a previously vaccinated person is not known then full post-exposure treatment is recommended.

FUTURE PERSPECTIVES

The nucleotide sequence of the mRNA encoding rabies virus glycoprotein was first reported in 1981[379]. All structural protein genes, except that coding for the L protein, have since been cloned[380] and the glycoprotein gene has been successfully inserted into *Escherichia coli*[381,382], *Saccharomyces cerevisiae*[382], vaccinia virus[383], and simian virus 40, adenovirus, and bovine papilloma virus for expression in mammalian cells[383]. Candidate vaccines produced by recombinant DNA technology have yet to be evaluated in man.

REFERENCES

1. Mantell, J. (1833). Letter to the *Sussex Advertiser*, 22 March
2. Babes, V. (1912). *Traité de la rage*. (Paris: Baillière et fils)
3. Lubinski, H. and Prausnitz-Breslau C. (1926). 1. *Lyssa. Ergebnisse der Hygiene Bakter Immun U Exp Therapie*, pp. 1–164. (Berlin: J. Springer)
4. Leach, C. N. and Johnson, H. N. (1940). Human rabies, with special reference to virus distribution and titer. *Am. J. Trop. Med.*, **20**, 335–40
5. Constantine, D. G. (1962). Rabies transmission by nonbite route. *Public Hlth. Rep.*, **77**, 287–9
6. Atanasiu, P. (1965). Transmission de la rage par la voie respiratoire aux animaux de laboratoire. *C. R. Acad. Sci. Paris*, **261**, 277–9
7. Hronovsky, V. and Benda, R. (1969). Experimental inhalation infection of laboratory rodents with rabies virus. *Acta Virol.*, **13**, 193–7
8. Hronovsky, V. and Benda, R. (1969). Development of inhalation rabies infection in suckling guinea pigs. *Acta Virol.*, **13**, 198–202
9. Irons, J. V., Eads, R. B., Grimes, J. E. and Conklin, A. (1957). The public health importance of bats. *Tex. Rep. Biol. Med.*, **15**, 292–8
10. Humphrey, G. L., Kemp, G. E. and Wood, E. G. (1960). A fatal case of rabies in a woman bitten by an insectivorous bat. *Public Hlth. Rep.*, **75**, 317–26
11. Winkler, W. G., Fashinell, T. R., Leffingwell, L., Howard, P. and Conomy, J. P. (1973). Airborne rabies transmission in a rabies worker. *J. Am. Med. Assoc.*, **226**, 1219–21
12. MMWR. (1977). Rabies in a Laboratory Worker New York. **26**, 183–4
13. Houff, S. A., Burton, R. C., Wilson, R. W., Henson, T. E., London, W. T., Baer, G. M., Anderson, L. J., Winkler, W. G., Madden, D. J. and Sever, J. L. (1979). Human to human transmission of rabies virus by corneal transplant. **300**, 603–4
14. MMWR. (1980). Human to human transmission of rabies via a corneal transplant, France 1980; **29**, 25–6
15. MMWR. (1981). Human to human transmission of rabies via a corneal transplant, Thailand, **30**, 473–4
16. Sureau, P., Portnoi, D., Rollin, P., Lapresle, C. and Chaouni-Berbich, A. (1981). Prevention

de la transmission inter-humaine de la rage aprés greffe de cornée. *C.R. Hebd. Seances Acad. Sci.*, **293**, 689–92

17. Greenwood, Mjr. (1945). Tenth report on data of anti-rabies treatments supplied by Pasteur Institutes. *Bull. WHO*, **12**, 301–64
18. Meyer, K. F. (1957). Man contracting rabies from man. *J. Am. Med. Assoc.*, **165**, 158–9
19. Anderson, J. A., Daly, F. T. and Kidd, J. C. (1966). Human rabies after antiserum and vaccine post-exposure treatment. *Ann. Intern. Med.*, **64**, 1297–1302
20. Emmons, R. W., Leonard, L. L., De Genaro, F., Protas, E. S., Bazely, P. L., Giammona, P. L. and Sturkow, K. (1973). A case of human rabies with prolonged survival. *Intervirology*, **1**, 60–72
21. MMWR. (1977). Human rabies, Texas, **26**, 31
22. Lintjorn, B. (1982). Clinical features of rabies in man. *Tropical Doctor*, **12**, 9–12
23. WHO. (1982). World survey of rabies XX for years 1980/81. *WHO/Rabies/* 82–193
24. MMWR. (1982). *Rabies – United States 1981*, **31**, 379–80
25. Horrenburger, R. (1952). Recherche du virus rabique chez les rats de la ville d'Alger. *Arch. Inst. Pasteur, Algerie*, **30**, 371–6
26. Winkler, W. G. (1972). Rodent rabies in the United States. *J. Infect. Dis.*, **126**, 565–67
27. Bögel, K., Posch, J., Quander, J., Kuwert, E. and Plichta, C. (1975). Antirabies treatment in man in relation to epidemiological conditions: Nordrhein-Westfalen 1972. *Zbl. Bakt. Hyg.* 1, *Abt. Orig.*, **A231**, 15–30
28. Bögel, K., Moegle, H., Knorpp, F., Arata, A., Dietz, K. and Dietheim, P. (1976). Characteristics of the spread of a wildlife rabies epidemic in Europe. *Bull. WHO*, **54**, 433–47
29. Förster, U., Wachendörfer, G. and Krekel, J. (1977). Testing of rodents and insectivores for rabies virus and antigen. *Berl. Münch. Tierärztl. Wschr*, **90**, 335–7
30. Botros, B. A. M., Lewis, J. C. and Kerkor, M. (1979). A study to evaluate non-fatal rabies in animals. *J. Trop. Med. Hyg.*, **82**, 137–41
31. Steck, F. and Wandeler, A. (1980). The epidemiology of fox rabies in Europe. *Epidemiol. Rev.*, **2**, 71–96
32. CDC. (1981). *Rabies Surveillance Annual Summary* 1979 (Issued October).
33. Bisseru, B. (ed.) (1972). *Rabies* (London: William Heinemann)
34. WHO (1977). World survey of rabies XVII for year 1975. *WHO/Rabies*/77183
35. WHO (1980). Rabies surveillance Europe 1979. *Wkly Epidem. Rec.*, **55**, 367
36. WHO (1976). Rabies surveillance 1974. *Wkly Epidem. Rec.*, **51**, 309–12
37. Schneider, H. P. (1985). Rabies in South West Africa/Namibia. In Kuwert, E., Mérieux, C. Koprowski, H. and Bögel, K. (eds), *Rabies in the Tropics*, pp. 520–35. (Berlin. Springer-Verlag)
38. Acha, P. N. and Arambulo, P. V. (1985). Rabies in the tropics — history and current status. In Kuwert, E., Mérieux, C., Koprowski, H. and Bögel, K. (eds), *Rabies in the Tropics*, pp. 343–59. (Berlin: Springer-Verlag)
39. Nikolic, M. and Jelesic, Z. (1956). Isolation of rabies virus from insectivorous bats in Yugoslavia. *Bull. WHO*, **14**, 801–4
40. Pitzschke, H. (1965). Tollwut bei einer breitflügel-fledermaus (*Eptesicus serotinus*) in Thüringen. *Zent. J. Bakt.*, 1 *Abt. Orig.*, **196**, 411–15
41. Smith, P. C., Lawhaswasdi, K., Vick, W. E. and Stanton, J. S. (1967). Isolation of rabies from fruit bats in Thailand. *Nature (London)*, **216**, 384
42. Pal, S. R., Arora, B., Chhuttani, P. N., Boor, S., Choudhury, S., Joshi, R. M. and Ray, S. D. (1980). Rabies virus infection of a flying fox bat, *Pteropus poliocephalus* in Chandigarh, Northern India. *Trop. Geogr. Med.*, **32**, 265–7
43. WHO (1970). Rabies in India. *WHO Chronicle*. **24**, 576
44. Sanmartin, C., Correa, P., Duenas, A. *et al.* (1967). Alguans consideraciones sobre 42 casos humanos de rabia. In *Memorias del Primer Seminaro Nacional Sobre Rabia. Medellin*, pp. 155–6 (Colombia: University of Medellin)
45. Anderson, L. J., Nicholson, K. G., Tauxe, R. V. and Winkler, W. G. (1984). Human rabies in the United States, 1960 to 1979: epidemiology, diagnosis, and prevention. *Ann. Intern. Med.*, **100**, 728–35
46. Foggin, C. M. and Swanepoel, R. (1979). Rabies in Rhodesia: the current situation. *Central African J. Med.*, **25**, 98–100

47. Benelmouffok, A., Belkaid, M. and Benhassine, H. (1979). Epidemiologie de la rage en Algerie. *Arch. l'Institut Pasteur d'Algerie*, **53**, 143–54
48. Fagbami, A. H., Anosa, V. O. and Ezabuiro, E. O. (1981). Hospital records of human rabies and antirabies prophylaxis in Nigeria 1969–78. *Trans. Roy. Soc. Trop. Med, Hyg.*, **75**, 872–6
49. PAHO (1981). Epidemiologic surveillance of rabies in the Americas. *Bull. Pan-Am Hlth Org.*, **15**, 271–8
50. Fekadu, M. (1982). Rabies in Ethiopia. *Am. J. Epidemiol.*, **115**, 266–73
51. Bjorvatin, B. and Gundersen, S. G. (1980). Rabies exposure among Norwegian missionaries working abroad. *Scand. J. Infect. Dis.*, **12**, 257–64
52. Bögel, K. and Motschwiller, E. (1986). Incidence of rabies and post-exposure treatment in developing countries. *Bull. WHO*, **64**, 883–7
53. Brown. F., Bishop, D. H. L., Crick, J., Franki, R. I. B., Holland, J. J., Hull, R., Johnson, K., Martelli, G., Murphy, F. A., Obijeski, J. F. Peters, D., Pringle, C. R., Reichmann, M. E., Schneider, L. G., Shope, R. E., Simpson, D. I. H., Summers, D. F. and Wagner, R. R. (1979). Rhabdoviridae. *Intervirology*, **12**, 1–7
54. WHO (1980). Report of consultation on rabies prevention and control. *WHO/Rabies*/80.188, 10
55. Shope, R. E. (1975). Rabies virus antigenic relationships. In Baer, G. M. (ed.) *The Natural History of Rabies*, Vol 1, pp. 141–54. (New York: Academic Press)
56. Wiktor, T. J. and Koprowski, H. (1978). Monoclonal antibodies against rabies virus produced by somatic cell hybridization: detection of antigenic variants. *Proc. Natl. Acad. Sci. USA*, **75**, 3938
57. Flamand, A., Wiktor, T. J. and Koproswki, H. (1980). Hybridoma antibody detects antigenic differences between rabies and rabies-related viruses. 1: Nucleocapsid antigens. *J. Gen. Virol.*, **48**, 97–104
58. Flamand, A., Wiktor, T. J. and Koprowski, H. (1980). Hybridoma antibody detects antigenic differences between rabies and rabies-related viruses. 2: Glycoprotein antigens. *J. Gen. Virol.*, **48**, 104–9
59. Wiktor, T. J., Flamand, A. and Koprowski, H. (1980). Use of monoclonal antibodies in diagnosis of rabies virus infection and differentiation of rabies and rabies-related viruses. *J. Virol. Methods*, **1**, 33–46
60. Schneider, L. G., Barnard, B. J. H., Schneider, H. P., Odegaard, O. A., Mueller, J., Selimov, M., Cox, J. H., Wandeler, A. I., Blancou, J. and Meyer, S. (1985). Application of monoclonal antibodies for epidemiological investigations and oral vaccination studies. In Kuwert, E., Mérieux, C., Koprowski, H. and Bögel, K. (eds), *Rabies in the Tropics*, pp. 47–59. (Berlin: Springer-Verlag)
61. Koprowski, H., Wiktor, T. J. and Abelseth, M. K. (1985). Cross-reactivity and cross-protection: rabies variants and rabies-related viruses. In Kuwert, E., Mérieux, C., Koprowski, H. and Bögel, K. (eds), *Rabies in the Tropics*, pp. 30–90. (Berlin: Springer-Verlag)
62. Wiktor, T. J. (1985). Is a special vaccine required against rabies-related viruses and variants of rabies? In Vodopija, I., Nicholason, K. G., Smerdel, S. and Bijok, U. (eds), *Improvements in Rabies Postexposure Treatment*, pp. 9–13. (Zagreb: Institute of Public Health)
63. Webster, L. T. and Dawson, J. R. (1935). Early diagnosis of rabies by mouse inoculation. Measurement of humoral immunity to rabies by mouse protection test. *Proc. Soc. Exp. Biol. (N.Y.)*, **32**, 570–3
64. Fitzgerald, E. A., Baer, G. M., Cabassao, V. J. and Vallancourt, R. J. (1975). A collaborative study on the potency testing of antirabies globulin. *J. Biol. Stand.*, **3**, 273–8
65. Kuwert, E. K., Thraenhart, O., Marcus, I., Werner, J., Atanasiu, P., Bahmanyar, M., Bögel, K., Cox, J. H., Schneider, L. G., Turner, G. and Wiktor, T. J. (1978). Comparative study on antibody determination by different methods in sera of persons vaccinated with HDCS rabies vaccine. *Dev. Biol. Stand.*, **40**, 221–9
66. Atanasiu, P. and Lépine, P. (1959). Multiplication du virus rabique des rues sur la tumeur ependymaire de la souris en coulture de tissus, effet cytolytique. *Ann. Inst. Pasteur*, **96**, 72–8
67. Fernandes, M. V., (1963). Mechanism of the cytopathic effect of rabies virus in tissue culture. *Virology*, **21**, 128–31
68. Kissling, R. E. and Reese, D. R. (1963). Antirabies vaccine of tissue culture origin. *J. Immunol.*, **91**, 362–8

69. Abelseth, M. K. Propagation of rabies virus in pig kidney cell culture. *Can. Vet. J.*, **5**, 84–7
70. Wiktor, T. J., Fernandes, M. V. and Koprowski, H. (1964). Cultivation of rabies virus in human diploid cell strain WI-38. *J. Immunol.*, **93**, 353–66
71. Yoshino, K., Tanigucji, S. and Arai, K. (1966). Autointerference of rabies virus in chick embryo fibroblasts. *Proc. Soc. Exp. Biol. Med.*, **123**, 387–92
72. Sedwick, W. D. and Wiktor, T. J. (1967). Reproducible plaquing system for rabies, lymphocytic choriomeningitis and other ribonucleic acid viruses in BHK-21/13S agarose suspensions. *J. Virol.*, **1**, 1224–6
73. Schneider, L. (1973). Cell monolayer plaque tests. In Kaplan, M. M. and Koprowski, H. (eds), *Laboratory Techniques in Rabies*, 3rd edn, pp. 339–42. (Geneva: WHO)
74. Smith, J. S., Yager, P. A. and Baer, G. M. (1973). A rapid reproducible test for determining rabies neutralising antibody. *Bull. WHO*, **48**, 535–41
75. Cho, H. C. and Fenje, P. (1975). Rabies neutralizing antibody determination in tissue culture by direct fluorescent antibody technique. *J. Biol. Stand.*, **3**, 101–5
76. Guillemin, F., Tixier, G., Soulebot, J. P. and Chappuis, G. (1981). Comparison de deux methodes de titrages de anticorps antirabique neutralisants. *J. Biol. Stand.*, **9**, 147–56
77. Atanasiu, P., Savy, V. and Perrin, P. (1977). Épreuve immunoenzymatique pour la détection rapide des anticorps antirabiques. *Ann. Microbiol. (Inst. Pasteur)*, **128A**, 489–98
78. Thraenhart, O. and Kuwert, E. K. (1977). Enzyme-immunoassay for demonstration of rabies-virus antibodies after immunisation. *Lancet*, **2**, 399–400
79. Nicholson, K. G. and Prestage, H. (1982). Enzyme-linked immunosorbent assay: a rapid reproducible test for the measurement of rabies antibody. *J. Med. Virol.*, **9**, 43–9
80. Wiktor, T. J., György, E., Schlumberger, H. D., Sokol, F. and Koprowski, H. (1973). Antigenic properties of rabies virus components. *J. Immunol.*, **110**, 269–76
81. Dietzschold, B., Wang, I., Rupprecht, C. E., Celis, E., Tollis, M., Ertl, H., Heber-Katz, E. and Koprowski, H. (1987). Induction of protective immunity against rabies by immunization with rabies virus ribonucleoprotein. *Proc. Natl. Acad. Sci.*, **84**, 165–9
82. Turner, G. S. (1978). Immunoglobulin (IgG) and (IgM) antibody responses to rabies vaccine. *J. Gen. Virol.*, **40**, 595–604
83. Habel, K. (1945). Seroprophylaxis in experimental rabies. *Public Hlth. Rep.*, **60**, 455–60
84. Koprowski, H., Van der Scheer, J. and Black, J. (1950). Use of hyperimmune antirabies serum concentrates in experimental rabies. *Am. J. Med.*, **8**, 412–20
85. Habel, K. and Koprowski, H. (1955). Laboratory data supporting the clinical trial of antirabies serum in persons bitten by a rabid wolf. *Bull. WHO*, **13**, 773–9
86. Winkler, W. G., Schmidt, R. C. and Sikes, R. K. (1969). Evaluation of human rabies immune globulin and homologous and heterologous antibody. *J. Immunol.*, **102**, 1314–21
87. Crick, J. (1973). The vaccination of man and other animals against rabies. *Postgrad. Med. J.*, **49**, 551–64
88. Nilsson, M. R., Sant'Anna, O. A., Siqueira, M., Nilsson, T. T. and Gennari, M. (1979). Rabies virus immunity in genetically selected high- and low-responder lines of mice. *Infect. Immun.*, **25**, 23–5
89. Sikes, R. K., Peacock, G. V., Acha, P., Arko, R. J. and Dierks, R. (1971). Rabies vaccines: duration of immunity study in dogs. *J. Am. Vetr. Med. Assoc.*, **159**, 1491–9
90. Bunn, T. O., Ridpath, H. D. and Beard, P. D. (1984). The relationship between rabies antibody titre in dogs and cats and protection from challenge. *Rabies Information Exchange*, **11**, 9–13
91. Sikes, R. K., Cleary, W. F., Koprowski, H., Wiktor, T. J. and Kaplan, M. M. (1971). Effective protection of monkeys against death from street virus by post-exposure administration of tissue-culture rabies vaccine. *Bull. WHO*, **45**, 1–11
92. Wiktor, T. J. (1971). New vaccines and the future of rabies prophylaxis. In: *International Conference on the Application of Vaccines Against Viral Rickettsial and Bacterial Diseases of Man*. Scientific Publication No. 226, pp. 66–75. (Washington DC: Pan American Health Organisation, WHO)
93. Baer, G. M., Moore, S. A., Shaddock, J. H. and Levy, H. B. (1979). An effective rabies treatment in exposed monkeys: a single dose of interferon inducer and vaccine. *Bull. WHO*, **57**, 807–13
94. Chowdhuri, A. N. R., Singh, G., Thomas, A. K. and Mondal, C. K. (1969). Trial of

combined serum vaccine treatment in the prophylaxis of rabies under field conditions in northern India. *Ind. J. Med. Res.*, **57**, 149–63

95. Yen, C. H. (1942). Protective value of antiviral serum in experimental rabies infection. *Proc. Soc. Exp. Biol. Med.*, **49**, 533–7
96. Koprowski, H. and Black, J. (1954). Studies on chick embryo adapted rabies virus. 5. Protection of animals with antiserum and living attenuated virus after exposure to street strain of rabies virus. *J. Immunol.*, **72**, 85–93
97. Baer, G. M. and Cleary, W. F. (1972). A model in mice for pathogenesis and treatment of rabies. *J. Infect. Dis.*, **125**, 520–27
98. Pasteur, L., Chamberland, C., Roux, E. and Thuiller, L. (1881). Sur la rage. *C. R. Acad. Sci.*, **92**, 1259–60
99. Pasteur, L., Chamberland, C. and Roux, E. (1884). Sur la rage. *Bull. Acad. Med.*, **13**, 661–4
100. Pasteur, L. (1885). Méthode pour prévenir la rage après morsure. *C. R. Hebd, Seanc. Acad. Sci.*, **101**, 765–74
101. Roux, E. (1887). Note sur une nouvel moyen de conserver les moelles rabique avec leur virulence. *Ann. Inst. Pasteur (Paris)*, **1**, 87
102. Calmette, A. (1891). Notes sur la rage en Indo-Chine et sur les vaccinations antirabique pratiquées a Saigon. *Ann. Inst. Pasteur (Paris)*, **5**, 633–38
103. Anonymous note. (1887). Pasteur's method simplified. *Lancet*, December, p. 1185
104. Puscariu, E. and Vesesco, M. (1895). Essais de vaccination antirabique avec le virus attenué par le chaleur. *Ann. Inst. Pasteur (Paris)*, **9**, 210–13
105. Babes and Lepp, (1889). Recherches sur la vaccination antirabique. *Ann. Inst. Pasteur*, **3**, 384–90
106. Fermi, C. (1908). Über die immunisierung gegen wutkrankheit. *Z. Hyg. Infekt.* **58**, 233–76
107. Semple, D. (1911). The preparation of a safe and efficent antirabies vaccine. Scientific memoirs by officers of the medical and sanitary departments of the government of India. No. 44. (Calcutta: Superintendent Government Printing)
108. Alvisatos, G. P. (1922). Die schutzimpfung gegen lyssa durch das mit aether behendelte virus fixe. *Deutsche Med Woch.*, **48**, 295–6
109. Hempt, A. (1925). Sur une method rapide de traitement antirabique. *Ann. Inst. Pasteur*, **39**, 632–40
110. Kelser, R. A. (1930). Chloroform-treated rabies vaccine. *J. Am. Vet. Med. Assoc.*, **71**, 595–603
111. Hempt, A. (1938). Über eine karbolisierte antirabische aether-vaccine und ihren schutzwert bei mensch und tier. *Berhringwerk Mitteil*, **9**, 150–209
112. Otten, L. (1947). Investigations in rabies. II. *Atonie van Leeuwenhoek J. Microbiol. Serol.*, **13**, 101–27
113. Webster, L. T. and Casals, J. (1942). An improved non-virulent rabies vaccine. *Am. J. Public Hlth.*, **32**, 268–70
114. Turner, G. S. (1969). Rabies vaccines. *Br. Med. Bull.*, **25**, 136–42
115. Bareggi, C. (1889). Su cinque casis di rabbia paralitica (de laboratorio) nell uomo. *Gazz Med. Lombarda*, **48**, 217–19
116. Cornwall, J. W. (1919). Anaphylactic reactions in the course of antirabic treatment. *Ind. J. Med. Res.*, **6**, 237–47
117. Horack, H. M. (1939). Allergy as a factor in the development of reactions to anti-rabic treatment. *Am. J. Med. Sci.*, **197**, 672–82
118. Remlinger, P. (1927). Les paralysies du traitement antirabique. In Rapports a la conference international de la rage. *League of Nations Report*, pp. 71–132
119. Remlinger, P. (1935). La rage dite de laboratoire. *Ann. Inst. Pasteur*, (Suppl.), pp. 35–68
120. Proca, G. and Bobes, S. (1940). Antirabic immunisation: living vaccines and killed vaccines. *Bull. Health Org.*, **9**, 79–117
121. Marinesco, G. (1908). La paralysie ascendante mortelle après le traitement antirabique. *C. R. Soc. Biol.*, **64**, 973–5
122. Rivers, T. M., Sprunt, D. H. and Berry, G. P. (1933). Observations on attempts to produce acute disseminated encephalomyelitis in monkeys. *J. Exp. Med.*, **58**, 39–53
123. Kabat, E. A., Wolf, A. and Bezer, A. E. (1947). The rapid production of acute disseminated encephalomyelitis in rhesus monkeys by injection of heterologous and homologous brain tissue with adjuvants. *J. Exp. Med.*, **85**, 117–29

124. Kabat, E. A., Wolf, A. and Bezer, A. E. (1948). Studies on acute disseminated encephalomyelitis produced experimentally in rhesus monkeys. *J. Exp. Med.*, **88**, 417–25
125. Lumsden, C. E. (1949). Experimental allergic encephalomyelitis. *Brain*, **72**, 198–226
126. Sellers, T. F. (1947). Complications of antirabic treatment. *J. Med. Assoc. Georgia*, **36**, 30–5
127. Shiraki, H., Otani, S., Tanthai, B., Chamuni, A., Chitondh, H. and Charuchiinda, S. (1962). Rabies postvaccinal encephalomyelitis and genuine rabies in human beings. *World Neurol.*, **3**, 125–48
128. Appelbaum, E., Greenberg, M. and Nelson, J. (1953). Neurological complications following antirabies vaccination. *J. Am. Med. Assoc.*, **151**, 188–91
129. Svet-Modavskij, G. J., Andjaparidze, O. G., Unanov, S. S., Karakajumcan, M. K, Svet-Modavskaja, I. A., Mucnik, L. S., Hieninson, M. A., Ravkina, L. I., Mtvarelidze, A. A., Volkova, O. F., Kriegshaber, M. R., Kalinkina, A. G., Salita, T. V., Klimovickaja, V. I., Bondeletova, I. N., Rojhel, V. M., Kiseleva, I. S., Levcenko, E. N., Marennikova, S. S. and Leonidova, S. L. (1965). An allergen-free antirabies vaccine. *Bull. WHO*, **32**, 47–58
130. Stuart, G. and Krikorian, K. S. (1933). Neuroparalytic accidents complicating antirabic treatment. *Br. Med. J.*, **1**, 501–4
131. McFadzean, A. J. S. and Choa, G. H. (1953). The neuroparalytic accidents of antirabies vaccination. *Trans. Roy. Soc. Trop. Med., Hyg.*, **47**, 372–85
132. Wilson, G. S. (1967). Allergic manifestations: complications, including paralysis after rabies vaccine. In *The Hazards of Immunisation*, pp. 179–91. (London: Athlone Press)
133. Hattwick, M. A. W. (1974). Human rabies. *Public Hlth. Rev.*, **3**, 229–74
134. Redewill, F. H. and Underwood, L. J. (1947). Neurological complications to treatment with rabies vaccine. *California Med.*, **66**, 360–3
135. Pait, C. F. and Pearson, H. E. (1949). Rabies vaccine encephalomyelitis in relation to the incidence of animal rabies in Los Angeles. *Am. J. Public Hlth.*, **39**, 875–7
136. Briggs, G. W. and Brown, W. M. (1960). Neurological complications of antirabies vaccine. Treatment with corticosteroids. *J. Am. Med. Assoc.*, **173**, 802–4
137. Assis, J. L. (1975). Neurologic complications of antirabies vaccination in Sao Paulo, Brazil. *J. Neurol. Sci.*, **26**, 593–8
138. Gibbs, F. A., Gibbs, D. L., Carpenter, P. R. and Spies, H. W. (1961). Comparison of rabies vaccines grown on duck embryo and on nervous tissue: and electroencephalographic study. *N. Engl. J. Med.*, **65**, 1002–3
139. Kirk, R. C. and Ecker, E. E. (1949). Time of appearance of antibodies to brain in the human receiving antirabies vaccine. *Proc. Soc. Exp. Biol. Med.*, **70**, 743–7
140. Koprowski, H., LeBell, I. (1950). The presence of complement fixing antibodies against brain tissue in sera of persons who had received antirabies vaccine treatment. *Am. J. Hyg.*, **51**, 292–9
141. Waksman, B. H. (1956). Further studies on skin reactions in rabbits with experimental allergic encephalomyelitis. *J. Infect. Dis.*, **99**, 258–69
142. Waksman, B. H. and Morrison, L. R. (1951). Tuberculin type sensitivity to spinal cord antigen in rabbits with isoallergic encephalomyelitis. *J. Immunol.*, **66**, 421–44
143. Paterson, P. Y. (1960). Transfer of allergic encephalomyelitis in rats by means of lymph node cells. *J. Exp. Med.*, **111**, 119–36
144. Astrom, K. E. and Waksman, B. H. The passive transfer of experimental allergic encephalomyelitis and neuritis with living lymphoid cells. *J. Pathol. Bacteriol.*, **83**, 89–106
145. Bell, J. F., Wright, I. T. and Habel, K. (1949). Rabies vaccines freed of the factor causing allergic encephalitis. *Proc. Soc. Exp. Biol. Med.*, **70**, 457–61
146. Paterson, P. Y., Pond, W. L., Warren, J. and Weil, M. L. (1953). Encephalitogenic property of crude and protamin treated rabbit and mouse brain preparations. *Proc. Soc. Exp. Biol. Med.*, **83**, 2787–81
147. Hottle, G. A. and Peers, J. J. (1954). Studies on the removal of the encephalitogenic factor from rabies vaccine. *J. Immunol.*, **72**, 236–42
148. Thomas, J. B., Ricker, A. S., Baer, G. M. and Sikes, R. K. (1965). Purification of fixed rabies virus. *Virology*, **25**, 271–5
149. Kaplan, C. and Turner, G. C. (1969). Removal of encephalitogenicity from extracts of normal rabbit central nervous system by treatment with fluorocarbon. *Nature*, **219**, 445–6

150. Webster, L. T. (1939). The immunizing potency of antirabies vaccines: a critical review. *Am. J. Hyg.*, **30**, 113–34
151. Rhodes, A. J. Anti-rabies treatment. A discussion in relation to recent experimental work. *Trop. Dis. Bull.*, **43**, 975–91
152. Semple, D. (1919). On the nature of rabies of antirabic treatment. *Br. Med., J.*, **2**, 333–6
153. Veeraraghavan, N. and Subrahmanyan, T. P. (1958). The value of 5 per cent Semple vaccine prepared in distilled water in human treatment: comparative mortality among the treated and untreated. *Ind. J. Med. Res.*, **46**, 518–24
154. Kitamoto, A., Otani, S., Nagano, Y., Shibuki, M. (1971) Postbite rabies prophylaxis in humans with ultraviolet ray inactivated vaccine. In Nagano Y. and Davenport, F. M. (eds), *Rabies*, pp. 127–35. (Baltimore: University Park Press)
155. Cornwall, J. W. (1923). Statistics of antirabic inoculations in India. *Br. Med. J.*, **2**, 298
156. Yu, T. F. (1941). Rabies. *Chinese Med. J.*, **59**, 326–8
157. Nikolic, M. (1952). Die ergebnisse der tollwutschutzimpfung beim menschen nach wolfverletzung. *Z. Tropenmed. Parasitol.*, **3**, 283–96
158. Gremliza, L. (1953). Kasuistik zum lyssa-problem. *Z. Tropenmed, Parasitol.*, **4**, 383–9
159. Baltazard, M. and Ghodssi, M. (1954). Prevention of human rabies. Treatment of persons bitten by rabid wolves in Iran. *Bull. WHO.*, **10**, 797–803
160. Bahmanyar, M. (1966). Success and failure of sero-vaccination as prophylactic treatment of individuals exposed to rabies. *Symp. Series Immunobiol. Stand.*, **1**, 307–12
161. Fathi, M., Sabeti, A. and Bahmanyar, M. (1970). Séroprophylaxie antirabique chez les sujets mordus pars loups enragés en Iran. *Acta Med. Iranica.*, **13**, 5–9
162. Fuenzalida, E. and Palacios, R. (1955). Rabies vaccine prepared from the brains of infected suckling mice. *Bol. Inst. Bacteriol. Chile*, **8**, 3–10
163. Gispen, R., Schmittmann, G. J. P. and Saathof, B. (1965). Rabies vaccine derived from suckling rabbit brain. *Arch. Ges. Virusforsch.*, **15**, 366–76
164. Fuenzalida, E., Palacios, R. and Borgono, J. M. (1964). Antirabies antibody response in man to vaccine made from suckling-mouse brains. *Bull. WHO*, **30**, 431–6
165. Gispen, R. and Saathof, B. (1965). Neutralising and fluorescent antibody response in man after antirabies treatment with suckling rabbit brain vaccine. *Arch. Ges Virusforsch.*, **15**, 377–86
166. Fuenzalida, E., Palacios, R. and Borgono, J. M. (1966). The use of rabies vaccine prepared in suckling mouse brain. *Symp. Ser. Immunobiol. Stand.*, **1**, 339–45
167. Held, J. R. and Adaros, H. L. (1972). Neurological disease in man following administration of suckling mouse brian antirabies vaccine. *Bull. WHO*, **46**, 321–7
168. Toro, G., Vergara, I. and Roman, G. (1979). Neuroparalytic accidents of antirabies vaccination with suckling mouse brain (SMB) rabies vaccine. Clinical and pathological study of 21 cases. *Arch. Neurol.*, **34**, 694–700
169. Escobar, A., Dauzon, F. L. and Romero, C. (1979). Meningoencefalomielitis por vacunacion antirabica con vacuna preparada en cerebro de ratón lactante. *Gac. Med. de Mexico*, **115**, 363–7
170. Vergara, I., Toro, G., Roman, G. and Mendoza, G. (1979). Fatal Guillain–Barré syndrome with reduced dose antirabies vaccination. *Arch. Neurol.*, **36**, 254
171. Sikes, R. K. and Larghi, O. P. (1967). Purified rabies vaccine: development and comparison of potency and safety with two human rabies vaccines. *J. Immunol.*, **99**, 545–53
172. Lavender, J. F. (1970). Purified rabies vaccine (suckling rat brain origin). *Appl. Microbiol.*, **19**, 923–7
173. Koprowski, H., Black, J. and Nelsen, D. J. (1954). Studies on chick embryo adapted rabies virus. Furher changes in pathogenic properties following prolonged cultivation in the developing chick embryo. *J. Immunol.*, **72**, 94–106
174. Koprowski, H. and Cox, H. R. (1948). Studies on chick embryo adapted rabies virus. 1. Culture characteristics and pathogenicity. *J. Immunol.*, **60**, 533–44
175. Koprowski, H. and Black, J. (1950). Studies on chick embryo adapted rabies virus. 2. pathogenicity for dogs and use of egg-adapted strains for vaccination purposes. *J. Immunol.*, **64**, 185–96
176. Koprowski, H. (1954). Biological modification of rabies virus as a result of its adaptation to chicks and developing embryos. *Bull. WHO*, **10**, 709–24
177. Schwab, M. P., Fox, D. P., Conwell, D. P. and Robinson, T. A. (1954).Avianised rabies virus vaccination in man. *Bull. WHO*, **10**, 823–35

178. Fox, J. P., Conwell, D. P. and Gerhardt, P. (1955). Immunization of man with living avianised rabies virus (Flury strain). *California Vet.*, **8**, 20–4

179. Fox, J. P., Koprowski, H., Conwell, D. P., Black, J. and Gelfand, H. M. (1957). Study of antirabies immunization of man. Observations of HEP Flury and other vaccines, with and without hyperimmune serum, in primary and recall immunizations. *Bull, WHO*, **17**, 869–904

180. Sharpless, G. R., Black, J., Cox, H. R. and Ruegsegger, J. M. (1957). Preliminary observations in primary antirabies immunization of man with different types of HEP Flury virus. *Bull. WHO*, **17**, 905–10

181. Ruegsegger, J. M., Black, J. and Sharples, G. R. (1961). Primary antirabies immunization of man with HEP Flury virus vaccine. *Am. J. Public Hlth.*, **51**, 704–16

182. Schnurrenberger, P. R., Anderson, G. R., Russell, J. H. and Wentworth, F. H. (1961). Avian embryo rabies immunisation. ii. A comparison of the antigenicity of high egg passage and duck embryo vaccine administered intradermally in man. *Am. J. Hyg.*, **74**, 1–6

183. Ruegsegger, J. M. and Sharpless, G. R. (1962). Flury rabies vaccine for human use. *Ann. Intern. Med.*, **110**, 260–3

184. Tierkel, E. A. and Sikes, R. K. (1967). Preexposure prophylaxis against rabies. Comparison of regimens. *J. Am. Med. Assoc.*, **201**, 911–14

185. WHO, Expert Committee on Rabies. (1966). Fifth Report. Technical Report Series No. 321. (Geneva: WHO)

186. Powell, H. M. and Culbertson, C. G. (1950). Cultivation of fixed rabies virus in embryonated duck eggs. *Public Hlth. Rep.*, **65**, 400–1

187. Peck, F. B., Powell, H. M. and Culbertson, C. G. (1955). A new antirabies vaccine for human use. Clinical and laboratory results using rabies vaccine made from embryonated duck eggs. *J. Lab. Clin. Med.*, **45**, 679–83

188. MacFarlane, J. O. and Culbertson, C. G. (1954). Attempted production of allergic encephalomyelitis with duck embryo suspension and vaccines. *Can. J. Public Hlth*, **45**, 28–9

189. LoGrippo, G. A. and Hartmann, F. W. (1955). Antigenicity of β-propiolactone virus vaccines. *J. Immunol.*, **75**, 123–8

190. Peck, F. B., Powell, H. M. and Culbertson, C. G. (1956). Duck embryo rabies vaccine. Study of fixed virus vaccine grown in embryonated duck eggs and killed with beta-propiolactone (BPL). *J. Am. Med. Assoc.*, **162**, 1373–6

191. Greenberg, M. and Childress, J. (1960). Vaccination against rabies with duck embryo and Semple vaccine. *J. Am. Med. Assoc.*, **173**, 333–7

192. Sikes, R. K. (1969). Rabies vaccines. *Arch. Env. Hlth.*, **19**, 862–7

193. Cabasso, V. J., Loofbourow, J. C., Roby, R. E. and Anuskiewicz, W. (1971). Rabies immune globulin of human origin: preparation and dosage determination in non-exposed volunteer subjects. *Bull. WHO*, **45**, 303–15

194. Kuwert, E., Marcus, I., Thraenhart, O. and Staudacher, H. (1972). Pre- and post-infection rabies immunization: development of neutralising antibodies after administration of different doses of a duck embryo vaccine in humans. *Dtsche Med. Woch.*, **97**, 1893–8

195. Crick, J. and Brown, F. (1970). Efficacy of rabies vaccine prepared from virus grown in duck embryo. *Lancet*, **1**, 1106–7

196. Ellenbogen, C. and Slugg, P. (1973). Rabies neutralising antibody: inadequate response to equine antiserum and duck embryo vaccine. *J. Infect. Dis.*, **127**, 433–6

197. Hattwick, M. A. W., Corey, L. and Creech, W. B. (1976). Clinical use of human globulin immune to rabies virus. *J. Infect. Dis.*, **133**, (Suppl.), A266–A272

198. Rubin, R. H., Dierks, R. E., Gough, P. Gregg, M. B., Gerlach, E. H. and Sikes, R. K. (1971). Immunoglobulin response to rabies vaccine in man. *Lancet*, **2**, 625–8

199. Grandien, M. and Espmark, A. (1974). Follow up of antibody response after post exposure rabies immunization. *Symp. Ser. Immunobiol. Stand.*, **21**, 243–52

200. Spiegelburg, H. Biological activities of immunoglobulins of different classes and subclasses. *Adv. Immunol.*, **19**, 259–94

201. Mims, C. A. (1976). In *The Pathogenesis of Infectious Disease*, (London: Academic Press)

202. Anderson, G. R., Schnurrenberger, P. R., Masterson, R. A. and Wentworth, F. H. (1960). Avian embryo rabies immunization. 1. Duck embryo vaccine administered intradermally in man. *Am. J. Hyg.*, **71**, 158–67

203. Dieterich, W. H., Shelton, D. H. and Jenevein, E. P. (1961). Pre-exposure rabies immunization in man using duck embryo vaccine. *J. Am. Med. Vet. Assoc.*, **139**, 999–1004
204. Farrar, W. E., Warner, A. R. and Vivona, S. (1964). Pre-exposure immunization against rabies using duck embryo vaccine. *Military Med.*, **1**, 960–5
205. Larsh, S. E. (1965). Indirect fluorecent antibody and serum neutralisation response in pre-exposure prophylaxis against rabies. *Ann. Intern. Med.*, **63**, 955–64
206. Smith, A. H. (1966). Prophylactic immunization against rabies with duck embryo vaccine. *S. African Med. J.*, **40**, 1125
207. Garner, W. R., Jones, D. O. and Pratt, E. (1976). Problems associated with rabies pre-exposure prophylaxis. *J. Am. Med. Assoc.*, **235**, 1131–2
208. Morgan, P., Willis, R., Wood, R. and Leavitt, J. (1978). A comparison of pre-exposure rabies prophylaxis regimens using duck embryo vaccine. *Bull. Pan. Am. Hlth. Org.*, **12**, 257–60
209. Dean, D. J. and Sherman, I. (1962). Potency of commercial rabies vaccine used in man. *Public Hlth. Rep.*, **77**, 705–10
210. Rubin, R. H., Sikes, R. K. and Gregg, M. B. (1973). Human rabies immune globulin. Clinical trials and effects on serum anti-gamma-globulins. *J. Am. Med. Assoc.*, **224**, 871–4
211. Prussin, G. and Katabi, G. (1964). Dorsolumbar myelitis following antirabies vaccination with duck embryo vaccine. *Ann. Intern. Med.*, **60**, 114–16
212. Kaiser, H. B., Sokol, A. and Beall, G. N. (1965). Unusual reaction to rabies vaccine. *J. Am. Med. Assoc.*, **193**, 369–70
213. Cowdrey, S. C. (1966). Sensitization to duck embryo rabies vaccine produced by prior yellow fever vaccination. *N. Engl. J. Med.*, **274**, 1311–13
214. Perrine, P. L., Harris, D. and Kirkpatrick, C. H. (1968). Immunologic reactions to duck embryo rabies vaccine. *J. Am. Med. Assoc.*, **205**, 559–62
215. Harrington, R. B. and Olin, R. (1971). Incomplete transverse myelitis following rabies duck embryo vaccination. *J. Am. Med. Assoc.*, **216**, 2137–8
216. Mozar, H. N., Finnigan, F. B., Petzold, H., Spitler, L. E., Emmons, L. E., Emmons, R. W. and Rothenberg, B. (1973). Myelopathy after duck embryo rabies vaccine. *J. Am. Med. Assoc.*, **224**, 1605–7
217. Schlenska, G. K. (1976). Neurological complications following rabies duck embryo vaccination. *J. Neurol.*, **214**, 71–4
218. Schell, K. R., Fürst, M., Haberstich, H. U., Mischler, R., Hoskins, J. M. and Wegmann, A., (1980). A highly purified and concentrated duck embryo rabies vaccine: a preliminary report. *J. Biol. Stand.*, **8**, 97–106
219. Glück, R., Wegman, A., Germanier, R., Keller, H., Hess, M. W., Kraus-Ruppert, R. and Wandeler, A. I. (1984). A new highly immunogenic duck embryo rabies vaccine. *Lancet*, **1**, 844–5
220. Glück, R. (1985). A highly immunogenic duck embryo rabies vaccine. In Vodopija, I., Nicholson, K. G., Smerdel, S. and Bijok, U. (eds), *Improvements in Rabies Postexposure Treatment*, pp. 139–42. (Zagreb: Zagreb Institute of Public Health)
221. Kissling, R. E. (1958). Growth of rabies virus in non-nervous tissue culture. *Proc. Soc. Exp. Biol. Med.*, **98**, 223–5
222. Fenje, P. (1960). A rabies vaccine from hamster kidney tissue cultures: preparation and evaluation in animals. *Can. J. Microbiol.*, **6**, 605–9
223. Ott, G. L. and Heyke, G. (1962). Preliminary trials of a new tissue culture rabies vaccine. *Vet. Med.*, **57**, 158–9
224. Ott, G. L. and Heyke, G. (1962). Propagation of rabies virus; evaluation of a vaccine. *Vet. Med.*, **57**, 613–16
225. Fenje, P. and Pinteric, L. (1966). Potentiation of tissue culture rabies vaccine by adjuvants. *Am. J. Publ. Health*, **12**, 2106–13
226. Fenje, P. (1974). Production and control of tissue culture rabies vaccines for human use. *Symp. Ser. Immunobiol. Stand.*, **21**, 148–56
227. Cho, H. C., Fenje, P. and Sparkes, J. D. (1972). Antibody and immunoglobulin response to antirabies vaccination in man. *Infect. Immun.*, **6**, 483–6
228. Devadason, C. (1976). Rabies antibody studies in New Brunswick. *Can. J. Public Hlth.*, **67**, 255–7

229. Selimov, M. A. and Aksenova, T. A. (1966). Tissue culture antirabies vaccine for human use. *Symp. Ser. Immunobiol. Stand.*, **1**, 377–80
230. Selimov, M. A. Aksenova, T. A., Klyueva, E., Gribencha, K. and Levedeva, I. (1978). Evaluation of the inactivated tissue culture rabies vaccine from the Vnukovo-32 strain. Results of its industrial production and field use for post-exposure immunization of man. *Dev. Biol. Stand.*, **40**, 57–62
231. Sinnecker, H., Apitzsch, L., Sinnecker, R., Selimov, M., Giard, W., Grimm, J., Mueller, B., Rasch, G. and Zilske, E. (1978). Serological investigations on rabies tissue culture vaccine (USSR) and development of short methods in postexposure treatment. *Dev. Biol. Stand.*, 40, 155–8
232. Fang-Tao, L., Xiaou-Zeng, L., Shu-Beng, C., Guao-Fu, W., Fan-Zhen, Z., Long- Mu, L., Nai-Min, C. and Ji-Zui, F. (1985). Further study on the stability and efficacy of the primary hamster kidney cell rabies vaccine. In Vodopija, I., Nicholson, K. G., Smerdel, S. and Bijok, U. (eds), *Improvements in Rabies Postexposure Treatment*. Zagreb: Zagreb Institute of Public Health)
233. Fang-Tao, L., Fan-Zhen, Z., Long- Mu, L., Xiaou-Zeng, L., Rong-Fang, Z., Yung-Rin, Y. and Nai-Min, C. (1983). The primary hamster kidney cell rabies vaccine: adaptation of viral strain production of vaccine and pre- and postexposure treatment. *J. Infect Dis.*, **147**, 467–73
234. Kondo, A., Takashima, Y. and Suzuki, M. (1974). Inactivated rabies vaccine of chick embryo cell culture origin. *Symp. Ser. Immunobiol. Stand.*, **21**, 182–9
235. Barth, R., Bijok, U, Gruschkau, H., Smerdel, S. and Vodopija, I. (1983). Purified chick embryo cell rabies vaccine for human use. *Lancet*, **1**, 700
236. Kondo, A. (1978). Pre-immunization and post-exposure treatment with inactivated rabies vaccine of chick embryo cell culture origin (CEC). *Dev. Biol. Stand.*, **40**, 147–53
237. Bijok, U. (1985). Purified chick embryo cell (PCEC) rabies vaccine: a review of the clinical development. In Vodopija, I., Nicholson, K. G., Smerdel, S. and Bijok, U. (eds), *Improvements in Rabies Postexposure Treatment*, pp. 103–11. (Zagreb: Zagreb Institute of Public Health)
238. Wasi, C., Chaiprasithikul, P., Chavanich, L., Puthavathana, P., Thongcharoen, P. and Trishanaanda, M. (1986). Purified chick embryo cell rabies vaccine. *Lancet*, **1**, 40
239. Nicholson, K. G., Farrow, P. R., Bijok, U. and Barth, R. (1987). Pre-exposure studies with purified chick embryo cell culture rabies vaccine and human diploid cell vaccine: serological and clinical responses in man. *Vaccine*, **5**, 208–10
240. Ljubicic, M., Vodopiji, I., Smerdel, S., Baklaic, Z., Svjetlicic, M. and Lojkic, M. (1985). Efficacy of PCEC vaccine in post-exposure rabies prophylaxis. In Vodopija, I., Nicholson, K. G., Smerdel, S. and Bijok, U. (eds), *Improvements in Rabies Postexposure Treatment*, pp. 95–101. (Zagreb: Zagreb Institute of Public Health)
241. Wasi, C. Chaiprasithikul, P., Puthavathana, P., Chavanich, L. and Thongcharoen, P. (1985). Immunogenicity and reactogenicity of the new tissue culture rabies vaccine for human use (purified chick embryo cell culture). In Vodopija, I., Nicholson, K. G., Smerdel, S. and Bijok, U. (eds), *Improvements in Rabies Postexposure Treatment*, pp. 85–94. (Zagreb: Zagreb Institute of Public Health)
242. Lavender, J. F. and Van Frank, R. M. (1971). Zonal centrifuged purified duck embryo cell culture rabies vaccine for human vaccination. *Appl. Microbiol.*, **22**, 358–65
243. Lavender, J. F. (1973). Immune response in primates vaccinated with duck embryo cell culture rabies vaccine. *Appl. Microbiol.*, **25**, 327–31
244. Atanasiu, P., Tsiang, H. and Gamet, A. (1974). A new rabies vaccine for human use prepared in primary tissue culture. *Ann. Microbiol. (Inst. Pasteur)*, **125B**, 419–32
245. Atanasiu, P., Tsiang, H., Recualrd, P., Aguilon, F., Lavergne, M. and Adamovicz P. (1978). Zonal centrifuge purification of human rabies vaccine obtained on bovine fetal kidney cells. Biological results. *Dev. Biol. Stand.*, **40**, 35–44
246. Van Wezel, A. L. and Van Steenis, G. (1978). Production of an inactivated rabies vaccine in primary dog kidney cells. *Dev. Biol. Stand.*, **40**, 69–75
247. Bektimirova, M. S., Osidze, D. F., Pille, E. R., Nadiachik, L. V., Matevosyan, K. Sh., Nagieva, F. G., Bogomolva, N. N., Boriskin, Yu. S. and Yanova, N. N. (1979). Properties of rabies virus (MNIIVP-74 strain) adapted to Japanese quail embryo cell culture. *Arch. Virol.*, **61**, 61–8
248. L'Institut Pasteur Production (1985). Characteristics of new rabies vaccines. In Vodiopija,

I., Nicholson, K. G., Smerdel, S. and Bijok, U. (eds), *Improvements in Rabies Postexposure Treatment.* (Zagreb: Zagreb Institute of Public Health)

249. Sureau, P., Rollin, P. E., Fritzell, B., Loucq, C., Marie, F. N., Courrier, A., Simonnet Ph, Arbogast, J. Fremont, J., Gaudiot, C. and Malo, J.-P. (1985). Reactogenicity and immunogenicity of primary fetal bovine kidney cell (FBKC) rabies vaccine: post-exposure treatment. In Vodopija, I., Nicholson, K. G., Smerdel, S. and Bijok, U. (eds), *Improvements in Rabies Postexposure Treatment.* (Zagreb: Zagreb Institute of Public Health)
250. Wiktor, T. J. and Koprowski, H. (1965). Successful immunisation of primates with rabies vaccine prepared in human diploid cell strain WI-38. *Proc. Soc. Exp. Biol. Med.*, **118**, 1069–73
251. Hayflick, L. and Moorhead, P. S. (1961). The serial cultivation of human diploid cell strains. *Exp. Cell. Res.*, **25**, 585–621
252. Plotkin, S. A. (1971). Vaccine production in human diploid cells. *Am. J. Epidemiol.*, **94**, 303–6
253. Plotkin, S. A., Farquhar, F. and Hornberger, E. (1976). Clinical trials of immunization with the Towne 125 strain of human cytomegalovirus. *J. Infect. Dis.*, **134**, 470–5
254. Takahashi, M., Okuno, Y., Otsuka, T., Osame, J., Takamizawa, A., Sasada, T. and Kubo, T. (1975). Development of a live attenuated varicella vaccine. *Biken J.*, **18**, 25–33
255. Wiktor, T. J., Plotkin, S. A. and Koprowski, H. (1978). Development and clinical trials of the new human rabies vaccine of tissue culture (human diploid cell) origin. *Dev. Biol. Stand.*, **40**, 3–9
256. Wiktor, T. J. and Clark, H. F. (1975). Growth of rabies virus in cell culture. In Baer, G. M. (ed.), *The Natural History of Rabies*, Vol 1, pp. 155–79. (New York: Academic Press)
257. Sokol, F., Kuwert, E., Wiktor, T. J., Hummeler, K. and Koprowski, H. (1968). Purification of rabies virus grown in tissue culture. *J. Virol.*, **2**, 836–49
258. Wiktor, T. J., Sokol, F., Kuwert, E. and Koprowski, H. (1969). Immunogenicity of concentrated and purified rabies vaccine of tissue culture origin. *Proc. Soc. Exp. Biol. Med.*, **131**, 799–805
259. Schlumberger, H. D., Wiktor, T. J. and Koprowski, H. (1970). Antigenic and immunogenic properties of components contained in rabies virus-infected tissue culture fluids. *J. Immunol.*, **105**, 291–8
260. Koprowski, H. (1971). Pre- and postexposure prophylaxis: present status and current trends. In Nagano, Y. and Davenport, F. M. (eds), *Proceedings of a Working Conference on Rabies, Tokyo*, 1970, pp. 111–26. (Univeristy of Tokyo Press)
261. Plotkin, S. A. (1980). Rabies vaccine prepared in human diploid cell cultures: progress and perspectives. *Rev. Infect. Dis.*, **2**, 433–47
262. Wiktor, T. J., Plotkin, S. A. and Grella, D. W. (1973). Human cell culture rabies vaccine. Antibody responses in man. *J. Am. Med. Assoc.*, **224**, 1170–1
263. Kaplan, M. (1974). Preliminary results on antibody profiles of humans receiving inactivated vaccine prepared in human diploid cells. *Symp. Ser. Immunobiol. Stand.*, **21**, 226–30
264. Bahmanyar, M. (1974). Preliminary results on antibody profiles of human receiving concentrated inactivated vaccine prepared in human diploid cells. *Symp. Ser. Immunobiol. Stand.*, **21**, 226–30
265. Bahmanyar, M., Fayaz, A., Nour-Salehi, S., Mohammadi, M. and Koprowski, H. (1976). Successful protection of humans exposed to rabies infection. Postexposure treatment with new human diploid cell rabies vaccine and antirabies serum. *J. Am. Med. Asso.*, **236**, 2751–54
266. Kuwert, E. K., Marcus, I., Werner, J., Scheiermann, N., Höher, P. G., Thraenhart, O., Hierhölzer, E., Wiktor, T. J. and Koprowski, H. (1977). Post-exposure use of human diploid cell culture rabies vaccine. *Dev. Biol. Stand.*, **37**, 273–86
267. Gardner, S. D. (1983). Prevention of rabies in man in England and Wales. In Pattison, J. R. (ed), *Rabies: a Growing Threat*, pp. 39–49. (Wokingham: Van Nostrand Reinhold)
268. Boe, E. and Nyland, H. (1980). Guillain-Barré syndrome after vaccination with human diploid cell rabies vaccine. *Scand. J. Infect. Dis.*, **12**, 231–2
269. Bernard, K. W., Smith, P. W., Kader, F. J. and Moran, M. J. (1982). Neuroparalytic illness and human diploid cell rabies vaccine. *J. Am. Med. Assoc.*, **248**, 3136–8
270. Aoki, F. Y., Tyrell, D. A. J., Hill, L. E. and Turner, G. S. (1975). Immunogenicity and acceptability of a human diploid cell culture rabies vaccine in volunteers. *Lancet*, **1**, 660–2

271. Nicholson, K. G. and Turner, G. S. (1978). Studies with human diploid cell strain rabies vaccine and human antirabies immunoglobulin in man. *Dev. Biol. Stand.*, **40**, 115–20
272. Turner, G. S., Nicholson, K. G., Tyrrell, D. A. J. and Aoki, F. Y. (1982). Evaluation of a human diploid cell strain rabies vaccine: final report of a three year study of pre-exposure immunization. *J. Hyg. (Camb)*, **89**, 101–10
273. Cox, J. H. and Schneider, L. G. (1976). Prophylactic immunization of humans against rabies by intradermal inoculation of human diploid cell culture vaccine. *J. Clin. Microbiol.*, **3**, 96–101
274. MMWR. (1984). Systemic allergic reactions following immunization with human diploid cell rabies vaccine. **33**, 185–7
275. Winkler, G. (1985). Current status of use of human diploid cell strain rabies vaccine in the US – May 1984. In Vodopija, I., Nicholson, K. G., Smerdel, S. and Bijok, U. (eds), *Improvements in Rabies Postexposure Treatment*, pp. 3–8. (Zagreb: Institute of Public Health)
276. Anonymous. (1985). Changes recommended in use of human diploid cell rabies vaccine. *J. Am. Med. Assoc.*, **254**, 14–15
277. Baer, H., Anderson, M. C. and Quinnan, G. (1985). Beta-propiolactone treated human serum albumin (BPL-HSA): an allergen for humans receiving rabies vaccine. *J. Allergy Clin. Immunol.*, **75**, 137
277a. Levenbook, I. S., Merritt, B. A., Fitzgerald, E. A. and Elisberg, B. L. (1986). Sensitization induced in guinea pigs with beta-propiolactone-treated serum albumin: experimental evidence for the cause of allergic reactions in humans receiving human diploid cell rabies vaccines. *Int. Arch. Allergy Appl. Immunol.*, **80**, 110–1
278. Turner, G. S., Aoki, F. Y., Nicholson, K. G., Tyrrell, D. A. J. and Hill, L. E. (1976). Human diploid cell strain rabies vaccine. Rapid prophylactic immunisation of volunteers with small doses. *Lancet*, **1**, 1379–81
279. Nicholson, K. G., Cole, P. J., Turner, G. S. and Harrison, P. (1979). Immune responses of humans to a human diploid cell strain of rabies virus vaccine: lymphocyte transformation, production of virus neutralizing antibody, and induction of interferon. *J. Infect. Dis.*, **140**, 176–82
280. Nicholson, K. G., Kuwert, E. K., Werner, J. and Harrison, P. (1979). Interferon reponse to human diploid cell strain vaccines in man. *Arch. Virol.*, **61**, 35–9
281. Nicholson, K. G., Prestage, H., Cole, P. J., Turner, G. S., Bauer, S. P. (1981). Multisite intradermal antirabies vaccination. Immune responses in man and protection of rabbits against death from street virus by post-exposure administration of human diploid cell rabies vaccine. *Lancet*, **2**, 915–18
282. Warrell, M. J., Warrell, D. A., Suntharasamai, P., Viravan, C., Sinhaseni, A., Udomsakdi, D., Phanfung, R., Xueref, C., Vincent-Falquet, J.-C., Nicholson, K. G., Bunnag, D. and Harinasuta, T. (1983). An economic regimen of human diploid cell strain anti-rabies vaccine for post-exposure prophylaxis. *Lancet*, **2**, 301–4
283. Warrell, M. J., Suntharasamai, P., Nicholson, K. G., Warrel, D. A., Chantavanich, P., Viravan, C., Sinhaseni, A., Phanfung, R., Xueref, C. and Vincent-Falquest, J.-C. (1984). Multi-site intradermal and multi-site subcutaneous rabies vaccination: improved economical regimens. *Lancet*, **1**, 874–6
284. Warrell, M. J., Nicholson, K. G., Warrel, D. A., Suntharasamai, P., Chantavanich, P., Viravan, C., Sinhaseni, A., Chiewbamroongkiat, M. K., Pouradier-Duteil, X., Xueref, C., Phanfung, R. and Udomsakdi, D. (1985). Economical multiple-site intradermal immunisation with human diploid-cell-strain vaccine is effective for post-exposure rabies prophylaxis. *Lancet*, **1**, 1059–62
285. Ratanavongsiri, J., Sriwanthana, B., Ubol, S. and Phanuphak, P. (1985). Cell-mediated immune response following intracutaneous immunisation with human diploid cell rabies vaccine. *Asian Pacific J. Allerg. Immunol.*, **3**, 187–90
286. Ubol, S. and Phanuphak, P. (1986). An effective economical intradermal regimen of human diploid cell rabies vaccination for post-exposure treatment. *Clin. Exp. Immunol.*, **63**, 491–7
287. Phanuphak, P., Khawplod, P., Sirivichayalkul, S., Siriprasomsub, W., Ubol, S. and Thaweepathomwat, M. (1987). Humoral and cell-mediated immune responses to various economical regimens of purified vero cell rabies vaccine. *Asian Pacific J. Allergy Immunol.*, **5**, 33–7

288. Smerdel, S., Vodopija, I., Svjetlicic, M., Baklaic, Z., Ljubicic, M., Pouradrier-Duteil, X., Xuref, C. and Zayet-Bechelet, M. (1985). A study in abbreviated regimens of rabies vaccinations with a standard (Merieux) HDCS vaccine. In Vodopija, I. *et al.* (eds), *Improvements in Rabies Postexposure Treatment.* (Zagreb: Institute of Public Health), pp. 171–7
289. Vodopija, I., Sureau, P., Lafon, M., Baklaic, Z., Ljubicic, M., Svejetlicic, M. and Smerdel, S. (1986). An evaluation of second generation tissue culture rabies vaccines for use in man: a four-vaccine comparative immunogenicity study using a pre-exposure vaccination schedule and an abbreviated 2–1–1 postexposure schedule. *Vaccine,* **4**, 245–8
290. WHO (1978). Application of rabies vaccines at reduced schedules. *Wkly. Epidem. Rec.,* **53**, 213–15
291. Anonymous (1984). Rabies prevention, United States, 1984. *J. Am. Med., Assoc.,* **252**, 883–93
292. MMWR. (1982). Supplementary statement on pre-exposure rabies prophylaxis by the intradermal route. **31**, 279–85
293. Bernard, K. W., Roberts, M. A., Sumner, J., Winkler, W.G., Mallonee, J., Baer, G. M. and Chaney, R. (1982). Human diploid cell rabies vaccine. Effectiveness of immunization with small intradermal or subcutaneous doses. *J. Am. Med. Assoc.,* **247**, 1138–42
294. Kuwert, E. K., Menzel, H., Marcus, I. and Majer, M. (1978). Antigenicity of low concentrated HDCS vaccine with and without adjuvant as compared to the standard fluid formulation. *Dev. Biol. Stand.,* **40**, 29–34
295. Klietman, W., Klietman, B., Cox, J. H., Biron, G. and Charbonnier, C. (1983). Comparative study of rabies immunization with HDCV (Mérieux) using reduced amounts of vaccine with and without adjuvant. In Kuwert, E. Mérieux, C., Koprowski, H. and Bögel, K., (eds), *Rabies in the Tropics,* pp. 153–61. (Berlin: Springer-Verlag)
296. Fishbein, D. B., Pacer, R. E., Holmes, D. F., Ley, A. B., Yager, P. and Tong,T C. (1987). Rabies preexposure prophylaxis with human diploid cell rabies vaccine: a dose-response study. *J. Infect. Dis.,* **156**, 50–5
297. MMWR. (1983). Field evaluations of pre-exposure use of human diploid cell rabies vaccine, **32**, 601–3
298. Bernard, K. W., Fishbein, D. B., Miller, K. D., Parker, R. A., Waterman, S., Sumner, J. W., Reid, F. L., Johnson, B. K., Rollins, A. J., Oster, C. N., Schonberger, L. B., Baer, G. M. and Winkler, W. G. (1985). Preexposure rabies immunization with human diploid cell vaccine: decreased antibody responses in persons immunized in developing countries. *Am. J. Trop. Med. Hyg.,* **34**, 633–47
299. Nicholson, K. G., Burney, M. I., Ali, S. and Perkins, F. T. (1983). Stability of human diploid-cell-strain rabies vaccine at high ambient temperatures. *Lancet,* **1**, 916–18
300. Fishbein, D. B., Sumner, J. W., Dressen, D. W. and Wagner, V. E. (1986). Human diploid cell rabies vaccine: retention of immunogenicity after reconstruction. *Trans. Roy. Soc. Trop. Med. Hyg.,* **80**, 172
301. Taylor, D. N., Wasi, C. and Bernard, K. (1984). Chloroquine prophylaxis associated with a poor antibody response to human diploid cell rabies vaccine. *Lancet,* **1**, 1405
302. Pappaioanou, M., Fishbein, D. B., Dressen, D. W., Schwartz, I. K., Campbell, G. H., Sumner, J. W., Patchen, L. C. and Brown, W. J. (1986). Antibody response to preexposure human diploid cell rabies vaccine given concurrently with chloroquine. *N. Engl. J. Med.,* **314**, 280–4
303. Shill, M., Baynes, R. D. and Miller, S. D. (1987). Fatal rabies encephalities despite appropriate post-exposure prophylaxis. *N. Engl. J. Med.,* **316**,1257–8
304. Fishbein, D. B., Sawyer, L. A., Reid-Sanden, F. L. and Weir, E. H. (1988). Administration of human diploid cell rabies vaccine in the gluteal area. *N. Engl. J. Med.,* **318**, 124–5
305. Hefti, J., Keller, H., Geiser, M., Gerber, H., Wandeler, A. and Steck, F. (1979). Antikörperbestimmung nach prophylaktischer und postexpositioneller tollwutschutzimpfung. *Schweiz Med. Woch.,* **109**, 509–16
306. Montagnon, B. J., Fournier, P. and Vincent-Falquet, J. C. (1985). Un nouveau vaccin antirabique a usage humain: rapport préliminaire. In Kuwert, E., Mérieux, C., Koprowski, H. and Bögel, K. (eds) *Rabies in the Tropics,* pp. 138–43 (Berlin: Springer-Verlag)
307. Fournier, P., Montagnon, B., Vincent-Falquet, J. C., Ajjan, N., Drucker, J., and Roumiantzeff, M. (1985). A new vaccine produced from rabies virus cultivated on vero cells. In

Vodopija, I., Nicholson, K. G., Smerdel, S. and Bijok, U. (eds), *Improvements in Rabies Postexposure Treatment*, pp. 115–21. (Zagreb: Zagreb Institute of Public Health)

308. Baer, G. M., Shaddock, J. H., Moore, S. A., Yager, P. A., Baron, S. S. and Levy, H. B. (1977). Successful prophylaxis against rabies in mice and rhesus monkeys: the interferon system and vaccine. *J. Infect. Dis.*, **136**, 286–91
309. Baer, G. M. and Yager, P. A. (1977). A mouse model for post-exposure rabies prophylaxis. The comparative efficacy of two vaccines and of antiserum administration. *J. Gen. Virol.*, **36**, 51–8
310. Fenje, P. and Postic, B. (1970). Protection of rabbits against experimental rabies by poly I – poly C. *Nature*, **226**, 171–2
311. Fenje, P. and Postic, B. (1971). Prophylaxis of experimental rabies with the polyriboinosinic–polyribocytidilic acid complex. *J. Infect. Dis.*, **123**, 426–8
312. Harmon, M. W. and Janis, B. (1975). Therapy of murine rabies after exposure: efficacy of polyriboinosinic-polyribocytidilic acid alone and in combination with three rabies vaccines. *J. Infect. Dis.*, **132**, 241–9
313. Hilfenhaus, J., Karges, H. E., Weinmann, E. and Barth, R. (1975). Effect of administered human interferon on experimental rabies in monkeys. *Infect. Immun.* **11**, 1156–8
314. Janis, B. and Habel, K. (1972). Rabies in rabbits and mice: protective effect of polyriboinosinic-polycytidilic acid. *J. Infect. Dis.*, **125**, 345–52
315. Kaplan, M., Cohen, D., Koprowski, H., Dean, D. and Ferrigan, L. (1962). Studies on the local treatment of wounds for the prevention of rabies. *Bull. WHO*, **26**, 765–75
316. Postic, B. and Fenje, P. (1971). Effect of administered interferon on rabies in rabbits. *Appl. Microbiol.*, **22**, 428–31
317. Turner, G. S. (1972). Rabies vaccines and interferon. *J. Hgy. (Camb.)*, **70**, 445–53
318. Vieuchange, J. (1967). Inteference entre le virus vaccinal et le virus rabique, role éventuel d'un interferon. *Arch. Ges. Virusforsch.*, **22**, 87–96
319. Vieuchange, J. and Fayaz, A. (1969). Essais de prévention de la rage expérimental du lapin par un extrait tissulaire de type 'interferon' injecté pendant la periode d'incubation. *C.R. Acad. Sci.*, **268**, 99–3
320. Wiktor, T. J., Postic, B., Ho, M. and Koprowski, H. (1972). Role of interferon induction in the protective efficacy of rabies vaccines. *J. Infect. Dis.*, **126**, 408–18
322. Pille, E. R. and Matevoysan, K. Sh. (1985). Inteferonogenicity of rabies vaccines as related to their therapeutic and prophylactic activities. *Acta Virol.*, **29**, 386–92
323. Baer, M., More, S. A., Shaddock, J. H. and Levy, B. (1979). An effective rabies treatment in exposed monkeys: a single dose of interferon inducer and vaccine. *Bull. WHO*, **57**, 807–13
324. Scheiermann, N., Baer, J., Hilfenhaus, J., Marcus, I. and Zoulek, G. (1987). Reactogenicity and immunogenicity of the newly developed purified chick embryo cell (PCEC)-rabies vaccine in man. *Zbl. Bakt. Hyg.*, **A265**, 439–50
325. Fermi, C. (1909). Wirkung der Antiwutimpstoffe und sera je nach der Tierspecies, aus welcher sie entstammen und welcher sie verabreicht werden. *Zbl Bakt.*, **49**, 452–7
326. Marie, A. (1908). Recherches sur le sérum antirabique. *Ann. Inst. Pasteur*, **22**, 271–88
327. Cabasso, V. J. (1976). Rabies immune globulin (human) in the prevention of rabies. *Am. J. Hosp. Pharm.*, **33**, 48–51
328. Proca, G. Bobes, S. and Jonnesco, D. (1934). Inoculation intracaudale du virus rabique et serotherapie de la rage. *C. R. Soc. Biol.*, **115**, 1313–15
329. Shortt, H. E., McGuire, J. P., Brooks, A. G. and Stephens, E. D. (1935). Anti-rabic immunization: probable lines of progress in improvement of methods. *Ind. J. Med. Res.*, **22**, 537–56
330. Covell, G., McGuire, J. P., Stephens, E. D., and Lahiri, B. N. (1936). Notes on antirabic immunization. *Ind. J. Med. Res.*, **24**, 373–88
331. Jonnesco, D. (1939). Recherches sur un sérum antirabique. *C. R. Soc. Biol.*, **130**, 1145–8
332. Proca, G. Bobes, S. and Jonnesco, D. (1934). Sur la serotherapie préventive de la rage. *C. R. Soc. Biol.*, **115**, 1001–3
333. Hoyt, A., Fisk, R. T., and Moore, F. J. (1935). Experimental rabies in white mice. Studies on passive immunization. *Proc. Soc. Exp. Biol. Med.*, **32**, 1560–1
334. Hoyt, A., Fisk, R. T. Moore, F. J. and Tracy, R. L. (1936). Experimental rabies in white mice. II Studies on passive immunization. *J. Infect. Dis.*, **59**, 152–8

335. Hoyt, A. and Gurley, M. K. (1937). Experimental street virus rabies in white mice. Studies on passive immunization. I. *Proc. Soc. Exp. Biol. Med.*, **37**, 454–5
336. Hoyt, A., Moore, F. J., Gurley, M. K. and Warner, D. (1938). Experiments on antirabic immunization. *J. Bacteriol.*, **36**, 287–8
337. Habel, K. (1954). Antiserum in the prophylaxis of rabies. *Bull. WHO*, **10**, 781–8
338. Habel, K. (1941). Tissue factors in antirabies immunity of experimental animals. *Public Hlth. Rep.*, **5**, 692–702
339. Gallardo, F. P., Zarzuelo, E. and Kaplan, M. M. (1957). Local treatment of rabies to prevent rabies. *Bull. WHO*, **17**, 963–78
340. Schindler, R. (1961). Protective effect of antirabies serum after intracerebral or intramuscular administration. *Bull. WHO*, **25**, 127–8
341. Soloviev, V. D. and Kobrinski, G. D. (1962). Local application of antirabies gamma globulin in dried form for the prevention of rabies. *Bull. WHO*, **26**, 777–82
342. Dean, D. J., Baer, G. M. and Thomson, W. R. (1963). Studies on the local treatment of rabies-infected wounds. *Bull. WHO*, **28**, 477–86
343. Kaplan, M. M. and Paccaud, M. F. (1963). Effectiveness of locally inoculated antirabies serum and gamma globulin in rabies infection of mice. *Bull. WHO*, **28**, 495–7
344. WHO, Expert Committee on Rabies (1957). Third Report. Technical Report Series No. 121. (Geneva: WHO)
345. Moynihan, N. H. (1955). Serum-sickness and local reactions in tetanus prophylaxis. *Lancet*, **2**, 264–6
346. Hosty, T. S. and Hunter, F. R. (1953). Incidence of reactions to antirabies horse serum. *Public Hlth. Rep.*, **68**, 789–91
347. Karliner, J. S. and Belaval, G. S. (1965). Incidence of reactions following administration of antirabies serum. *J. Am. Med. Assoc.*, **193**, 109–12
348. Anderson, G. R. and Sgouris, J. T. (1966). The preparation of rabies immune globulin and use in monkeys following virus challenge. *Symp. Ser. Immunobiol. Stand.*, **1**, 319–32
348a. Veeraraghaven, N., Subrahmanyan, T.P., Rangasami, R. and Kulla, A. (1958). Studies on antirabies serum. Pasteur Institute of Southern India, Coonoor. *Annual Report of the Director* (1956) *and Scientific Report* (1957). pp. 44–60. Madras
349. Archer, B. G. and Dierks, R. E. (1968). Effects of homologous or heterologous antiserum on neutralizing-antibody response to rabies vaccine. *Bull. WHO*, **39**, 407–17
350. Babes, and Cerchez (cited in ref. 351)
351. Semple, D. (1908). On the preparation and use of antirabic serum, and on the rabicidal properties of the serum of patients after undergoing antirabic treatment; also a note on the blood of a patient suffering from hydrophobia. *Lancet*, **1**, 1611–18
352. Proca, G., Bobes, S. and Jonnesco, D. (1937). Sérothérapie de la rage. *C.R. Soc. Biol.*, **2**, 609–17
353. Smith, R. O. A. (1937). Antirabic vaccine enquiry. *Rep. Sci. Adv. Bd. Ind. Res. Fund Assoc.*, **ST-567**, 64–8
354. Koprowski, H. and Cox, H. R. (1951). Recent developments in the prophylaxis of rabies. *Am. J. Public Hlth.*, **41**, 1483–9
354a. Koprowski, H., Van der Scheer and Black, J. (1950). Use of hyperimmune antirabies serum concentrates in experimental rabies. *Am. J. Med.*, **8**, 412–20
355. Baltazard, M., Bahmanyar, M., Ghodssi, M., Sabeti, A., Gajdusek, C., and Rouzbehi, E. (1955). Essai pratique du sérum antirabique chez les mordus par loups enragés. *Bull. WHO*, **13**, 747–72
356. Selimov, A., Boltucij, L., Semenova, E., Kobrinskij, G. and Zmusco, L. (1959). Anwendung des antirbies-gammaglobulins bei menschen, die von tollwütigen wölfen oder anderen tieren schwer gebissen wurden. *J. Hyg. Epidemiol. Microbiol. Immunol.*, **3**, 168–80
357. Atanasiu, P., Bahamanyar, M., Baltazard, M., Fox, J. P., Habel, K., Kaplan, M. M., Kissling, R. E., Komarov, A., Koprowski, H., Lépine, P., Pérez Gallardo, F. and Schaeffer, M. (1956). Rabies neutralizing antibody response to different schedules of serum and vaccine in non-exposed persons. *Bull. WHO*, **14**, 593–611
358. Atanasiu, P., Bahamanyar, M., Baltazard, M., Fox, J. P., Habel, K., Kaplan, M. M., Kissling, R. E., Komarov, A., Koprowski, H., Lépine, P., Pérez Gallardo, F. and Schaeffer, M. (1957). Rabies neutralizing antibody response to different schedules of serum and vaccine in non-exposed persons: Part II. *Bull. WHO*, **17**, 911–32

359. Atanasiu, P., Cannon, D. A., Dean, D. J., Fox, J. P., Habel, K., Kaplan, M. M., Kissling, R. E., Koprowski, H., Lépine, P., Pérez Gallardo, F. (1961). Rabies neutralizing antibody response to different schedules of serum and vaccine in non-exposed persons: Part III. *Bull. WHO*, **25**, 103–14

360. Atanasiu, P., Dean, D. J., Habel, K., Kaplan, M. M., Koprowski, H., Lépine, P. and Serie, C. (1967). Rabies neutralizing antibody response to different schedules of serum and vaccine in non-exposed persons: Part IV. *Bull. WHO*, **14**, 593–611

361. Rubin, R. H., Gregg, M. B. and Sike, R. K. (1969). Rabies in citizens in the United States, 1963–68: Epidemiology, treatment, and complications of treatment. *J. Infect. Dis.*, **120**, 268–73

362. Dehner, L. P. (1970). Human rabies encephalitis in Vietnam, *Ann. Intern. Med.*, **72**, 375–8

363. Hattwick, M. A. W., Hochberg, F. H., Landrigan, P. J. and Gregg, M. B. (1972). Skunk associated human rabies. *J. Am. Med. Assoc.*, **22**, 44–7

364. Shah, U. and Jaswal, G. S. (1976). Victims of a rabid wolf bite in India: effect of severity and location of bites on development of rabies. *J. Infect. Dis.*, **134**, 25–9

364a. Anderson, J. A., Daly, F. T. and Kidd, J. C. (1966). Human rabies after antiserum and vaccine post-exposure treatment. *Ann. Intern. Med.*, **64**, 1297–302

365. Hosty, T. S., Kissling, R. E., Schaeffer, M., Wallace, G. A. Dibble, E. H. (1959). Human rabies gamma globulin. *Bull. WHO*, **20**, 1111–19

366. Cohn, E. J., Strong, L. E., Hughes, W. H., Mulford, D. J., Ashworth, J. N., Melin, M. and Taylor, H. L. (1946). Preparation and properties of serum and plasma proteins, IV. A system for the separation into fractions of the protein and lipoprotein components of biological tissues and fluids. *J. Am. Chem. Soc.*, **68**, 459–75

367. Oncley, J. L., Melin, M., Richert, D. A., Cameron, J. W. and Gross, P. M. (1949). The separation of the antibodies, isoagglutinins, plasminogen, and β1-lipoprotein into subfractions of human plasma. *J. Am. Chem. Soc.*, **71**, 541–50

368. Smolens, J., Vogt, A. B. and Crawford, M. N. (1961). The persistence in the human circulation of horse and human tetanus antitoxins. *J. Pediatr.*, **59**, 899–902

369. Sikes, R. K. (1969). Human rabies immune globulin. *Public Hlth. Rep.*, **84**, 797–801

370. Loofbourow, J. C. Cabasso, V. J., Roby, R. E. and Anuskiewicz, W. (1971). Rabies immune globulin (human). Clinical trials and dose determination. *J. Am. Med. Assoc.*, **217**, 1825–31

371. Dierks, R. E., Gough, P. M. and Rubin, R. H. (1974). Comparative studies of the immunological response to duck embryo vaccine and/or human rabies immune globulin in man. *Symp. Ser. Immunobiol. Stand.*, **21**, 267–76

372. Hafkin, B., Alls, M. E. and Baer, G. M. (1978). Human rabies globulin and human diploid vaccine dose determinations. *Dev. Biol. Stand.*, **40**, 121–7

372a. Kuwert, E.K., Werner, J., Marcus, I. and Cabasso, V.J. (1978). Serovaccination by human immunoglobulin and HDLS vaccine against rabies. *Devel. Biol. Stand.*, **40**, 129–36

373. Mertz, G. J., Nelson, K. E., Vithayasai, V., Makornakwkeyoon, S., Rosanoff, E. I., Tint, H., and Wiktor, T. J. (1982). Antibody responses to human diploid cell vaccine with and without rabies immune globulin. *J. Infect. Dis.*, **145**, 720–7

374. Keller, H., Hauser, R., Wandeler, A. and Steck, F. (1977). Versuche zur postexpositionellen aktiven und passiven immunisierung gegen tollwut beim menschen. *Schweiz. Med. Woch.*, **107**, 1857–9

374a. Nicholson, K. G. Turner, G. S. and Aoki, F. Y. (1978). Immunization with a human diploid cell strain of rabies virus vaccine. Two year results. *J. Infect. Dis.*, **137**, 783–8

375. Steck, F., Spengler, G. A., Hauser, R., Keller, H. and Wandeler, A. I. (1978). IgM and IgG antibody profiles after immunization of man with a HDCS-vaccine (preliminary communication). *Dev. Biol. Stand.*, **40**, 137–9

376. Méan, F, Steck, F. and Tanner, F. (1978). Humoral immunity conferred by the HDCS rabies vaccine Merieux administered after exposure. 151 cases with and without specfic immune globulin of human origin. *Dev. Biol. Stand.*, **40**, 159–61

377. Méan, F. (1980). La rage, données pour la prevention et le traitement prococé, et contribution a l'évaluation immunologique et epidémiologique du vaccin antirabique cultivé sur céllules diploides humaines dans l'emploi aprés exposition. MD thesis, University of Lausanne, 1980

378. Klietman, W., Schöttle, A., Klietman, B. and Cox, J. (1981). A lare scale antirabies immunization study in humans using HDCS vaccine: prophylactic vaccination using different routes of application and post exposure treatment combined with and without simultaneous serum administration. In Kuwert, E. K., Wiktor, T. J. and Koprowski, H. (eds). *Cell Culture Rabies Vaccines and their Protective Effect in Man*, pp. 330–7. (Geneva: International Green Cross)
379. Anilionis, A., Wunner, W. H. and Curtis, P. J. (1981). Structure of the glycoprotein gene in rabies virus. *Nature*, **294**, 275–78
380. WHO (1984). Expert Committee on Rabies, Seventh Report. Technical Report Series 709, (Geneva: WHO).
381. Yelverton, E., Norton, S., Obijeski, J. F. and Goeddel, D. V. (1983). Rabies virus glycoprotein analogs: biosynthesis in *Escherichia coli*. *Science*, **219**, 614–20
382. Lathe, R., Kieny, M. P., Schmitt, D., Curtis, P. and Lecocq, J. P. (1984). M13 bacteriophage vectors for the expression of foreign proteins in Escherichia coli: the rabies glycoprotein. *J. Molec. Appl. Gen.* **2**, 331–42
383. Kieny, M. P., Lathe, R., Drillien, R., Lemoine, Y., Wiktor, T. and Lecocq, J. P. (1985). Rabies protectin via genetic engineering: expression of the surface glycoprotein in vaccinia virus and other vectors. In Vodopija, I., Nicholson, K. G., Smerdel, S. and Bijok, U. (eds), *Improvements in Rabies Postexposure Treatment*, pp. 195–9. (Zagreb: Zagreb Institute of Public Health)
384. Trejos, A., Lewis, V., Fuenzalida, E. and Larghi, O. P. (1971). Laboratory investigations of neuroparalytic accidents associated with suckling mouse brain rabies vaccine. *Ann. Immunol.* (*Inst. Pasteur*), **125C**, 917–24
385. Hattwick, M. A. W., Rubin, R. H., Music, S., Sikes, R. K., Smith, J. S. and Gregg, M. B. (1974). Postexposure rabies prophylaxis with human rabies immune globulin. *J. Am. Med. Assoc.*, **227**, 407–410

9
Rubella vaccines

J. E. BANATVALA and J. M. BEST

Immunization against rubella is unique since, in contrast with vaccination against other diseases, its aim is not to prevent a severe disease or its complications in the recipient, because postnatally acquired rubella is generally mild and complications rare. Rubella vaccination programmes are directed towards protecting fetuses from congenitally acquired disease; it is the only vaccine directed specifically towards preventing the consequences of an intrauterine infection.

HISTORICAL BACKGROUND

Recognition of teratogenic effects caused by rubella virus

Historical milestones are listed in Table 1. The association between maternal rubella and congenitally acquired anomalies was first observed by an Australian ophthalmologist, N. McAlistar Gregg[1] who noted cataract, retinopathy and cardiac defects in infants whose mothers gave a history of rubella-like illness in early pregnancy. Seventy-eight infants, all of whom had a similar type of cataract, were born in New South Wales following an extensive rubella epidemic in 1940; all but ten of the mothers gave a history of rubella, usually in the first and second months of pregnancy. Cardiac defects were also detected in 44 of the 67 infants whose cardiac condition was recorded. These findings were soon confirmed in Australia by Swan and his colleagues[2] who noted that many congenitally infected infants were also deaf, and some had microcephaly. Further confirmation was soon forthcoming not only from Australia, but also from other countries (reviewed in ref. 3).

Early prospective studies

These first studies, being retrospective, demonstrated a high incidence of defects following maternal rubella. However, prospective studies conducted during the 1950s and early 1960s, in which the outcome of pregnancy in

Table 1 Main historical events

1941	Teratogenic effects of rubella first recognized by Gregg in Australia.
1962	Rubella virus isolated in cell cultures. Neutralization test developed.
1963–64	Extensive epidemics of rubella in USA and Europe.
1965–67	Development of attenuated vaccine stains and first vaccine trials.
1969	*USA*: HPV77.DE5 and Cendehill vaccine strains licensed. Vaccination offered to all pre-school children.
1970	*UK*: Cendehill vaccine strain licensed. Vaccination offered to all 11–14-year-old schoolgirls.
1971	*USA*: MMR1[a] licensed.
1972	*UK*: Rubella vaccination extended to all susceptible adult women of child-bearing age including women attending antenatal clinics. Susceptible pregnant women offered vaccination in the immediate post-partum period.
1977	*USA*: National Childhood Immunization initiative – intensification of rubella vaccination of teenagers and susceptible adult women.
1978–79	*UK*: Rubella epidemics; 124 cases of congenitally acquired rubella and 1405 terminations of pregnancy due to rubella or rubella contact.
1979	*USA*: RA27/3 replaced other vaccine strains.
1980	*UK*: Intensification of vaccination programme.
1983	*UK*: Rubella epidemic. Further intensification of vaccination campaign.
1988	*UK*: Vaccination policy augmented by offering MMR to pre-school children of both sexes. MMR[b] licensed.

[a]MMRI contained measles virus (Moraten strain), mumps virus (Jeryl Lynn) and rubella virus (HPV77.DE5).
[b]MMR vaccines licensed in the UK contain measles virus (Schwartz strain), mumps virus (Urabe AM/9) and rubella virus (RA27/3 strain).

women with a history of rubella at different gestational ages was assessed, showed that the incidence of developmental anomalies was much less than in retrospective enquiries. The risks of major malformation after maternal infection in the first trimester ranged from 10.4 to 54.2% (reviewed in ref. 4). Defects were frequently multiple and severe when maternal rubella was acquired prior to fetal organogenesis, i.e. during the first 8 weeks of gestational life. After the first trimester the risks of severe congenital malformations were shown to decline markedly.

However, these early prospective studies underestimated the true incidence of congenitally acquired malformations. They were conducted before laboratory diagnosis was available, and may have included women who did not have rubella and who were delivered of normal babies. Some investigations also varied considerably in the duration and quality of follow-up studies on 'at-risk' babies. Further progress was hindered until the development of techniques to isolate rubella virus and detect serological responses to it (see below). Subsequent studies showed that rubella during the first trimester of pregnancy usually resulted in generalized and persistent fetal infection, this being associated with multisystem disease. It was also recognized that many infants, although apparently normal at birth, may, when followed up over a period of many years, be found to have such defects as perceptive deafness or minor CNS anomalies (reviewed in ref. 4).

Isolation of rubella virus and development of serological techniques

Rubella virus was first isolated in 1962[5,6]. The growth of the virus in cell cultures allowed the development of tests to detect specific antibodies. A number of studies showed that following postnatally acquired rubella, neutralizing antibodies developed rapidly after the onset of rash, persisted at a variable level, probably for life, and were associated with a very high level of protection against rubella[7]. Seroepidemiological studies showed that the prevalence of rubella antibodies was related to age and social class, but in general some 15–20% of women of child-bearing age living in urban communities in western countries were susceptible to rubella[8,9]. Serological studies showed that a past history of rubella was an unreliable index of previous infection.

It was also shown that virus could be recovered from the nasopharyngeal secretions, blood, urine and stools of patients with postnatally acquired rubella, virus being present in the nasopharynx for 7–10 days before, and up to 10–14 days after, onset of rash. Viraemia could be detected for 5–7 days prior to onset of rash, but once this appeared neutralizing antibodies developed and viraemia ceased. Virus isolation studies also showed that rubella virus could be isolated from 90–100% of the products of conception following spontaneous abortion or termination of pregnancy resulting from maternal rubella in the first trimester of pregnancy[10,11].

Results of the rubella epidemic in the USA, 1963–64

In 1963–64 one of the most extensive epidemics of rubella in recent times occurred in the USA. Many workers exploited the newly developed laboratory techniques and the findings led to a greater understanding of the pathogenesis and clinical and virological features of congenitally acquired infection. Inevitably many pregnant women were infected, and it was estimated that about 30000 rubella-damaged babies were born[12]. Multisystem involvement was common, and the range of abnormalities was much wider than hitherto observed. The range of abnormalities described as a result of the epidemic, and from follow-up studies on congenitally infected infants, is shown in Table 2. It was shown that, despite active synthesis of rubella antibodies, many infected babies excreted virus for prolonged periods, and often transmitted infection to susceptible contacts[13,14].

More recent developments

True incidence of rubella-associated defects following maternal rubella

Although many of the early prospective studies failed to assess the risks of congenitally acquired disease following maternal rubella accurately, recent studies have shown that the incidence of defects following maternal rubella in the first trimester is much higher than had hitherto been realized. These studies followed up infants whose mothers acquired virologically confirmed infection, but who elected to continue with their pregnancies. Although the number of infants whose mothers had first-trimester rubella is therefore inevitably small, almost all infants had serological evidence of intrauterine infection and most infants had one or more congenital defects[15,16]. Thus, Miller and her colleagues[15] showed that rubella defects occurred in all nine infants infected before the 11th week of gestation, most infants having

Table 2 Clinical features associated with congenitally acquired rubella

	Common	*Uncommon*
Transient	Low birthweight Thrombocytopenic purpura Hepatosplenomegaly Bone lesions Meningoencephalitis	Cloudy cornea Hepatitis Generalized lymphadenopathy Haemolytic anaemia Pneumonitis
Developmental	Sensorineural deafness Peripheral pulmonary stenosis Mental retardation Central language defects Diabetes mellitus	Severe myopia Thyroiditis Hypothyroidism Growth hormone deficiency 'Late-onset disease'
Permanent	Sensorineural deafness Peripheral pulmonary stenosis Pulmonary valvular stenosis Patent ductus arteriosus Ventricular septal defect Retinopathy Cataract Microphthalmia Psychomotor retardation Microcephaly Cryptorchidism Inguinal hernia Diabetes mellitus	Severe myopia Thyroid disorders Dermatoglyptic abnormalities Glaucoma Myocardial abnormalities

Adapted from Banatvala and Best (1984)[4].

congenital heart disease and deafness. These findings are consistent with reports that rubella virus may usually be detected in the products of conception when maternal rubella occurred in the first trimester.

Risks of maternal rubella after the first trimester

Rubella virus is seldom isolated from infants whose mothers acquired rubella after the first trimester, although serological studies confirm that a high proportion of infants are infected. Cradock–Watson and his colleagues[17] detected rubella-specific IgM in 25–33% of infants whose mothers had rubella between the 16th and 20th week of pregnancy. Such infants rarely have severe or multiple anomalies, because organogenesis is complete by 12 weeks and in more mature fetuses immune responses may limit or terminate infection. Most surveys have shown that deafness and retinopathy, which *per se* does not affect vision, are likely to be the only anomalies commonly associated with post-first-trimester rubella[15,16,18,19]. Deafness is usually the sole clinical manifestation of fetal infection occurring between 13 and 16 weeks, and is relatively common, but deafness or any other defect is only rarely encountered after this time.

Risks of preconceptual rubella

Although occasional case reports, not always documented with adequate virological data, suggested that if acquired preconception, rubella virus may occasionally cause fetal damage (reviewed in ref. 4), it is encouraging that more recent studies conducted in the Federal Republic of Germany and Britain indicate that preconceptual rubella does not result in transmission of rubella virus to the fetus. Thus, there was no serological or clinical evidence of intrauterine infection in 38 infants whose mothers' rash appeared before or within 11 days after their last menstrual period (LMP). However, an interval of 12–21 days between LMP and rash resulted in fetal infection in four of 13 cases and all of 10 women who developed rash 3–6 weeks after their LMP transmitted infection to their fetuses[20].

Development of serological tests

A number of serological techniques have been developed which are of value in assessing immune responses. The earliest test to be employed was the neutralization test, and although this still represents a sensitive and specific assay, it is labour-intensive, cumbersome and now seldom used. It was replaced initially by haemagglutination inhibition (HAI), which was used for diagnosis and screening purposes[21]. However, when it was realized that incomplete removal of the serum lipoprotein inhibitors of haemagglutination led to false-positive results in rubella antibody screening tests, HAI was replaced by other assays, such as single radial haemolysis (SRH), enzyme immunoassay (EIA), passive haemagglutination and latex agglutination (LA) (reviewed in ref. 22). Some of these assays have been adapted for detecting class-specific antibody responses to rubella, and have been of value for comparing immune responses following naturally acquired and vaccine induced rubella infection[23,24].

DEVELOPMENT OF RUBELLA VACCINES AND EARLY VACCINE TRIALS

The extensive rubella epidemic in the USA in 1963–64, which resulted in the delivery of many thousands of rubella-damaged infants, emphasized the importance of attempting to prevent rubella by vaccination. Initial attempts to induce immunity with inactivated vaccines were disappointing, since they were poorly antigenic and conferred little protection following experimental challenge with rubella virus[25]. There were no further attempts to develop an inactivated rubella vaccine, because it was soon reported that a live attenuated rubella vaccine showed considerable promise, and as unusually severe measles occurred following exposure to infection months or years after the administration of inactivated measles vaccine.

Attenuation of rubella virus is achieved by multiple passage in cell cultures of strains isolated from patients with rubella. The first attenuated strains were prepared by attenuation of strains of rubella isolated from a US military recruit in 1961 (M33) and a child with postnatally acquired rubella in 1964 (ML). Attenuation was achieved by multiple passage in vervet monkey kidney to give the prototype vaccine known as high passage virus-77 (HPV77)[26,27]. This attenuated strain was given a further five passages in duck embryo fibroblasts, since avian cells are less likely to contain extraneous agents than are monkey kidney cells. This vaccine, which was designated HPV77.DE5[28,29], was licensed for use in the USA and many parts of Europe in 1969–70. Another HPV-derived vaccine was produced by giving the HPV77 strain an additional 12 passages in dog kidney cell cultures (HPV77.DK12)[30]. However, its use was discontinued, since it was associated with an unacceptable number of reactions. Additional vaccines were soon developed, attenuation being achieved by passage in primary rabbit kidney cultures (Cendehill strain), in human diploid fibroblasts (WI-38) at temperatures ranging from 35° to 30°C (RA27/3 strain) or in primary guinea-pig kidney followed by rabbit kidney cell cultures (TO-336 strain). The RA27/3 strain was isolated in the USA from the kidney of a rubella-infected fetus. The name RA27/3 is derived from 'rubella abortus, 27th specimen, third explant'[31]. Table 3 shows the origin and passage levels of these strains, as well as some other strains which are now available in Japan[32].

The aim of most of the early vaccine trials was not only to assess reactogenicity and immune responses, but also to determine whether transmission to susceptible contacts occurred. This was of considerable import-

Table 3 Attenuated rubella virus vaccines

Vaccine	*Strain derivation*	*Attenuation*	*Reference*
HPV77	Army recruit with rubella (1961)	VMK(77)[a]	Parkman *et al.*[26] Meyer *et al.*[28]
HPV77.DE5	As above	VMK(77); duck embryo (5)	Buynak *et al.*[33]
Cendehill	Urine from a case of post-natally acquired rubella (1963)	VMK(3)primary rabbit kidney (51)	Peetermans and Huygelen[34] Martin du Pan *et al.*[35]
RA27/3	Kidney of rubella-infected fetus (1964)	Human embryonic kidney (4); WI-38 fibroblasts (17–25)	Plotkin *et al.*[31,36]
MEQ11	Throat washing from patient in Osaka (1966) – Matsuura strain	VMK(14); Chick amnion(65); quail embryo fibroblast cells(11)	Minekawa *et al.*[37]
TO-336	Pharyngeal secretion from child with postnatally acquired rubella, Toyama, Japan (1967)	VMK(7); primary guinea-pig kidney(20); primary rabbit kidney(3)	Hoshino *et al.*[38]
DCRB 19	Throat swab from patient in Tokyo (1967)	VMK(1); bovine kidney(53); rabbit kidney(3)	Reviewed in Shishido and Ohtawara[32]
KRT	Throat swab from patient in Matsue city (1968) – Takahashi (MAT) strain	VMK(4); primary rabbit testicle(36); primary rabbit kidney(1)	Ohwada *et al.*[39]
SK	Throat washing from patient in Kumamato (1969) – Matsuba strain	VMK(1); swine kidney(60); rabbit kidney (6)	Ueda *et al.*[40]

VMK = vervet monkey kidney
[a]Number of passages in parentheses.

ance, since at the time the teratogenic potential of attenuated rubella virus strains was unknown. The risk of transmission to susceptible contacts, some of whom might be pregnant, needed to be excluded before trials could be conducted in the general community. Thus, experimental trials which employed rhesus monkeys were followed by a large number of vaccine trials in institutional communities, and later, when lack of transmission had been clearly shown, in 'open' communities.

Rhesus monkeys were used because following inoculation with rubella virus they exhibited patterns of virus excretion and antibody responses similar to those observed in humans, although not developing clinically apparent disease[41]. When responses following intravenous and intramuscular inoculation of attenuated HPV77 (high passage) and non-attenuated (low passage) strains were compared, it was shown that the proportion of rhesus monkeys developing neutralizing antibody responses and the range of titres obtained were comparable. When challenged intravenously and intramuscularly with non-attenuated rubella virus, the monkeys were protected against reinfection. Although animals given low passage rubella virus strains transmitted infection to susceptible cage contacts, those given the attenuated strains did not[26].

Trials with HPV77 were then extended to children living in cottages in residential institutions in the USA. These trials confirmed that the HPV77 strain was attenuated and immunogenic, neutralizing antibody responses developing some 20–27 days post-vaccination. No rubella-like features occurred in the recipients after vaccination. Some of the children excreted virus, usually 10–20 days after vaccination, but did not transmit infection to susceptible unvaccinated control children living in the same cottage. By chance, during these trials, naturally acquired rubella was introduced into a single cottage, and this allowed for comparison to be made between vaccine induced and naturally acquired immune responses and virus excretion patterns[28]. Viraemia could be detected consistently in those with naturally acquired infections but was not detected in vaccinees. The amount of virus excreted from the nasopharynx was approximately 100-fold less among vaccinees, who also developed 100-fold lower concentrations of neutralizing antibodies. In due course the accumulated data from a number of vaccine trials conducted in institutional communities confirmed lack of transmission to susceptible contacts and more extensive studies were then conducted in 'open' communities.

In November 1968 and February 1969, two international conferences were held in London and Washington, respectively. Data presented at these conferences confirmed that vaccines were generally well tolerated, induced antibody responses, as measured by neutralization and haemagglutination inhibition, which appeared to persist and protect against rubella, and were safe to use in open communities[42,43]. Presentations and discussion at these conferences paved the way for product licences to be given for HPV77.DE5 and Cendehill vaccines in the USA in 1969, and in Britain for Cendehill in 1970 and RA27/3 in 1972.

LICENSED VACCINES

The HPV77.DE5 vaccine obtained a product licence in the USA in 1969. It was incorporated in the combined measles, mumps and rubella (MMR) vaccine, which was licensed in the USA in 1971 and has been widely used there. The antibody response to each of the components of MMR is quantitatively similar to that achieved by the monovalent vaccines[44,45]. MMR vaccine is generally well tolerated, although occasional reactions may include fever, malaise, anorexia, rash and very occasionally a febrile convulsion[46]. These reactions are associated with the measles, rather than the other components of this vaccine. The HPV77.DE5 strain of rubella in MMR was replaced with RA27/3 in 1979, since a number of workers felt that the pattern of development of antibodies produced by RA27/3, and the protection it afforded, was superior. The RA27/3 strain is now the most widely used rubella vaccine strain (Table 4).

ADMINISTRATION OF RUBELLA VACCINES

Dose and route of administration

Rubella vaccines are usually administered subcutaneously. A dose of not less than 1000 $TCID_{50}$ is given in an 0.5 ml volume. Unlike HPV-derived and Cendehill vaccines, RA27/3 will induce an immune response when administered intranasally (i.n.)[36,48]. However, as some degree of expertise is required by the vaccinator, and because the recipient must be cooperative

Table 4 Availability of rubella vaccines in 1984 (reproduced with permission from Perkins[47])

Manufacturer	*Virus strain*	*Cell substrate*	*Countries/regions where vaccine licensed*
Merck Sharpe & Dohme, United States	RA27/3	WI-38	Western Pacific, American Region, Europe, South Africa
Smith Kline-RIT, Belgium	Cendehill RA27/3	Rabbit kidney MRC-5	Far East, Europe Weestern Pacific, Europe
Swiss Serum and Vaccine Institute, Switzerland	RA27/3	MRC-5	Western Pacific, North and Central Africa, Southeast Asia, Europe
Institut Mérieux, France	RA27/3	WI-38 (MRC-5)	South America, Europe, North Africa
Sclavo, Italy	RA27/3	WI-38	Southeast Asia, South America, Greece
Wellcome, United Kingdom	RA27/3	MRC-5	Western Pacific, Americas, Europe, North Africa
Institute of Immunology, Yugoslavia	RA27/3	MRC-5	Far East
Chemo-sero-therapeutic Research Institute, Japan	Matsuba	Rabbit kidney	Japan
Chiba Serum Institut, Japan	DCRB 19	Rabbit kidney	Japan
The Kitasato Institute, Japan	Takahashi	Rabbit kidney	Japan
Osaka University, Japan	Matsuura	Quail-embryo fibroblast	Japan
Takeda Chemical Industries, Japan	TO-336	Rabbit kidney	Japan

and free from respiratory infection and obstruction, the i.n. route of vaccination was not considered suitable for routine use.

Contraindications

Since the rubella vaccine virus may be transmitted transplacentally, pregnancy is an absolute contraindication and should be avoided for 1 month after vaccination (see below). As with other live vaccines, it is better to postpone rubella vaccination if the patient is suffering from a febrile illness. It should not be given to patients whose immunological response is deficient, whether as a result of disease (e.g. malignancy) or of treatment with immunosuppressive drugs. When it is necessary to give another live vaccine at the same time, the two vaccines should be given simultaneously but at different sites; alternatively the two vaccinations should be separated by an interval of at least 3 weeks. A 3-week interval should also be allowed between the administration of live vaccines, such as rubella, and BCG. The manufacturer's leaflet should be carefully studied before patients with known hypersensitivity are vaccinated, since rubella vaccines contain traces of antibiotics (neomycin and/or kanamycin or polymyxin). Vaccination should be delayed for about 3 months after a blood transfusion or a dose of human immunoglobulin, since passively acquired antibodies might interfere with the immune response. Although, previous administration of anti-D immune globulin is not a contraindication to post-partum vaccination, it is advisable to confirm seroconversion 8–12 weeks later.

Virus excretion

Many of the early vaccine trials showed that a variable but significant proportion of recipients excreted virus via the nasopharynx, usually some 1–4 weeks after vaccination. However, if particular care is taken to ensure that adequate specimens are collected and sensitive methods for virus isolation are used, the proportion of vaccinees excreting virus, regardless of which vaccine is given, ranges between 65 and 100%[49]. However, the risk of infecting women in the early stages of pregnancy is negligible, as the accumulated data obtained from numerous trials have shown that virus transmission is very rare.

Although it is believed that lack of communicability may be related to the small amount of virus excreted by vaccinees, some may excrete amounts comparable with that detected in naturally acquired infection. Thus, following the administration of RA27/3 vaccine to susceptible adults, Harcourt and her colleagues[50] showed that 24 of 26 (96%) vaccinees excreted virus with virus isolated from 34 of the 44 (77%) nasopharyngeal swabs obtained at titres which ranged from $10^{0.5}$ to $10^{3.5}$ $TCID_{50}$/0.1 ml the upper range being comparable with the amounts excreted by those with naturally acquired infection. Over a short time there may be considerable variation in the amount of virus excreted by vaccinees. Thus, specimens collected by a less skilled person from individual vaccinees showed variation in titres of more than 1000-fold over a 4-h period. No association was found between HLA antigens of the A and B locus and excretion of high and low titres of attenuated virus[50]. The above findings suggest that lack of transmission of attenuated virus may not be due to the relatively low titres of virus excreted by vaccinees. It is possible that attenuation results in some alteration of the biological properties of the virus whereby it fails to replicate in the respiratory mucosae of susceptible contacts.

Vaccine-induced reactions

Rubella vaccines are generally very well tolerated. However, lymphadenopathy, rash, arthralgia (painful joints) or arthritis (joint swelling or limitation of movement) may occur some 2–4 weeks after vaccination. Such reactions are usually considerably less severe than those following naturally acquired disease. Lymphadenopathy is seldom noticed, although very occasionally vaccinees may complain of enlarged and tender lymph nodes. Rash is uncommon, but if it does occur it is usually macular, faint and fleeting. Reactions, particularly joint involvement, are commonly encountered in post-pubertal females but are rare in children. Weibel and his colleagues[51], in a study of 653 females aged between 8 months and 41 years given HPV77.DE5 vaccine, observed that joint reactions increased markedly with age. Joint symptoms did not occur in children under 12, whereas they occurred in 7.5% of persons aged 12–25, and 58.3% in those aged 26–41. Knees, finger joints, wrists and ankles are most frequently involved, but symptoms are generally mild, do not usually persist for longer than 3–4 days and rarely result in time lost from work[49]. Cendehill and the Japanese vaccine TO-336 are less likely to induce joint reactions in adult women than are RA27/3 and HPV77.DE5 vaccines, which may cause arthralgia or arthritis in 35–40% of vaccinees[49]. However, joint reactions following vaccination with HPV77-derived vaccines tend to be more severe.

The HPV77.DK12 vaccine, which was soon withdrawn, induced particularly severe joint reactions, even in children, some experiencing an intermittent arthritis over a period which occasionally extended to 3 years[52,53]. There have also been rare reports of persons who were vaccinated as adults with currently licensed vaccines experiencing recurrent joint symptoms over periods extending to 1 or more years. Generally only a single joint is involved, usually the knees, and because investigations fail to identify any other cause of recurrent arthritis, it is assumed to be vaccine-related.

Joint involvement may result from direct invasion of the synovium, since rubella virus has been isolated from joint aspirates of vaccinees with vaccine-induced arthritis[54]. Furthermore, attenuated virus strains have been shown to replicate in human synovial membrane cell cultures, the HPV77 vaccine strain growing to higher titres than Cendehill[55]. However, immune mechanisms may play a role in the pathogenesis of vaccine-induced arthritis for, in addition to virus, joint aspirates have also been shown to contain rubella-specific IgG[56], which suggests that joint symptoms may be mediated by immune complexes. This is supported by the findings that the presence of immune complexes in the sera of vaccine recipients is associated with a high incidence of joint symptoms[57,58].

Hormonal factors may also play a role, for in addition to being common in post-pubertal females, the development of joint symptoms appears to be related to the menstrual cycle; after rubella vaccination joint involvement is significantly more likely to occur within 7 days after the onset of the cycle[50]. It might therefore be possible to reduce the incidence of joint symptoms by vaccinating women during the last 7 days of their cycle. The incidence of joint symptoms does not appear to be related to oral contraception[49] or to HLA antigens of the A and B loci[50].

Rubella virus has been suggested as a possible cause of chronic inflammatory joint disease. Rubella virus has been isolated from peripheral blood and synovial mononuclear cells from a small number of persons a number of years after acute infection or immunization[59,60]. This group of workers also isolated rubella virus from the mononuclear cells of seven of 19 (35%) children with chronic rheumatic disease[61] and have suggested that chronic joint manifestations may be the result of persistence of rubella virus in circulating lymphocytes or within the joints. Most of these subjects, however, had received the HPV77.DE5 vaccine. These results may perhaps be explained by the persistence of this attenuated strain, since rubella-specific IgM responses have been detected for up to 3 years after immunization with this vaccine, suggesting continued antigenic stimulation[24].

Although the development of a petechial or purpuric rash is a rare complication of natural but not vaccine-induced infection, a study on a small number of adult volunteers given the RA27/3 vaccine showed that they developed sharp reductions in platelet counts between the 7th and 14th day after vaccination, followed by some compensating increase in counts in the 3rd week[62]. Mild thrombocytopenia has also been recorded among Cendehill vaccinees[63].

IMMUNE RESPONSES

Antibody responses

Vaccine trials have shown that approximately 95% of susceptible vaccinees develop an HAI antibody response following vaccination[42,43]. Although most vaccinees develop antibodies between 10 and 28 days after vaccination[24,64,65], responses may occasionally be delayed, and it is therefore advisable to delay conducting tests to determine whether seroconversion has occurred until at least 8 weeks after immunization.

Vaccine-induced HAI titres are usually 4–8-fold lower than those resulting from naturally acquired infection. The Cendehill vaccine generally produces lower antibody concentrations than other vaccines[66,67]. RA27/3 induces an antibody response that resembles most closely that following natural infection[24,66], which is one of the reasons it is now used so widely.

Cusi and colleagues[68] have examined the antibody response to the viral structural proteins by immunoblotting, following immunization wth RA27/3. Antibodies specific for all three major structural proteins, E1, E2 and C, could be detected 1 month after immunization. Results on sera obtained after an extended interval following immunization have not yet been published.

Duration of antibody responses

It is now more than 20 years since the first rubella vaccine trials, and the results of studies on the long-term persistence of vaccine-induced antibodies show that more than 96% of vaccinees had detectable antibodies when tested 9–21 years after vaccination (Tables 5 and 6). However, several different serological techniques were used to measure rubella antibodies in these studies, the sensitivity of which would have influenced the results. Thus, using HAI, a relatively insensitive technique, Horstmann and her colleagues[70] found that 16% of HPV77.DE5 vaccinees were seronegative 11–12 years after vaccination. When more sensitive techniques, such as EIA and LA, were used to detect antibody levels as low as 7000 IU/l, a much smaller percentage of vaccinees were found to be seronegative[67,72,74].

Studies in the UK, where 15 000 IU/l is regarded as a protective level of antibody, showed that 96% of 117 vaccinees had antibody concentrations

Table 5 Long-term persistence of antibodies following vaccination of seronegative persons

Study and country	*Vaccine*	*Years after vaccination*	*No. seronegative/ no. tested (percentage seronegative)*
Hoshino *et al.*[38] (1982), Japan	TO-336	9	0/25
Zealley and Edmund (personal	RA27/3	12	1/94 (1%)
communication) (1983) UK	Cendehill		3/145 (2%)
Hillary and Griffith[69] (1984) Eire	RA27/3	15	1/21 (4.7%)
Horstmann *et al.*[70] (1985) USA	RA27/3	11	0/35
	HPV77.DE5	11–12	13/79 (16%)
Just *et al.*[71] (1985) Switzerland	Cendehill	15	3/319 (1%)
Orenstein *et al.*[72] (1986) USA	HPV77.DE5	10–14	26[a]/302 (8.7%)
Chu *et al.*[67] (1988) USA	Cendehill	16	18[a]/400 (4.5%)
	HPV77.DE5	16	18/385 (4.7%)
Enders and Nickerl[73]	RA27/3	14	0/115
(1988) Germany	Cendehill	14–17	2/102 (2%)
	HPV77.DE5	14	0.15
O'Shea *et al.*[74] (1988) UK	RA27/3	10–21	1/48 (2.1%)
	Cendehill	10-21	1[b]/40 (2.5%)
	HPV77.DE5	10–21	1/18 (5.5%)
	TO-336	12–13	0/11
Total		9–21	88/2154 (4.1%)

[a] <7000 IU/l

[b] This vaccinee was seronegative by SRH and HAI, but had antibodies detectable by EIA and LA

Table 6 Persistence of antibodies 10–21 years after immunization of seronegative persons – comparison of four vaccines

Vaccine	*No. tested*	*No. (%) seropositive*
RA27/3	313	310 (94.0%)
Cendehill	1006	979 (97.3%)
HPV77.DE	799	741 (92.7%)
TO-336	36	36 (100%)

>15 000 IU/l when tested 10–21 years after immunization[74] However, 10% of vaccinees had antibody concentrations <15 000 IU/l 5–8 years after vaccination, the proportion with low titres decreased in subsequent years (S O'Shea, J. M. Best and J. E. Banatvala, unpublished results). This suggests that low titres may have been boosted by reinfection. In general, those vaccinated with Cendehill and HPV77-derived vaccines are more likely to have low antibody concentrations, become seronegative and exhibit booster antibody responses[73,74].

Class-specific serum and nasopharyngeal antibody responses

Following the administration of rubella vaccines the major classes of rubella-specific antibodies can be detected in the serum of most vaccinees. Provided sensitive techniques are employed, rubella-specific IgM antibodies can be detected between 3 and 8 weeks after immunization[24,75,76]. Although such responses are usually of relatively short duration, persistent IgM responses may occur, although only at low concentrations, particularly among those given HPV77.DE5 vaccine[24]. This should be remembered when interpreting low levels of rubella-specific IgM in pregnant women.

Specific IgG antibodies may not be at maximum levels until about 6 months after vaccination, and persist for more than 12 years in most recipients[24].

Serum and nasopharyngeal IgA responses can be detected following the administration of rubella vaccines as well as after naturally acquired infection[24,77,78]. In the serum there is apparently a transient oligomeric (10S) IgA response[79] and a persistent 7S IgA response, which may be detected in some vaccinees at a low level for 10–12 years after immunization provided sensitive techniques are used[24]. Using radioimmunoassay, O'Shea and her colleagues[24] found that specific IgA concentrations declined more rapidly than specific-IgG, only 45.5% of the vaccinees tested have detectable IgA antibody 10–12 years after immunization. There was little difference in the responses following the subcutaneous and intranasal administration of RA27/3.

O'Shea and her colleagues[24] also detected nasopharyngeal IgA antibodies in 80% of vaccinees 6 weeks after immunization. These antibodies were detected for up to 5 years in RA27/3 vaccinees, but only for 2–3 years among Cendehill, HPV77.DE5 and TO-336 vaccinees. IgA antibody concentrations were also higher following immunization with RA27/3. Nasopharyngeal IgG antibodies were detected in only 40% of vaccinees at 6 weeks after immunization.

Cell-mediated immunity

There have been few studies on cell-mediated immune responses to rubella virus. Lymphoproliferative responses are lower after immunization than after natural infection, and may be difficult to detect[80–82].

VACCINE EFFICACY AND REINFECTION

Both naturally acquired and vaccine-induced infection are followed by a very high order of protection against reinfection. However, significant 'booster' antibody responses may occur after close and prolonged exposure to naturally acquired infection or experimental challenge with rubella virus, and following challenge some of those with vaccine-induced immunity may even excrete small amounts of virus via the nasopharynx[83]. Booster antibody responses are more likely to occur when immunity is vaccine-induced, their frequency being higher among those given HPV77-derived and Cendehill vaccines than those incorporating the RA27/3 strain[23,83]. Specific-IgM responses have also been detected following challenge of those with vaccine-induced immunity when sensitive assays have been used. Rubella-specific IgM may also be detected in reinfection resulting from natural exposure to rubella. In general its concentration is lower, and the duration of response shorter, than following primary infection[83,84]. Reinfection is not usually accompanied by any clinical symptoms.

Despite these observations it is important to emphasize that should reinfection with rubella occur in early pregnancy it is unlikely to provide a threat to the fetus. Thus, studies conducted in patients with carefully documented serological evidence of reinfection in early pregnancy, associated in some cases with rubella-specific IgM, failed to reveal evidence of transmission of rubella virus to the fetus[84,85]. These findings are supported by the fact that viraemia is seldom detected following intranasal challenge of volunteers with low levels of rubella antibody with high titre RA27/3. Thus, O'Shea and her colleagues[83], using very sensitive techniques, detected a transient viraemia in only one of 19 vaccinees following challenge. Schiff and his colleagues[86] also detected viraemia in three of six vaccinees with low or undetectable antibodies, following intranasal challenge with an enormous dose ($\sim$1000 $TCID_{50}$) of an unattenuated strain of rubella virus (Howell). All six of those challenged shed virus and developed a significant rise in antibody titre, while four developed lymphadenopathy and a low-grade fever.

Despite the results of the above studies, a small number of apparently well-documented cases of virologically confirmed reinfection, in which such clinical features as rash, arthralgia and fetal infection and damage were reported, suggest that viraemia may occur following both naturally acquired and vaccine-induced infection (reviewed in ref. 87). Some of the reports must be interpreted with caution, particularly when evidence of pre-existing immunity was from the detection of HAI 'antibody' in an earlier serum, since this finding may result from failure to remove non-specific inhibitors adequately[88]. However, there can be little doubt that genuine cases of reinfection associated with viraemia have been reported, although it must be stressed that this is an extremely rare occurrence. There are five well-documented cases in the literature where there is evidence of transmission of virus to the fetus in women who had been shown to have rubella antibodies before the affected pregnancy[89–93] and five or six others have been documented in England and Wales between 1985 and 1988 (J. M. Best, P. Morgan-Capner and E. Miller, unpublished observations). Six of these 11 cases had a history of rubella vaccination. It is possible that this phenomenon is host-related, being due to a specific defect in a patient's immune response to rubella. With the reduction in circulation of wild rubella, which will hopefully result from the augmented rubella vaccination programme in Britain, the incidence of this problem will become even more rare.

RISKS OF RUBELLA VACCINATION IN PREGNANCY

Rubella vaccination has always been contraindicated during pregnancy since, when vaccines were first licensed, it was not known whether virus would be transmitted to the fetus following vaccination during pregnancy and whether transmission would result in congenital anomalies. Early studies gave cause for concern, since rubella virus was recovered from the placenta and such fetal organs as the kidney and bone marrow (reviewed in ref. 4). Furthermore, the finding that rubella virus could be isolated from fetal organs for as long as 3 months after vaccination suggested that, in common with naturally acquired infection, rubella vaccine strains induced persistent infections. These reports related to pregnant women inadvertently vaccinated with Cendehill and HPV77.DE5 vaccine strains, since they were more widely used. Somewhat surprisingly, RA27/3, despite having a shorter passage history and producing an immune response which more closely resembles that induced by naturally acquired infection than other vaccines, has only rarely been recovered from the products of conception[94].

Despite transmission of vaccine strains transplacentally, fetal damage has not been reported. Clinical follow-up studies on women who elected to go to term following inadvertent vaccination in early pregnancy, revealed no abnormalities compatible with congenital rubella among babies delivered of 449 women. However, there was virological evidence of congenital infection in nine of the 372 babies tested (Table 7)[95,96] (also S. Shepherd, personal communication; M. Forsgren, personal communication). In the US series 170 of 264 women received the RA27/3 vaccine strain (Table 8). However, if rubella vaccines were to induce congenital defects, it may only be over a much shorter interval than after naturally acquired infection. It should therefore be noted that only 55 (32%) of these women were vaccinated at about the time of conception, between 1 week before and 4 weeks after conception[96] (Table 8).

Using the above observations it has been calculated that the theoretical maximum risk of rubella-induced major malformations among infants born to susceptible mothers is 1.4%[94,95]. This risk is less than the risk of major malformation among unselected pregnancies (2–3%). It is not known whether the lack of teratogenic effects following rubella vaccination is because there is less virus transmitted to the fetus following vaccination as compared with naturally acquired infection, or to the reduced teratogenicity of attenuated vaccine strains.

As a result of this reassuring information, inadvertent vaccination of a pregnant woman is, now, not normally a reason for termination of pregnancy, although the decision should be made by the patient and her obstetrician.

Table 7 Pregnancy outcome in susceptible women going to term following rubella vaccination during pregnancy or within the 3 months before conception (adapted from J. M. Best and J. E. Banatvala (1987) In *Principles and Practice of Clinical Virology*, by permission of John Wiley and Sons, Ltd., Chichester)

Country	*No. live births in women receiving*					
	HPV77.DE5 Cendehill	*RA27/3*	*NK*[a]	*Total*	*Evidence of infection*	*Abnormalities compatible with CRS*
USA	94	172[b]	1	267[b]	6/197[c] (3.0%)	0/267[d]
Federal Republic of Germany	115	24		139	2/139[e] (1.4%)	0/139
Sweden		5		5	0/4	0/5
UK	2	24	12	38	1[f]/32 (3.1%)	0/38
Total	211	225	13	449	9[f]/372 (2.4%)	0/449

[a]Not known
[b]Include two sets of twins
[c]No. positive/no. tested
[d]No. cases with CRS abnormalities/no. examined
[e]Two of 115 Cendehill vaccinees
[f]Received RA27/3

Table 8 Consequences of rubella vaccination during pregnancy or within the 3 months before conception, USA 1971–6[96,97] (adapted from J. M. Best and J. E. Banatvala (1987) In *Principles and Practice of Clinical Virology*, by permission of John Wiley and Sons, Ltd., Chichester)

	Pregnancy outcome in susceptibles going to term			
Vaccine	*No. going to term*	*No. vaccinated between 1 week before and 4 weeks after conception/no. with date of conception known*	*Evidence of infection*[a]	*Abnormalities*[b]
HPV77.DE5/ Cendehill	94	33/86 (38.4%)	3/61[c]	0/94[d]
RA27/3	170	55/170 (32%)	3/136[e]	0/172
Total	264	88/256 (34%)	6/197 (3.1%)	0/266

[a]IgM present, IgG persisting beyond 6 months or isolation of rubella virus
[b]Compatible with congenital rubella
[c]Five of 45 infants tested, born to women of unknown immune status also had evidence of subclinical infection
[d]Now aged 2–10.5 years
[e]Two of 156 infants born to mothers of unknown immune status had serological evidence of infection, but no defects compatible with CRS

Nevertheless, as the number of women vaccinated during the critical period is still relatively small (approximate total 150), it is therefore still necessary to exercise caution and continue to collect further data.

Most adult women who are vaccinated will have been previously screened and shown to be susceptible to rubella. However, in cases where a woman is inadvertently vaccinated during pregnancy without prior screening, it is often possible to determine her previous immune status retrospectively. Thus, rubella-specific IgM can usually be detected in serum samples taken within 8 weeks after vaccination[75,76].

Vaccine failures

Rubella is a relatively labile virus and failure to follow the manufacturer's instructions for storage and reconstitution of the vaccine may result in inactivation of the vaccine. A small proportion of recipients (about 5%) fail to seroconvert after vaccination with any of the licensed vaccines, but usually respond when revaccinated. Occasional vaccinees experience a delayed response, antibodies appearing a month or more later than usual. Vaccine failure may be due to a concurrent infection or to a low level of pre-existing antibody, which may be undetectable by the less sensitive antibody screening techniques, such as HAI or SRH[98,99]. If an antibody response is not detected, sera should be retested by a more sensitive technique, such as EIA or LA. Some women fail to produce antibody concentrations >15000 IU/l as detected by SRH, even after several vaccinations. Therefore, many laboratories consider women with a well-documented history of two or more vaccinations to be immune if a low level of antibody is detectable by both SRH and another assay. Passively acquired antibody may interfere with vaccine uptake. This may occur if rubella vaccine is given shortly after blood transfusion[100–102], or when infants are vaccinated at too young an age, when maternal antibodies are still present[103].

VACCINATION PROGRAMMES

A national vaccination strategy is dependent on such factors as the age of acquisition of rubella, accessibility of the target population for rubella vaccination, vaccine coverage attainable and the availability of serologic testing, both for identifying susceptible adult women and to monitor change in the epidemiology of rubella following the introduction of rubella vaccination. It is also important to initiate and maintain a congenital rubella surveillance programme to determine whether the rubella vaccination programme is effective, since the main aim of all programmes is to reduce and eventually eliminate congenitally acquired rubella.

Vaccination strategy in the USA

In the USA, universal immunization of pre-pubertal children of both sexes was introduced in 1969[94]. The aim of this programme was to interrupt transmission of rubella virus from young children to susceptible pregnant women. This strategy also avoided the risk of inadvertently vaccinating adult women who might be pregnant or become pregnant during the post-vaccination period. Furthermore, by vaccinating children, the incidence of vaccine-induced reactions, particularly joint symptoms, would be low, since they occur most commonly in post-pubertal females (see p. 164). In the USA, rubella vaccines are now usually administered with measles and mumps as a combined vaccine (MMR) (p. 161–2). Because high vaccination uptake rates have been achieved among children, this being in part a reflection of legislation in all states requiring children to be vaccinated before entering primary school, there has been a dramatic decline in both postnatally and congenitally acquired rubella (Figure 1). However, in the late 1970s it was observed that there was still a high proportion of adolescents and young adults who were susceptible, despite a marked reduction in susceptibility and incidence of rubella among pre-school children. This was reflected in reports of outbreaks among university students, and military and hospital personnel (reviewed in ref. 94), which led to an increase in the number of reported rubella cases from 12400 in 1976 to 20300 in 1977. However, as a result of a vigorous vaccination programme directed at adolescents and susceptible adult women who missed rubella vaccination in childhood, the incidence of rubella has been reduced substantially. Only 551 cases of rubella were reported in 1986, a 99% decrease from 1969, when rubella vaccines were first given product licences[104].

Vaccination strategies in the UK

In the UK a selective vaccination programme was introduced in 1970. Initially, this was directed towards 11–14-year-old schoolgirls without prior rubella antibody screening. As a result of this programme it was anticipated that most women of child-bearing age would be immune to rubella in due course, since those who had escaped naturally acquired infection would acquire vaccine-induced immunity. However, this strategy would not affect circulation of wild rubella virus in the community. Thus, many persons

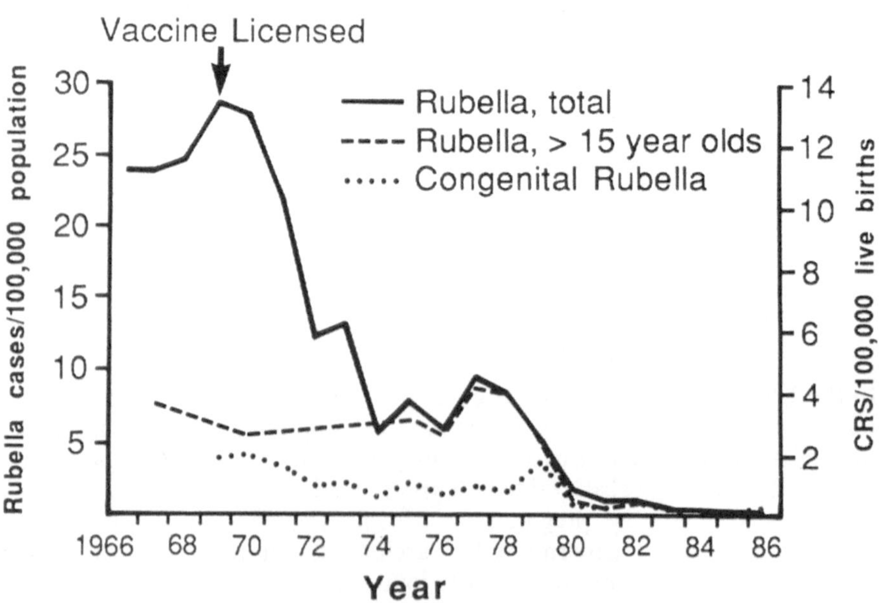

Figure 1 Declining incidence of postnatally acquired and congenital rubella in the USA, 1966–86

would continue to acquire immunity via natural infection and some with low levels of antibody might experience 'booster' responses. It was appreciated that this strategy would not result in a substantial decline in congenitally acquired rubella for a decade or more[105]. In order to reduce rubella susceptibility among women in the high-risk age groups, the programme was extended in 1972 to women at special risk, such as nurses, doctors and schoolteachers. However, in order to obviate the risk of inadvertently vaccinating women who were already pregnant, or might become pregnant post-vaccination, it was recommended that adult women should be tested for rubella antibodies before vaccination. Since approximately 80% would already be immune, the risk of vaccinating pregnant women would be markedly reduced. In 1974 the programme was extended to women attending antenatal and family planning clinics. Susceptible pregnant women were offered rubella vaccine in the immediate post-partum period. General practitioners were advised to encourage all adult female patients of child-bearing age to be screened and, if susceptible, offered rubella vaccine.

Intensification of the rubella vaccination programme in the mid-1980s resulted in uptake rates approaching 90% among schoolgirls and a marked reduction in susceptibility among women of child-bearing age. Thus, between 1984 and 1986 only 2.3–5.8% of women attending antenatal clinics in different parts of England and Wales were found to be susceptible, and in Scotland and Northern Ireland the proportion of susceptibles was as low as 1.7%[106]. A lower rate of susceptibility among multiparous women suggested that post-partum vaccination was effective in reducing susceptibility[107]. However, despite these encouraging trends, and the fact that the number of cases of congenital rubella showed some decline[108], rubella still continued to infect remaining susceptible pregnant women. Thus, although the proportion of women attending antenatal clinics in Manchester, who were susceptible to rubella, fell from 6.4% in 1979 to 2.7% in 1984, rubella was confirmed in 57 pregnant women between 1983 and 1984, representing 2% of susceptibles[109]. In 1986, 173 cases of laboratory-confirmed rubella were reported in England and Wales during the first 16 weeks of pregnancy[107]; many of these pregnancies were terminated (Figure 2).

It must be considered that those cases of maternal rubella which continue to occur are the result of failure to implement the vaccination policy adequately. Thus, an analysis of 99 cases of maternal rubella in England and Wales in 1987–88 showed that 33% of these women were of an age to have been offered vaccination at school, and 62% had been eligible for post-partum vaccination following a previous pregnancy (E. Miller, personal communication). Eighteen of 27 (67%) proven cases of maternal rubella in Edinburgh in 1979 occurred in women who had been shown to be rubella-susceptible in a previous pregnancy[110].

Seronegative pregnant women are often exposed to their own children with rubella. A study in London in 1986 showed that 27% had been exposed to their own children, and that 79% of the contacts reported had been children under the age of 10[111]. Since it is unrealistic to believe that the 2–3% susceptibility rate among women of child-bearing age will be substantially improved, and because the continued circulation of rubella still results in

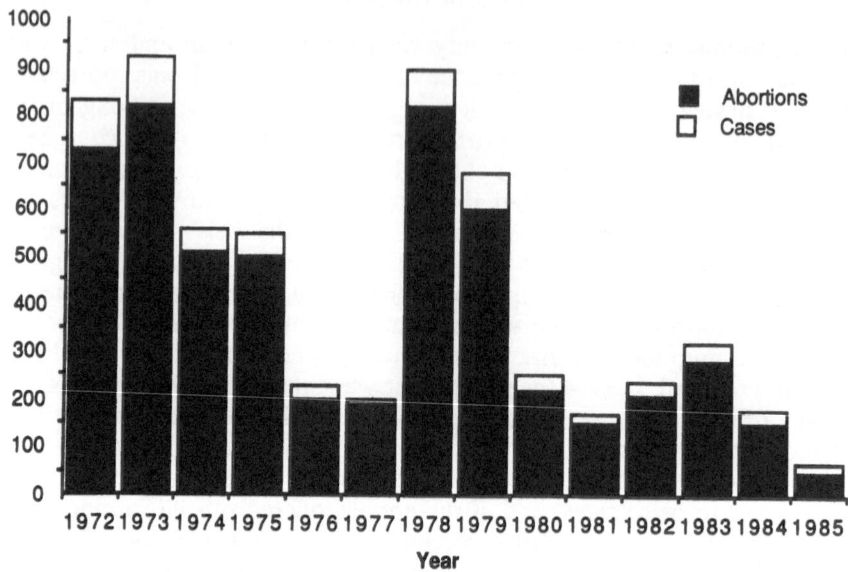

Figure 2 Cases of congenitally acquired rubella and terminations of pregnancy due to rubella, in the UK, 1972–85 (from the PHLS Communicable Disease Surveillance Centre)

infection occurring among the few remaining susceptible women, the rubella vaccination programme has now been augmented. From 1 October 1988 the single-antigen measles vaccine was replaced by MMR for children aged 13–15 months, of both sexes. As part of a 'catch-up' programme to continue for 3–4 years, MMR is also being given to children aged 4–5 years at the time of their pre-school diphtheria/tetanus/polio booster, regardless of a history of previous measles vaccine or a history of measles, mumps or rubella infection[112,113]. However, the programme of vaccination of schoolgirls and susceptible adult women must continue for several years, until rubella virus no longer circulates and 90-95% of adolescents are immune. This programme is directed towards the eradication of congenitally acquired rubella, since not only will high levels of immunity be maintained among schoolgirls and adult women, but by vaccinating infants and young children, transmission of wild virus to pregnant women will be prevented. The success of this vaccination programme depends on a high uptake of MMR among pre-school children. Knox[114], and Anderson and May[115], used mathematical models to show that failure to immunize a very high proportion of pre-school children would result in a delay in the age at which rubella is acquired, which in turn might result in infection occurring more frequently among adolescents and young adults, as previously occurred in the USA. Anderson and Grenfell[116] calculated that only uniform vaccination rates of greater than 80–85% among pre-school children would in the long term eradicate rubella virus. The target has been set at 90% coverage by 1990.

Monitoring the new programme

In order to monitor the uptake of MMR vaccine, the COVER (Cover of Vaccinations Evaluated Rapidly) programme, plans to obtain quarterly reports on vaccine uptake, which will allow quick identification of districts where implementation is poor[113]. The monitoring process will also include surveillance of measles, mumps and rubella, continued surveillance of rubella in pregnancy and serological surveillance of susceptibility in different age groups[117].

Vaccination programmes in other countries

In the early 1980s Sweden, Norway and Finland extended their existing programme of vaccinating pre-pubertal girls by offering MMR vaccination to pre-school children[46,118]. This has resulted in improvements of vaccine coverage. However, recent data from Finland have identified an 'immunity gap' among girls aged 11–13 years[119], which emphasized the need for surveillance and the need to continue to vaccinate girls in this age group. In Iceland, a small country with an accessible target population, the policy of screening all women aged 12–40 years and vaccinating the susceptibles has been shown to be cost-effective[120].

A recent survey of rubella vaccination policies in 17 European countries showed that several different strategies are being used, and warned that this could be dangerous for young migrants and pregnant women who travel to countries where rubella virus continues to circulate[121]. A harmonization of immunization policies is therefore advisable. Problems of this nature were experienced in Canada, where two different immunization policies were adopted in 1969 by the 10 provinces. In 1982 a combined policy of mass vaccination of pre-school children and selective vaccination of pre-pubertal girls was introduced in all provinces[122].

REFERENCES

1. Gregg, N. McA. (1941). Congenital cataract following German measles in the mother. *Trans. Ophthal. Soc. Aust.*, **3**, 35–46
2. Swan, C., Tostevin, A. L., Moore, B., Mayo, H. and Black, G. H. B. (1943). Congenital defects in infants following infectious diseases during pregnancy, with special reference to relationship between German measles and cataract, deaf-mutism, heart disease and microcephaly, and to period of pregnancy in which occurrence of rubella is followed by congenital abnormalities. *Med. J. Austr.*, **2**, 201–10
3. Hanshaw, J. B., Dudgeon, J. A. and Marshall, W. C. (1985). *Viral Diseases of the Foetus and Newborn*, 2nd edn. (Philadelphia: W. B. Saunders)
4. Banatavala, J. E. and Best, J. M. (1984). Rubella. In Brown, F. and Wilson, Sir G (eds), *Topley and Wilson's Principles of Bacteriology, Virology and Immunity*, Vol. 4, pp. 271–302. (London: Edward Arnold)
5. Parkman, P. D., Buescher, E. L. and Artenstein, M. S. (1962). Recovery of rubella virus from army recruits. *Proc. Soc. Exp. Biol. Med.*, **111**, 225–30
6. Weller, T. H. and Neva, F. A. (1962). Propagation in tissue culture of cytopathic agents from patients with rubella-like illness. *Proc. Soc. Exp. Biol. Med.*, **111**, 215–25
7. Parkman, P. D., Buescher, E. L., Artenstein, M. S., McCowan, J. M., Mundon, F. K. and Druzd, A. D. (1964). Studies of rubella. 1. Properties of the virus. *J. Immunol.*, **93**, 595–607
8. Givan, K. F., Rozee, K. R. and Rhodes, A. J. (1965). Incidence of rubella antibodies in female subjects. *Can. Med. Assoc. J.*, **92**, 126–8
9. Rawls, W. E., Melnick, J. L., Bradstreet, C. M. P., Bailey, M., Ferris, A. A., Lehmann, N. I., Nagler, F. P., Furesz, J., Kono, R., Rohtawara, M., Halonen, P., Stewart, J., Ryan, J.

M., Strauss, J., Zdrazilek, J., Leerhoy, J., Von Magnus, H., Sohier, R. and Ferreira, W. (1967). WHO collaborative study on the sero-epidemiology of rubella. *Bull. WHO*, **37**, 79-88

10. Rawls, W. E. (1968). Congenital rubella: the significance of virus persistence. *Prog. Med. Virol.*, **10**, 238–85
11. Thompson, L. M. and Tobin, J.O'H. (1970). Isolation of rubella virus from abortion material. *Br. Med. J.*, **2**, 264-6
12. Cooper, L. Z. (ed.) (1975). *Infections of the Fetus and the Newborn Infant. Congenital Rubella in the United States*, Vol. 3, pp. 1–21. (New York: A. R. Liss)
13. Plotkin, S. A., Oski, F. A., Hartnett, E. M., Hervada, A. R., Friedman, S. and Gowing, J. (1965). Some recently recognized manifestations of the rubella syndrome. *J. Pediatr.*, **67**, 182–91
14. Rubella Symposium (1965). *Am. J. Dis. Child.*, **110** (4)
15. Miller, E., Cradock-Watson, J. E. and Pollock, T. M. (1982). Consequences of confirmed maternal rubella at successive stages of pregnancy. *Lancet*, **2**, 781–4
16. Grillner, L., Forsgren, M., Barr, B., Böttinger, M., Danielsson, L. and De Verdier, C. (1983). Outcome of rubella during pregnancy with special reference to the 17–24 weeks of gestation. *Scand. J. Infect. Dis.*, **15**, 321–5
17. Cradock-Watson, J. E., Ridehalgh, M. K. S., Anderson, M. J., Pattison, J. R. and Kangro, H. O. (1980). Fetal infection resulting from maternal rubella after the first trimester of pregnancy. *J. Hyg. (Camb.)*, **85**, 381-91
18. Peckham, C. S. (1972). Clinical and laboratory study of children exposed in utero to maternal rubella. *Arch. Dis. Child.*, **47**, 571-7
19. Munro, N. D., Sheppard, S., Smithells, R. W., Holzel, H. and Jones, G. (1987). Temporal relations between maternal rubella and congenital defects. *Lancet*, **2**, 201–4
20. Enders, G., Nickerl-Pacher, U., Miller, E. and Cradock-Watson, J. E. (1988). Outcome of confirmed periconceptional maternal rubella. *Lancet*, **1**, 1445–6
21. Stewart, G. L., Parkman, P. D., Hopps, H. E., Douglas, R. D., Hamilton, J. P. and Meyer, H. M. (1967). Rubella-virus hemagglutination-inhibition test. *N. Engl. J. Med.*, **276**, 554–7
22. Best, J. M. and O'Shea, S. (1988). Togaviridae: *Rubella Virus*, In Lennette, E. H., Halonen, P. and Murphy, F. A. (eds) *Laboratory Diagnosis of Infectious Diseases: Principles and Practice* Togaviridae: Vol. II, pp. 435–50 (New York: Springer)
23. Harcourt, G. C., Best, J. M. and Banatvala, J. E. (1980). Rubella-specific serum and nasopharyngeal antibodies in volunteers with naturally acquired and vaccine induced immunity following intranasal challenge. *J. Infect. Dis.*, **142**, 145–55
24. O'Shea, S., Best, J. M., Banatvala, J. E. and Shepherd, W. M. (1985). Development and persistence of class-specific antibodies in the serum and nasopharyngeal washings of rubella vaccinees. *J. Infect. Dis.*, **151**, 89–98
25. Sever, J. L., Schiff, G. M. and Huebner, R. J. (1963). Inactivated rubella virus vaccine. *J. Lab. Clin. Med.*, **62**, 1015
26. Parkman, P. D., Meyer, H. M., Kirschstein, B. L. and Hopps, H. E. (1966). Attenuated rubella virus. I. Development and laboratory characterization. *N. Engl. J. Med.*, **275**, 569-74
27. Meyer, H. M., Parkman, P. D., Hobbins, T. E. and Ennis, F. A. (1968). Clinical studies with experimental live rubella virus vaccine (strain HPV-77). *Am. J. Dis. Child.*, **115**, 648–54
28. Meyer, H. M., Parkman, P. D. and Panos, T. C. (1966). Attenuated rubella virus. II. Production of an experimental live-virus vaccine and clinical trials. *N. Engl. J. Med.*, **275**, 575–80
29. Hilleman, M. R., Buynak, E. B., Whitman, J. E., Weibel, R. W. and Stokes, J. (1969). Live attenuated rubella virus vaccines. Experiments with duck embryo cell preparations. *Am. J. Dis. Child.*, **118**, 166–71
30. Parkman, P. D. and Meyer, H. M. (1969). Prospects for a rubella virus vaccine. *Progr. Med. Virol.*, **11**, 80–106
31. Plotkin, S. A., Farquhar, J., Katz, M. and Ingalls, T. H. (1967). A new attenuated rubella virus grown in human fibroblasts: evidence for reduced nasopharyngeal excretion. *Am. J. Epidemiol.*, **86**, 468–77
32. Shishido, A. and Ohtawara, M. (1976). Development of attenuated rubella virus vaccines in Japan. *Jpn. J. Med. Sci. Biol.*, **29**, 227–53

33. Buynak, E. B., Hilleman, M. R., Weibell, R. E. and Stokes, J. (1968). Live attenuated rubella virus vaccines, prepared in duck embryo cell culture I. Development and clinical testing. *J. Am. Med. Assoc.*, **204**, 195–200
34. Peetermans, J. and Huygelen, C. (1967). Attenuation of rubella virus by serial passage in primary rabbit kidney cell cultures. I. Growth charateristics *in vitro* and production of experimental vaccines at different passage levels. *Arch. Ges. Virusforsch.*, **21**, 133–42
35. Martin du Pan, R., Huygelen, C., Peetermans, J. and Prinzie, A. (1968). Clinical trials with a live attenuated rubella virus vaccine. *Am. J. Dis. Child.*, **115**, 658-62
36. Plotkin, S. A., Ingalls, T. H., Farquhar, J. D. and Katz, M. (1968). Intranasally administered rubella vaccine. *Lancet*, **2**, 934
37. Minekawa, Y., Suzuki, M., Osame, J., Ueda, S., Yamanishi, K., Takahashi, M. and Okuno, Y. (1973). Studies on live rubella vaccine. IV. Comparative field trials with attenuated vaccines at different passage levels in Japanese quail embryo fibroblast cells. *Biken J.*, **16**, 155–60
38. Hoshino, M., Oka, Y., Deguoji, M., Hirajama, M. and Kono, R. (1982). The ten year follow-up of the persistence of humoral antibody to rubella virus acquired by vaccination with the Japanese TO-336 vaccine. *J. Biol. Stand.*, **10**, 213-19
39. Ohwada, Y., Yamane, Y., Nagashima, T., Adachi, A., Ikumi, H., Hashimoto, T. and Mizunoe, K. (1973). Studies on the live attenuated rubella virus vaccine. II. Research concerning attenuation of 'Takahashi strain' isolated in Japan. *Kitasato Arch. Exp. Med.*, **46**, 93-113
40. Ueda, K., Nagayama, T., Kanemitsu, T., Kyoshoin, F., Katsuta, M., Istii, K., Kanimori, T., Yashikawa, H., Ohhashi, T. and Nonaka, J. (1974). Clinical studies on an attenuated rubella virus vaccine (Matsuba strain GMK_3 SK_{60} RK_6). *Jpn. Med. J.*, **2616**, 29–32
41. Parkman, P. D., Phillips, P. E., Kirschstein, R. L. and Meyer, H. M. (1965). Experimental rubella virus infection in the rhesus monkey. *J. Immunol.*, **95**, 743-52
42. Regamey, R. H., De Barbieri, A., Hennessen, W., Ikic, D. and Perkins, F. T. (eds) (1969). International Symposium on Rubella Vaccines, London. *Symp. Series Immunobiol. Stand.* (Basel/New York: Karger)
43. Proceedings of the International Conference on Rubella Immunisation (1969). *Am. J. Dis. Child.*, **118**
44. Weibel, R. E., Buynak, E. B., McLean, A. A., Roehm, R. R. and Hilleman, M. R. (1980). Persistence of antibody in human subjects for 7–10 years following administration of combined live attenuated measles, mumps and rubella virus vaccines. *Proc. Soc. Exp. Biol. Med.*, **165**, 260–3
45. Robertson, C. M., Bennett, V. J., Jefferson, N. and Mayon-White, R. T. (1988). Serological evaluation of a measles, mumps and rubella vaccine. *Arch. Dis. Child.*, **63**, 612-16
46. Böttiger, M., Christenson, B., Romanus, V., Taranger, J. and Strandell, A. (1988). Swedish experience of two dose vaccination programme aiming at eliminating measles, mumps and rubella. *Br. Med. J.*, **295**, 1264–7
47. Perkins, F. T. (1985). Licensed vaccines. *Rev. Infect. Dis.*, **7** (Suppl. 1), S73–76
48. Plotkin, S. A., Farquhar, J. D. and Ogra, P. L. (1973). Immunologic properties of RA27/3 rubella vaccine. *J. Am. Med. Assoc.*, **225**, 585–90
49. Best, J. M., Banatvala, J. E. and Bowen, J. M. (1974). New Japanese rubella vaccine: comparative trials. *Br. Med. J.*, **3**, 221–4
50. Harcourt, G. C., Best, J. M. and Banatvala, J. E. (1979). HLA antigens and responses to rubella vaccination. *J. Hyg.* (*Camb.*), **83**, 405–12
51. Weibel, R. E., Stokes, J., Buynak, E. B. and Hilleman, M. R. (1972). Influence of age on clinical response to HPV-77 duck rubella vaccine. *J. Am. Med. Assoc.*, **222**, 805–7
52. Spruance, S. L., Klock, L. E., Bailey, A., Ward, J. R. and Smith, C. B. (1972). Recurrent joint symptoms in children vaccinated with HPV-77. DK12 rubella vaccine. *J. Pediatr.*, **80**, 413–17
53. Thompson, G. R., Weiss, J. J., Shillis, J. L. and Brackett, R. G. (1973). Intermittent arthritis following rubella vaccination. *Am. J. Dis. Child.*, **125**, 526–30
54. Stokes, J. Jr., Weibel, R. E., Buynak, E. B. and Hilleman, M. R. (1969). Clinical laboratory findings in adult women given HPV-77 rubella vaccine. International Symposium on Rubella Vaccines, London. *Symp. Series Immunobiol. Stand.*, **11**, 415–22. (Basel/New York: Karger)

55. Grayzel, A. I. and Beck, C. (1970). Rubella infection of synovial cells and the resistance of cells derived from patients with rheumatoid arthritis. *J. Exp. Med.*, **131**, 367–73
56. Ogra, P. L. and Herd, J. K. (1971). Arthritis associated with induced rubella infection. *J. Immunol.*, **107**, 810–13
57. Vergani, D., Morgan-Capner, P., Davies, E. T., Anderson, A. W., Tee, D. E. H. and Pattison, J. R. (1980). Joint symptoms, immune complexes and rubella. *Lancet*, **2**, 321–2
58. Coyle, P. K., Wolinsky, J. S., Buimovici-Klein, E., Moucha, R. and Cooper, L. Z. (1982). Rubella-specific immune complexes after congenital infection and vaccination. *Infect. Immun.*, **36**, 498–503
59. Chantler, J. K., Ford, D. K. and Tingle, A. J. (1981). Rubella-associated arthritis: rescue of rubella virus from peripheral blood lymphocytes two years post vaccination. *Infect. Immun.*, **32**, 1274–80
60. Chantler, J. K., Ford, D. K. and Tingle, A. J. (1982). Persistent rubella infection and rubella-associated arthritis. *Lancet*, **1**, 1323–5
61. Chantler, J. K., Tingle, A. J. and Petty, R. E. (1985). Persistent rubella virus infection associated with chronic arthritis in children. *N. Engl. J. Med.*, **313**, 1117–22
62. Freestone, D. S., Prydie, J., Smith, S., Hamilton, G. and Laurence, G. (1971). Vaccination of adults with Wistar RA27/3 rubella vaccine. *J. Hyg. (Camb.)*, **69**, 471–7
63. Forrest, J. M., Honeyman, M. C. and Louric, V. A. (1974). Rubella vaccination and thrombocytopenia. *Aust. N.Z. J. Med.*, **4**, 352–5
64. Meegan, J. M., Evans, B. K. and Horstmann, D. M. (1983). Use of enzyme immunoassays and the latex agglutination test to measure the temporal appearance of immunoglobulin G and M antibodies after natural infection or immunization with rubella virus. *J. Clin. Microbiol.*, **18**, 745–8
65. Enders, G., Knotek, F. and Pacher, U. (1985). Comparison of various serological methods and diagnostic kits for the detection of acute, recent, and previous rubella infection, vaccination and congenital infections. *J. Med. Virol.*, **16**, 219–32
66. Banatvala, J. E. (1977). Rubella vaccines. In Waterson, A. P. (ed.), *Recent Advances in Clinical Virology*, pp. 171–190. (Edinburgh: Churchill Livingstone)
67. Chu, S. Y., Bernier, R. H., Stewart, J. A., Herrmann, K. L., Greenspan, J. R., Henderson, A. K. and Liang, A. P. (1988). Rubella antibody persistence after immunization. Sixteen-year follow-up in the Hawaiian islands. *J. Am. Med. Assoc.*, **259**, 3133–6
68. Cusi, M. G., Rossolini, G. M., Cellesi, C. and Valensin, P. E. (1988). Antibody response to wild rubella virus structural proteins following immunization with RA27/3 live attenuated vaccine. *Arch. Virol.*, **101**, 25–33
69. Hillary, I. B. and Griffith, A. H. (1984). Persistence of rubella antibodies 15 years after subcutaneous administration of Wistar 27/3 strain live attenuated rubella virus vaccine. *Vaccine*, **2**, 274–76
70. Horstmann, D. M., Schluederberg, A., Emmons, J. E., Evans, B. K., Randolph, M. F. and Andiman, W. A. (1985). Persistence of vaccine-induced immune responses to rubella: comparison with natural infection. *Rev. Infect. Dis.*, **7** (Suppl. 1), S80–85
71. Just, M., Just, V., Berger, R., Burkhardt, F. and Schilt, U. (1985). Duration of immunity after rubella vaccination: A long term study in Switzerland. *Rev. Infect. Dis.*, **7** (Suppl. 1), S91–93
72. Orenstein, W. A., Herrmann, K. L., Holmgreen, P., Bernier, R., Bart, K. J., Eddins, D. L. and Fiumara, N. J. (1986). Prevalence of rubella antibodies in Massachusetts schoolchildren. *Am. J. Epidemiol.*, **124**, 290–8
73. Enders, G. and Nickerl, U. (1988). Rubella vaccination: persistence of antibodies for 14–17 years and immune status of women with and without vaccination history. *Immun. Infect.*, **16**, 58–64
74. O'Shea, S., Woodward, S., Best, J. M., Banatvala, J. E., Holzel, H. and Dudgeon, J. A. (1988). Rubella vaccination: Persistence of antibodies for 10–21 years. *Lancet*, **2**, 909
75. Banatvala, J. E., Druce, A., Best, J. M. and Al-Nakib, W. (1977). Specific IgM responses after rubella vaccination potential application following inadvertent vaccination during pregnancy. *Br. Med. J.*, **2**, 1263–4
76. Mortimer, P. P., Edwards, J. M. B., Porter, A. D., Tedder, R. S. and Haslehurst, J. (1984). The immunoglobulin M response to rubella vaccine in young adult women. *J. Hyg. (Camb.)*, **92**, 277–83

77. Ogra, P. L., Kerr-Grant, D., Umana, G., Dzierba, J. and Weintraub, D. (1971). Antibody response in serum and nasopharynx after naturally acquired and vaccine-induced infection with rubella virus. *N. Engl. J. Med.*, **285**, 1333–9
78. Cradock-Watson, J. E., MacDonald, H., Ridehalgh, K. S., Bourne, M. S. and Vandervelde, E. M. (1974). Specific immunoglobulin responses in serum and nasal secretions after administration of attenuated rubella vaccine. *J. Hyg. (Camb.)*, **73**, 127–41
79. Inouye, S., Kono, R. and Takeuchi, Y. (1978). Oligomeric immunoglobulin A antibody response to rubella virus infection. *J. Clin. Microbiol.*, **8**, 1–6
80. Honeyman, M. C., Forrest, J. M. and Dorman, D. C. (1974). Cell-mediated immune response following natural rubella and rubella vaccination. *Clin. Exp. Immunol.*, **17**, 665–71
81. Rossier, E., Phipps, P. H., Polley, J. R. and Webb, T. (1977). Absence of cell-mediated immunity to rubella virus 5 years after rubella vaccination. *Can. Med. Assoc. J.*, **116**, 481–4
82. Buimovici-Klein, E. and Cooper. L. Z. (1985). Cell-mediated immune response in rubella infections. *Rev. Infect. Dis.*, **7** (Suppl. 1), S123–8
83. O'Shea, S., Best, J. M. and Banatvala, J. E. (1983). Viremia, virus excretion and antibody responses after challenge in volunteers with low levels of antibody to rubella virus. *J. Infect. Dis.*, **148**, 639–47
84. Morgan-Capner, P., Hodgson, J., Hamblin, M. H., Dulake, C., Coleman, J. J., Boswell, P. A., Watkins, R. P., Booth, J., Stern, H., Best, J. M. and Banatvala, J. E. (1985). Detection of rubella specific IgM in subclinical rubella reinfection in pregnancy *Lancet*, **1**, 244–6
85. Cradock-Watson, J. E., Ridehalgh, M. K. S., Anderson, M. J. and Pattison, J. R. (1985). Rubella re-infection and the fetus. *Lancet*, **2**, 1039
86. Schiff, G. M., Young, B. C., Stefanovic, G. M., Stamler, E. F., Knowiton, D. R., Grundy, B. J. and Dorsett, P. H. (1985). Challenge with rubella virus after loss of detectable vaccine-induced antibody. *Rev. Infect. Dis.*, **7** (Suppl. 1), S157–63
87. Morgan-Capner, P. (1986). Does rubella reinfection matter? In Mortimer, P. P. (ed.), *Public Health Virology*, 12 *Reports*. (London: Public Health Laboratory Service)
88. Banatvala, J. E. and Best, J. M. (1973). Rubella reinfections. *Lancet*, **1**, 1452
89. Forsgren, M., Carlström, G. and Strangert, K. (1979). Congenital rubella after maternal reinfection. *Scand. J. Infect. Dis.*, **11**, 81–3
90. Bott, L. M. and Eizenberg, D. H. (1982). Congenital rubella after successful vaccination. *Med. J. Aust.*, **1**, 514–15
91. Enders, G., Calm, A. and Schaub, J. (1984). Rubella embryopathy after previous maternal rubella vaccination. *Infection*, **12**, 96–8
92. Forsgren, M. and Soren, L. (1985). Subclinical rubella reinfection in vaccinated women with rubella-specific IgM response during pregnancy and transmission of virus to the fetus. *Scand. J. Infect. Dis.*, **17**, 337–41
93. Hornstein, L., Levy, U. and Fogel, A. (1988). Clinical rubella with virus transmission to the fetus in a pregnant woman considered to be immune. *N. Engl. J. Med.*, **319**, 1415–16
94. Bart, K., Orenstein, W. A., Preblud, S. R. and Hinman, A. R. (1985). Universal immunization to interrupt rubella. *Rev. Infect. Dis.*, **7** (suppl. 1), S177–84
95. Enders, G. (1985). Rubella antibody titres in vaccinated and nonvaccinated women and results of vaccination during pregnancy. *Rev. Infect Dis.*, **7** (Suppl. 1), S103–107
96. Centers for Disease Control (1987). Rubella vaccination during pregnancy – United States 1971–1986. *Morbid. Mortal. Weekly Rep.*, **36**, 457–61
97. Preblud, S. R., Stetler, H. C., Frank, J. A., Greaves, W. L., Hinman, A. R. and Herrmann, K. L. (1981). Fetal risk associated with rubella vaccine. *J. Am. Med. Assoc.*, **246**, 1413–17
98. Best, J. M., Harcourt, G. C., Druce, A., Palmer, S. J., O'Shea, S. and Banatvala, J. E. (1980). Rubella immunity by four different techniques: results of challenge studies. *J. Med. Virol.*, **5**, 239–47
99. Buimovici-Klein, E., O'Beirne, A. J., Millian, S. J. and Cooper, L. Z. (1980). Low level rubella immunity detected by ELISA and specific lymphocyte transformation. *Arch. Virol.*, **66**, 321–7
100. Grillner, L. and Forssmann, L. (1974). Post-partum rubella vaccination, anti-D immunoglobulins and blood transfusion. *Br. Med. J.*, **4**, 47
101. Watt, R. W. and McGucken, R. B. (1980). Failure of rubella immunization after blood transfusion: birth of congenitally infected infant. *Br. Med. J.*, **281**, 977–8

102. Drabu, Y. J., Walsh, B., Huber, T. J., Schlesinger, P., Vigerathnam, S. and Hicks, L. (1987). Maternal rubella: one problem in diagnosis and another in prevention. *Lancet*, **2**, 561–2
103. Balfour, H. H. and Amren, D. P. (1978). Rubella, measles and mumps antibodies following vaccination of children. A potential rubella problem. *Am. J. Dis. Child.*, **132**, 573–7
104. Rubella and congenital rubella – United States 1984–1986 (1987). *Morbid. Mortal. Weekly Rep.*, **36**, 664–75
105. Dudgeon, J. A. (1985). Selective immunization: protection of the individual. *Rev. Infect. Dis.*, **7** (Suppl. 1), S185–90
106. Noah, N. D. and Fowle, S. E. (1988). Surveillance of immunity to rubella in women of childbearing age in the UK 1984–1986. *Br. Med. J.*, **297**, 1301–4
107. Miller, C. L., Miller, E. and Waight, P. A. (1987). Rubella susceptibility and the continuing risk of infection in pregnancy. *Br. Med. J.*, **294**, 1277–8
108. Holzel, H., Jones, G., Smithells, R. W. and Sheppard, S. (1988). National congenital rubella surveillance programme report: 1987. *Comm. Dis. Rep.*, **15**
109. Miller, C. L., Miller, E., Sequeira, P., Cradock-Watson, J. E., Longson, M. and Wiseberg, E. C. (1985). Effect of selective vaccination on rubella susceptibility and infection in pregnancy. *Br. Med. J.*, **291**, 1398–1401
110. Edmond, E. and Zealley, H. (1986). The impact of a rubella prevention policy on the outcome of rubella in pregnancy. *Br. Med. J.*, **93**, 563–7
111. Best, J. M., Welch, J. M., Baker, D. A. and Banatvala, J. E. (1987). Maternal rubella at St. Thomas' Hospital in 1978 and 1986: support for augmenting the rubella vaccination programme. *Lancet*, **2**, 88–90
112. Badenoch, J. (1988). Big bang for vaccination. *Br. Med. J.*, **297**, 750-1
113. Begg, N. T. (1988). Measles/mumps/rubella vaccine/MMR-implementation. *Comm. Dis. Rep.*, **29**
114. Knox, E. G. (1980). Strategy for rubella vaccination. *Int. J. Epidemiol.*, **9**, 13–23
115. Anderson, R. M. and May, R. M. (1983). Vaccination against rubella and measles: quantitative investigations of different policies. *J. Hyg. (Camb.)*, **90**, 259–325
116. Anderson, R. M. and Grenfell, B. T. (1986). Quantitative investigations of different vaccination policies for the control of congenital rubella syndrome (CRS) in the United Kingdom. *J. Hyg. (Camb.)* **96**, 305–33
117. Miller, C. L., Miller, E., Begg, N. T. and Morgan-Capner, P. (1987). Rubella vaccination policy: a note of reassurance. *Lancet*, **2**, 210
118. Peltola, H., Karanko, V., Kurki, T., Hukkanen, V., Virtanen, M., Penttinen, K., Nissinen, M. and Heinonen, O. P. (1986). Rapid effect on endemic measles, mumps and rubella of nationwide vaccination programme in Finland. *Lancet*, **1**, 137–9
119. Ukkonen, P. and von Bonsdorff, P. (1988). Rubella immunity and morbidity: effects of vaccination in Finland. *Scand. J. Infect. Dis.*, **20**, 255–9
120. Gudnadöttir, M. (1985). Cost-effectiveness of different strategies for prevention of congenital rubella infection: a practical example from Iceland. *Rev. Infect. Dis.*, **7** (Suppl. 1), S200–9
121. Mata, I. de la and Wals, P. de la (1988). Policies for immunization against rubella in European countries. *Eur. J. Epidemiol.*, **4**, 175–80
122. Furesz, J., Varughese, P., Acres, S. E. and Davies, J. W. (1985). Rubella immunization strategies in Canada. *Rev. Infect. Dis.*, **7** (Suppl. 1), S191–3

10
Hepatitis B and A vaccines

R. W. ELLIS and P. J. PROVOST

INTRODUCTION

Hepatitis has been recognized as a serious disease throughout recorded history. Outbreaks of jaundice came to be recognized over time as potentially infectious in nature. The confirmation of a viral aetiology to certain forms of hepatitis was established in the early 1940s in studies in human volunteers to whom hepatitis could be transmitted by a non-bacterial filterable agent[1]. In 1947 MacCallum first coined the terms hepatitis A for infectious hepatitis and hepatitis B for serum hepatitis, terms whose use has stood the test of time.

Over the past 25 years appropriate clinical specimens have been used to initiate either transmissible infection of cells in culture or transmissible infection and disease in appropriate simian species. Such biological studies, when coupled with the development of serological assays for detecting viral antigens and virally-induced antibodies, led to the identification of at least six distinct replication-competent viral agents which cause hepatitis in man[1]. Two of these, cytomegalovirus and Epstein–Barr virus, are members of the herpesvirus family, which are primarily lymphotropic in host range and which cause hepatitis in only a small percentage of people with primary infections. The two or more non-A, non-B (NANB) hepatitis viruses are serologically undefined agents, antigenically non-crossreactive with hepatitis A virus (HAV) or hepatitis B virus (HBV), and thought to be primarily hepatotropic. NANB viruses cause both infectious and blood-borne hepatitis[2]. Infectious NANB appears to be caused by a small enveloped virus[3]. Blood-borne NANB, a disease with a high frequency for developing chronic infections and with a morbidity and mortality from chronic disease generally more severe than that associated with chronic hepatitis B, is caused by one or more hitherto undefined viral agents which appear to be small and enveloped. The other two agents, HAB and HBV, are primarily hepatotropic. This chapter will focus upon the successful and ongoing development of vaccines against infection by these two agents.

Following the development of serum enzyme assays diagnostic for clinical hepatitis, the Willowbrook studies of the late 1950s and 1960s confirmed and extended the earlier definitions for hepatitis A and hepatitis B through epidemiological, clinical and serological analyses[4,5]. The 'MS-1' type of hepatitis fitted MacCallum's designation of hepatitis A, and the 'MS-2' type fitted that of hepatitis B. In particular, the incubation period for hepatitis A was less than 5 weeks, while being longer for hepatitis B. Hepatitis A could be transmitted by filtered stool extracts, while hepatitis B could be transmitted by intimate body contact. Furthermore, acquired immunity to reinfection by one agent did not prevent infection by the other agent.

The Australia (Au) antigen was originally proposed to be a serological marker of leukaemia[6,7]. Subsequently, Au was linked by Blumberg to the development of viral hepatitis, then by Prince, Krugman and co-workers[8,9] specifically to hepatitis B. Electron microscopic examination of plasma from hepatitis B carriers revealed spheres or tubules 22 nm in diameter[10], as well as double-shelled spheres 42 nm in diameter[11]. The 42-nm enveloped particle, or Dane particle (Figure 1A), became identified as the HBV virion by virtue of its containing a core antigen, surface antigen, DNA molecule and DNA polymerase[12]. Ths virus is the prototype of the hepadnavirus family, whose other members discovered to date are associated with hepatitis in ducks, ground squirrels and woodchucks[13]. The 22-nm particle became known as hepatitis B surface antigen (HBsAg), consisting of excess surface protein of HBV lacking DNA and assembled into non-infectious lipoprotein particles. Both types of particles became the central focus for the development of vaccines against hepatitis B due to the lack of replication of the virus in standard cell cultures.

Following the Willowbrook studies the transmissible nature of hepatitis A was confirmed by serial passage of the viral agent to marmosets[14,15] and to chimpanzees[16]. A key study was the visualization, by means of immune electron microscopy using antibodies from convalescent sera, of virions in the stools of volunteers who had been injected with HAV[17]. Serological studies defined a single major antigen of HAV which defined antibodies of diagnostic significance[18]. The HAV virion is a non-enveloped spherical

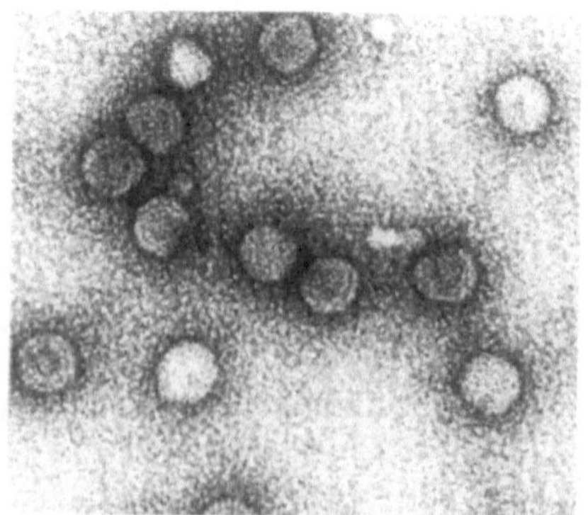
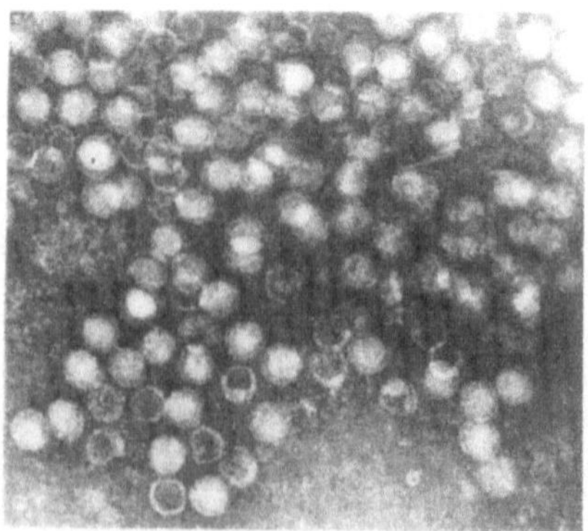

Figure 1 Electron microscopy of (**A**) hepatitis B virus, and (**B**) hepatitis A virus. (Magnification × 200 000)

particle with a diameter of 27 nm and icosahedral symmetry (Figure 1B). It has been assigned within the picornavirus family to the enterovirus genus, whose other members include polioviruses, coxsackieviruses, and echoviruses[19]. The HAV genome is a single-stranded RNA molecule[20].

Consistent with the contrasting physical properties of HAV and HBV (Table 1), the hepatitides caused by each virus contrast both epidemiologically and clinically, as described below. Moreover, the strategies for developing vaccines for each disease have proceeded along very different lines. In this regard the successful development and licensure of two different hepatitis B vaccines, one plasma-derived and the other recombinant yeast-derived, stand in contrast to the ongoing development and clinical testing of two different hepatitis A vaccines, one live attenuated and the other chemically inactivated whole virus.

HEPATITIS B

Epidemiology

HBV infection is one of the world's most widespread public health problems. Chronic infection with this virus is endemic in many parts of the world. Rates of chronic infection are greater than 5% of the population in southeast Asia and sub-Saharan Africa, 3–5% in other parts of Asia, the Middle East and northern Africa and 1–2% in Japan, eastern and southern Europe, Central America and South America[21]. Chronic infections in these populations are the primary human reservoir for HBV. In these populations the most common modes of transmission are from chronically infected mothers to their newborn infants and children, and from close physical contact. Neonates exposed to the virus in this fashion develop chronic hepatitis B infections at a high rate, even though they tend not to develop clinically recognizable acute infections. Such chronic infections can last throughout the lifetime of the infected individual. In developed countries, where rates of

Table 1 Comparative properties of HBV and HAV

	HBV	*HAV*
Family	Hepadnaviridae	Picornaviridae
Diameter	42 nm	27 nm
Lipid envelope	+	–
Design	Spherical	Spherical
Symmetry	Complex	Icosahedral
Genomic nucleic acid	DNA	RNA
Genomic length (nt)	3182–3215	7457
Virion polymerase	+	–
Structural proteins	HBsAg, HBcAg	VPO, VP1, VP2, VP3, VP4
Density (g/cm^3)	1.40	1.34
Other particles	22 nm HBsAg (density = 1.20)	–
Derived vaccines	1. Plasma-derived 2. Recombinant yeast-derived	1. Live attenuated virus 2. Chemically inactivated virions

chronic carriage are lower than in less developed countries, there are two modes of transmission – one being perinatal transmission to newborns from chronically infected mothers (many of whom were born in areas of high endemicity), the other being percutaneous through intimate physical contact or exposure to blood. High-risk adult groups include the sexually promiscuous, illicit users of intravenous drugs who share needles, residents of institutions, those of lower socioeconomic status, and health-care workers exposed to blood. Up to 50% of adults and adolescents exposed to HBV develop recognizable acute infection. While most exposed adults and adolescents completely recover, up to 1% die of fulminant hepatitis, and 5–10% develop chronic hepatitis B. The number of chronic hepatitis B carriers worldwide has been estimated[22] at over 250 million. Beyond the severe morbidity suffered by many of these individuals, hundreds of thousands of these carriers die annually from long-term sequelae of chronic hepatitis B, namely cirrhosis and hepatocellular carcinoma[23]. Unfortunately, there is no understanding of the factors that influence the probability of perinatal exposure or acute infection leading to chronic infection, or of chronic infection developing into chronic active hepatitis, cirrhosis or carcinoma. Since there is no effective treatment available for acute or chronic hepatitis B, prevention becomes paramount.

Successful vaccine development

The initial lead for developing a hepatitis B vaccine emerged from the Willowbrook studies. MS-2 serum, having been shown to contain both HBsAg and HBV, was diluted in water and boiled[24]. As expected, the infectivity of the preparation was destroyed. However, the heat-inactivated serum unexpectedly retained its immunogenicity. Moreover, vaccination of subjects with this boiled preparation resulted in partial protection against HBV infection following exposure[25]. The result demonstrated that HBsAg particles in plasma, whose immunogenicity was resistant to heat treatment, represented a candidate hepatitis B vaccine. The observed protection against disease was proposed to be mediated by antibodies to HBsAg (anti-HBs). This proposal was demonstrated by numerous studies in the 1970s with hepatitis B immune globulin (HBIG), prepared from anti-HBs$^+$ serum, which showed that passive immunization with HBIG could prevent or attenuate hepatitis B infections[26].

Thus, a hepatitis B vaccine candidate was identified. The strategy to develop this candidate into a safe and effective vaccine involved the use of techniques to purify HBsAg from plasma while inactivating HBV that coexisted with HBsAg and which might contaminate final HBsAg preparations[27]. This strategy was facilitated by the development of a chimpanzee model for HBV infections[28,29]. The chimpanzee is one of the few species outside of man which is known to be susceptible to HBV infection. In this species a typical acute infection, which appears 6–18 weeks post-inoculation with standardized HBV preparations, results in the appearance of HBsAg, antibodies to hepatitis B core antigen (anti-HBc), elevations in serum levels of liver enzymes, and histopathological changes of hepatitis in liver biopsies.

As a model for testing the efficacy of a hepatitis B vaccine candidate, a chimpanzee can be vaccinated and then challenged with an inoculum of HBV known to consistently cause the above-mentioned signs of infection. If the animal remains free of these signs for 24 weeks following challenge, the vaccine is deemed effective at preventing infection.

Another critical development during the 1970s was the establishment of sensitive, specific and rapid serological tests for the detection of HBsAg and anti-HBs. Among tests for the detection and quantitation of HBsAg, radioimmunoassays (RIA) and related enzyme-linked immunosorbent assays have been used most commonly[30]. Similarly, the RIA tests are most commonly used for the detection and quantitation of anti-HBs in patients recovered from HBV infection and in vaccinees.

Early testing of HBsAg from a wide range of specimens revealed that all HBsAg preparations possessed the *a* serological determinant, which thus became identified as group-common epitopes[31]. In addition, allelic type-specific determinants were defined, that is *d*/*y* and *r*/*w*, such that the major subtypes of HBsAg, and HBV by inference, are *adr*, *adw*, *ayr* and *ayw*[32]. The existence of the group-common *a* epitopes raised the possibility that a vaccine consisting of HBsAg might protect against all HBV subtypes, which indeed turned out to be the case, as described in the following section.

Plasma-derived vaccine

Source of vaccine antigen

During the course of active HBV infections, either acute or chronic, large amounts of HBsAg, the major viral surface protein, are synthesized in infected liver cells in vast excess over those necessary for physical incorporation into virions. In the rough endoplasmic reticulum and secretory vesicles this excess HBsAg is assembled with cellular lipids into non-infectious 22-nm diameter HBsAg particles. Following secretion from cells these lipoprotein particles circulate in plasma at very high levels (up to 100–500 μg/ml), at a ratio to infectious HBV[29] of up to ($10^4:1$). Since HBV has not been demonstrated to be capable of replicating in cells in culture, plasma containing high levels of HBsAg was exploited as a source material for the successful development of a safe and effective hepatitis B vaccine.

Production process

The process for manufacturing the plasma-derived vaccine in the United States (Heptavax B® or H-B VAX®, Merck Sharp & Dohme)[27] is summarized in Figure 2. The starting material for purification is plasma from chronic hepatitis B carriers who are asymptomatic. Plasma donors are selected for having the highest available titres of HBsAg. Following collection by plasmapheresis the HBsAg is concentrated. Then the purification phase of the process exploits the physical ability to separate low-density 22-nm HBsAg particles from high-density 42-nm HBV particles by two sequential ultracentrifugation techniques. The inactivation phase of the process is designed to kill any residual HBV or other adventitious agents present.

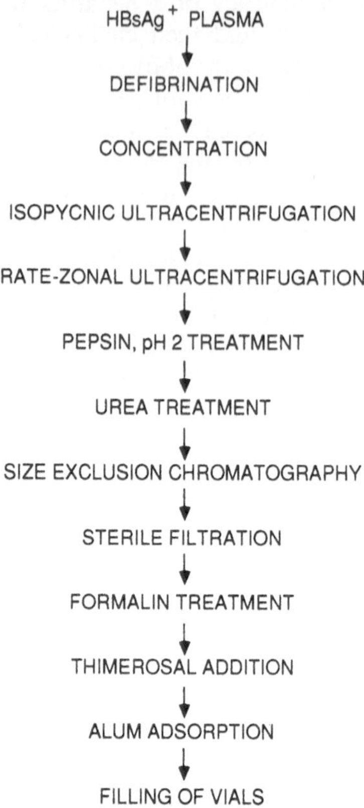

Figure 2 Process for the manufacture of the plasma-derived hepatitis B vaccine, Heptavax B® or H-B-VAX® (Merck, Sharp & Dohme)

Three inactivation steps are used: 1 μg/ml pepsin at pH 2 for 18 h at 37°C, 8 mol/l urea for 4 h at 37°C, and 0.025% (w/v) formalin for 72 h at 37°C[27]. Each of these three steps is capable of inactivating 10^5 chimpanzee infectious doses (ID_{50})/ml of HBV[33]. Furthermore, these steps are capable of inactivating the infectivity of representative agents from all known groups of viruses[33], including human immunodeficiency virus[34]. The product of this entire manufacturing process is a purified preparation of 22-nm HBsAg particles (Figure 3A).

Preclinical testing

The most important preclinical testing of the plasma-derived hepatitis B vaccine was conducted in chimpanzees[29]. This animal model for HBV infection was used to establish two principles – safety and efficacy.

The safety of the vaccine was assured by demonstrating that the manufacturing process for the vaccine resulted in the inactivation of HBV infectivity. As mentioned above, treatment of 10^5 ID_{50} of HBV with any one of the three inactivation procedures used during manufacture resulted in a preparation incapable of inducing infection upon intravenous injection into

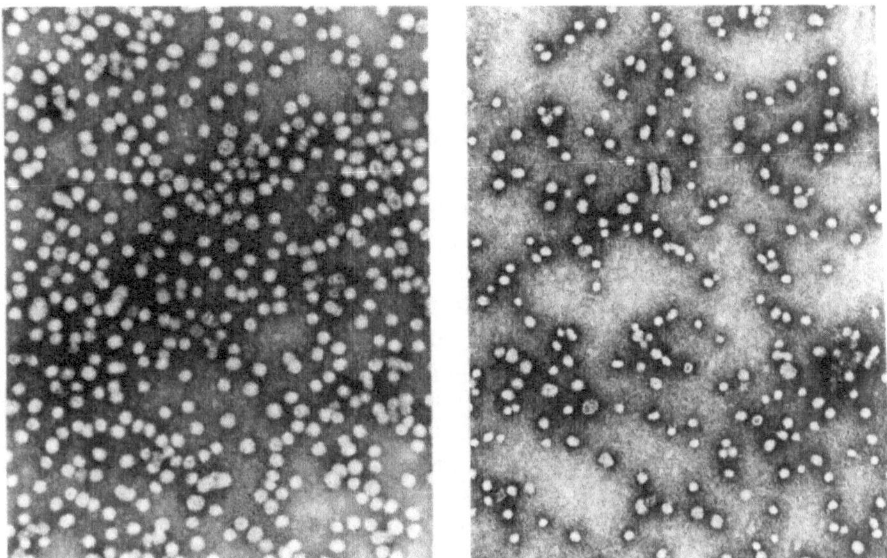

Figure 3 Elecron microscopy of hepatitis B vaccine derived from (**A**) plasma, or (**B**) recombinant yeast. (Magnification × 160000)

chimpanzees[29]. Furthermore, the injection of 1, 10, or 20 doses of purified vaccine antigen failed to induce HBV infection[35,36]. Such safety testing has become standard for hepatitis B vaccines worldwide.

The protective efficacy conferred by injections with the plasma-derived vaccine was demonstrated in chimpanzees. Initially, standardized HBV inocula of subtypes *adr*, *adw* and *ayw* were prepared by United States government laboratories and titrated for infectivity in chimpanzees[28,29]. In the first successful protection experiment reported[37], six chimpanzees were vaccinated with three 20-μg doses of Heptavax B® (mostly *adw*); five of these animals produced high titres of anti-HBs. Following challenge with 10^3 ID_{50} of HBV, none of the six vaccinated animals developed any sign of HBV infection (HBsAg, anti-HBc or elevated levels of liver enzymes in serum), while the five unvaccinated animals injected with the same HBV inocula all developed signs of HBV infection. Thus, plasma-derived HBsAg was proven to be a protective antigen. Furthermore, cross-protection of animals could be demonstrated, in that chimpanzees recovered from infection by a particular HBV subtype (*ayw*) were protected against challenge with HBV of a different subtype (*adr*)[35]. These studies reaffirmed the importance of the *a* epitopes as the group-specific serological determinants which elicit antibodies protective against all HBV subtypes. Recent studies have shown that the *a* epitopes map to amino acids 124–137 in the HBsAg polypeptide[38]. Moreover, a monoclonal antibody (MAB) directed against one particular *a* epitope, when mixed *in vitro* with HBV, neutralized the infectivity of HBV for chimpanzees[39].

Clinical testing

The first stage of clinical testing for Heptavax B® was a phase I clinical trial in which safety and tolerability were confirmed in healthy volunteers. These studies also provided initial data on the immunogenicity of the vaccine. Subsequently, phase II trials were conducted, during which optimal doses were selected for all age groups and the immunogenicity of the vaccine in man was confirmed. Phase III studies then tested the ability of the vaccine to protect against clinical infection. Volunteers seronegative for HBsAg, anti-HBs and anti-HBc were vaccinated intramuscularly at 0, 1 and 6 months. Sera taken at 0, 1, 3, 6 and 7–9 months were tested for anti-HBs. Similarities in the immune responses of adults to three 20–40 μg doses[40,41] led to the selection of a 20-μg dose for adults and, by similar analysis, a 10-μg dose for children 10 years of age or younger. These phases of clinical testing encompassed vaccination of over 10000 volunteers.

Two protective efficacy trials of the vaccine were conducted among sexually active homosexuals, a group which had a high attack rate of hepatitis B. Both studies were double-blind placebo-controlled trials in which volunteers were randomized to vaccinated and control groups receiving either the plasma-derived vaccine or an alum placebo control. In one study[42] using three 40-μg doses of vaccine, the 25.6% attack rate for HBV infection in the control group contrasted with the 3.2% rate among vaccinees. This represented an 87% efficacy rate for vaccination. In another study using three 20 μg doses of vaccine[43], a similar efficacy rate was observed; 85% of vaccinees made anti-HBs after receiving the three doses of vaccine. In both studies, most cases of HBV infection occurred in vaccinees who produced little or no anti-HBs. In light of these studies, Heptavax B® was licensed in the United States in November 1981.

These studies demonstrated that the protection afforded by vaccination against clinical hepatitis B could be correlated with the levels of anti-HBs elicited in vaccinees. Specifically, a protective level of anti-HBs has been considered to be greater than 10 sample ratio units[43,44], that is, $S/N \geq 10$. This level is approximately equal to 10 milli-International Units (mIU)/ml, which has been defined relative to an internationally accepted reference standard[45]. Thus, ≥ 10 mIU anti-HBs/ml has become the target for immunogenicity in developing both plasma-derived and non-plasma-derived hepatitis B vaccines.

Despite the excellent safety profile of the plasma-derived vaccine used in millions of recipients worldwide, acceptance has been less than anticipated. Furthermore, the human source for HBsAg has been a limiting factor in the production of sufficient quantities of vaccine for worldwide use. Therefore, a need has developed for a second-generation hepatitis B vaccine.

Recombinant DNA (rDNA) technology was emerging to the forefront as a research tool in the late 1970s. The relaxation of guidelines for biological and physical containment, coupled with early breakthroughs in several research areas, made rDNA technology attractive as a means for providing such a second-generation vaccine, in particular one which would be efficient in eliciting ≥ 10 mIU anti-HBs/ml in vaccinees.

Recombinant yeast-derived vaccine

The yeast-derived hepatitis B vaccine is the first recombinant-derived vaccine approved for human use; it remains the only one approved at the time of publication of this volume. Unless referenced otherwise, this section will describe the development of the recombinant yeast-derived vaccine known as Recombivax HB® or H-B-VAX II® (Merck Sharp & Dohme).

Identifying the S gene

In order to utilize rDNA technology to produce a hepatitis B vaccine it was necessary to insert the gene for HBsAg into an expression vector capable of directing the synthesis of large quantities of HBsAg in heterologous host cells. The early studies of the molecular biology of HBV had been hampered by the failure to demonstrate that the virus could replicate in cell cultures, as mentioned earlier. Therefore, in the late 1970s the HBV genome, a partially double-stranded DNA molecule within virions, was cloned[46–48]. DNA sequence analyses of several cloned genomes revealed the presence of four open reading frames (ORFs) capable of encoding large polypeptides. In order to identify which of these four ORFs encoded HBsAg, the amino acid sequence imputed from the nucleotide sequence of each of the ORFs was compared to the N-terminal amino acid sequence of plasma-derived HBsAg[49]. By virtue of the identity by this comparison of 14 consecutive N-terminal amino acids, the gene designated as S was identified as encoding HBsAg (Figure 4A). The S gene is actually a part of a larger ORF that is divided into three domains, each of which begins with an in-frame ATG codon that is capable of functioning as a translational initiation site. These domains are referred to as preS1, preS2 and S respective to their 5′ to 3′ order in the gene[12]. Thus, these domains define three polypeptides referred to as S or HBsAg (226 amino acids), PreS2 + S (281 amino acids), and preS1 + preS2 + S (389–400 amino acids depending on HBV subtype). The 681-nucleotide S gene encodes the 24-kilodalton (kd) polypeptide which is the predominant protein in 22-nm particles from human plasma. Therefore, the S gene became the gene of choice for expressing a hepatitis B vaccine in a heterologous host cell.

Since *Escherichia coli* was the best-developed heterologous expression system in the late 1970s, early attempts at expression of the S gene focused on *E. coli* as a host cell. However, all such attempts were unsuccessful, due to the instability of the S polypeptide and the lack of its assembly into 22 nm particles in this bacterium. Subsequently, satisfactory levels of expression were achieved both in bakers' yeast *Saccharomyces cerevisiae*[50] and in mammalian cells. Both host cell systems produce HBsAg polypeptides assembled into 22-nm lipoprotein particles which are highly immunogenic for eliciting anti-HBs and are highly related antigenically to plasma-derived HBsAg. All yeast-derived HBsAg contains only non-glycosylated polypeptides; approximately 25% of mammalian-derived HBsAg is composed of glycosylated polypeptides[51] with a single asparagine-linked complex-type oligosaccharide at amino acid residue 146[52]. Nevertheless, this biochemical difference is reflected neither in the antigenicity of the different particles nor

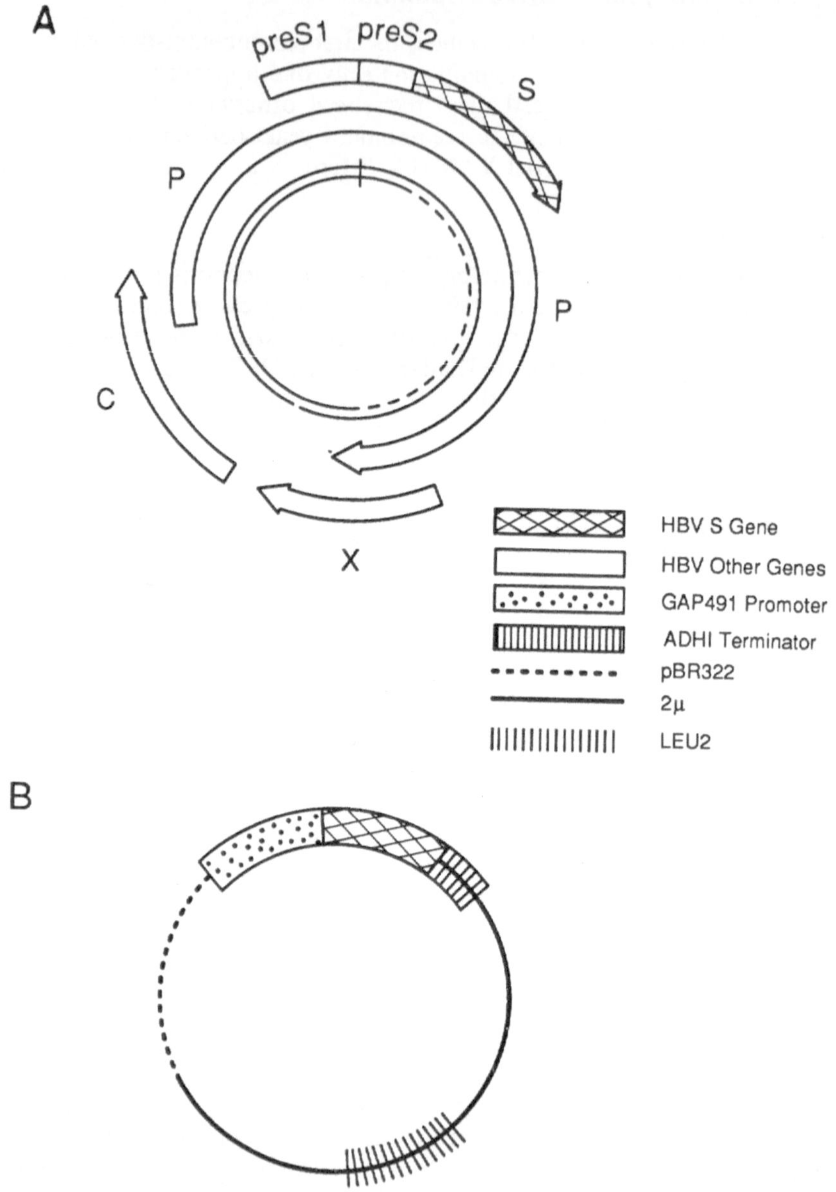

Figure 4 A: Structure of the HBV genome. HBV DNA has a single nick in one strand (near the end of the X gene) and a single-stranded region of variable size (––––). Nucleotide 1 of the 3.2 kilobase pair molecule is marked at the top of the circle (vertical slash). The four large ORFs (P, C, X, preS1 + preS2 + S) are indicated. Arrows point in the direction of translation of each of the ORFs, beginning at the ATG translational initiation codon and ending at the termination codon of the respective ORF. Each of the three domains of the preS1 + preS2 + S ORF is demarcated by its respective ATG codon. **B**: structure of the plasmid which directs the expression of HBsAg in yeast

in their ability to elicit virus-neutralizing antibodies. In addition, the yeast-derived antigen is expressed intracellularly, while the mammalian-derived antigen is secreted from expressor cells.

Yeast production system

Since both *S. cerevisiae* and mammalian cells produce HBsAg, scientists had to select which system was more desirable for producing a second-generation hepatitis B vaccine[53]. There are three general considerations that are important for making a decision regarding the system of expression for most recombinant-derived biological products: these are the biological activity of the expressed protein, the scalability of the production process, and the potential concern for safety of the final product relative to its host cell for production[54].

As discussed above, the biological activities, i.e., immunogenicities, of both the yeast-derived and mammalian-derived HBsAg are comparable. This presents no *a priori* reason for choosing one system over the other. Yeast cultures can be scaled up readily using experience gained over centuries of fermentation at an industrial scale, while scale-up of mammalian cell cultures has been accomplished relatively recently. The molecular stability of recombinant yeast cells during fermentation can be controlled much more precisely than that of recombinant mammalian cells. Recombinant proteins can be produced in yeast cells at higher yields and correspondingly lower costs than in mammalian cells. While these factors should be considered in general, they apply to HBsAg in particular. Therefore, yeast is the preferred expression system for scalability of the production process.

The eventual worldwide use of a hepatitis B vaccine in hundreds of millions of healthy individuals, especially newborns, is the most important consideration in selecting a host cell for expression[53]. There has been concern that mammalian cells used for expressing foreign genes generally are continuous cell lines, which possess one or more properties associated with *in vivo* tumorigenicity or *in vitro* transformation, and which harbour endogenous mammalian proto-oncogenes and retroviruses, properties that can be associated with residual mammalian DNA in a product. It is essentially impossible to demonstrate the complete removal of all DNA from vaccine preparations. In contrast, yeast cells are not associated with these risk factors, so that the presence of minute quantities of yeast DNA in a vaccine is of little concern[53]. Therefore, for reasons of perceived safety and production, yeast is the preferred host for the expression of recombinant-derived hepatitis B vaccines.

Intracellular HBsAg expression in yeast is directed by a high-copy number plasmid (Figure 4B). The *GAP*491 gene provides one of the strongest promoters for the constitutive expression of HBsAg in yeast; the *GAP*491 gene product, glyceraldehyde-3-phosphate dehydrogenase, represents about 5% of total yeast protein[55]. Besides the promoter and the S gene, the other regulatory element in the expression cassette is the transcriptional termination region from the *ADH*I gene[56]. In addition, the plasmid contains the complete yeast 2 μ sequences (Figure 4B) which enable plasmid amplification to about

100 copies per cell in *cir*^{0} yeast hosts[57], while the *LEU*2 gene permits selection for plasmid retention in leu$^-$ host strains.

Production and preclinical testing

Recombinant yeast cells expressing HBsAg are grown in stirred tank fermenters inoculated from stored vials of a stable production master seed. Since the HBsAg accumulates intracellularly, the yeast cells are harvested, washed and disrupted by high pressure. The antigen is then purified by conventional biochemical techniques (Figure 5)[58] to >99% purity with respect to protein, and is formulated into a vaccine by adsorption to aluminium hydroxide, a commonly used adjuvant. The final vaccine antigen is a particle about 22 nm in diameter which is similar in morphology to plasma-derived HBsAg (Figure 3B). Numerous chemical, biochemical and physical assays are performed as quality controls on the final product to assure a thorough characterization and a lot-to-lot consistency for the product[58]. In light of the importance of the group-specific *a* epitopes in eliciting anti-*a* antibodies which react with all HBV subtypes, provide protection against different subtypes[35,39], and are the most abundant elicited

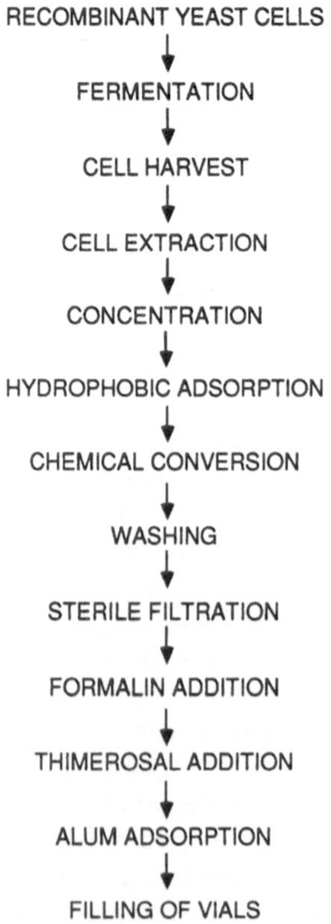

Figure 5 Process for the manufacture of the recombinant-derived hepatitis B vaccine, Recombivax HB® or H-B-VAX II® (Merck, Sharp & Dohme)

by HBsAg[59,60], appropriate quantitative immunoassays using anti-*a*-MABs assure the continued presence of high levels of these key epitopes on yeast-derived HBsAg.

A commonly used test for the immunogenicity of hepatitis B vaccines is the mouse potency assay, in which graded quantities of each vaccine lot are inoculated in a single intraperitoneal injection into groups of 10 mice. Six weeks after immunization, the mice are bled, and the sera are assayed for anti-HBs by a commercially available test. For each lot of vaccine the effective dose capable of seroconverting 50% of the mice in a given group (ED_{50}) is calculated[59]. The advantage of the one-dose mouse potency assay over other animal assays for immunogenicity is the availability of large numbers of mice of a single inbred strain: this assures statistical validity and reproducibility of the test. A consistent process can provide vaccines with ED_{50} levels that fall within a reproducible range, typically <1.5 μg. Immunogenicity tests also have been performed in grivet monkeys in a multiple dose regimen similar to that used in humans[61].

As for the plasma-derived vaccine, efficacy in chimpanzees is the most important preclinical immunological test for the yeast-derived vaccine. Chimpanzees received three doses of the vaccine at monthly intervals[58,59]. Vaccinated animals were shown to produce anti-HBs titres of 800–3000 mIU/ml. Following intravenous challenge with a titred HBV inoculum, none of the animals receiving the vaccine showed any signs of hepatitis B throughout the entire 24-week observation period. In contrast, all placebo-injected animals developed typical signs of infection. As observed with the plasma-derived vaccine, the yeast-derived vaccine (subtype *adw*) protected against HBV challenges of subtypes *adr* or *ayw*, thus highlighting the protective effect *in vivo* of anti-*a* antibodies. This test established yeast-derived HBsAg as a protective antigen and a product candidate for testing in human clinical trials.

Clinical testing

The yeast-derived hepatitis B vaccine has been studied to date in over 8000 individuals in clinical trials using protocols similar to those described above for Heptavax B®. The vaccine has been generally very well tolerated[62,63]. Mild and transient clinical complaints, such as headache, fatigue, nausea, and malaise, or those related to the injection site, have been observed. Initial dose-ranging studies evaluated 20-, 10-, 5- and 2.5-μg doses of the vaccine in adults[62,64,65]. Even though the kinetics of the immune response and the percentage of individuals seroconverting were similar for all four doses, the 10- and 20-μg doses elicited much higher geometric mean titres (GMTs) than the lower doses. Consequently, the 10-μg dose was chosen for adults. By comparative testing of 5-, 2.5-, and 1.25-μg doses of vaccine in children 1–10 years of age the 5-μg dose was selected for children 10 years of age and younger[62]. As also was observed for Heptavax B®, seroconversion in children, as compared to adults, is more rapid and frequent, and GMTs are invariably much higher even after receiving lower dosage levels of vaccine.

Since the plasma-derived and yeast-derived vaccines are biochemically distinct, it was important to compare the serological properties of vaccine-induced antibodies to each[59,60]. Both vaccines elicit antibodies which (1) have similar immunoglobulin isotype and avidity, (2) have similar kinetics of appearance following vaccine inoculation, (3) are capable of binding to plasma-derived HBsAg with equivalent avidities, (4) can be absorbed totally by either yeast- or plasma-derived vaccine antigen, (5) are capable of binding with equivalent affinities and titres to a synthetic peptide containing an *a* epitope, and (6) protect chimpanzees against challenge with HBV (subtype *adw* or *ayr*). By these criteria the two vaccines are immunologically comparable *in vivo*.

The introduction into the manufacturing process of a second more highly productive yeast master seed, and improvements made to the original purification process itself, resulted in a more highly purified vaccine as well as a higher-yielding production process[58]. As a result of these changes the vaccine was shown to elicit peak GMTs of about 1850 mIU/ml in young adults, a significant increase relative to those elicited by the product of the original master seed and production process[58,63].

The final proof of the efficacy of the yeast-derived vaccine lay in demonstrating its effectiveness in preventing clinical infection in humans. Even though the yeast-derived vaccine is comparable immunologically to the plasma-derived vaccine, it has been considered important to directly demonstate the protective effect in man of anti-HBs elicited by the yeast-derived vaccine in controlled clinical trials. However, due to the changed epidemiology of hepatitis B in other high-risk groups, it was deemed necessary to carry out efficacy studies in high-risk newborn children born to chronic carrier mothers[66]. In earlier studies it had been shown that infants born to viraemic carrier mothers positive for both HBsAg and HBeAg (hepatitis *e* antigen, a marker of HBV replication) had a 70–90% rate of infection as well as a very high risk of becoming chronic carriers[67]. In such infants, passive immunization at birth with one dose of HBIG reduced the rate of infection by approximately half[68]. Combined passive immunization with HBIG plus active immunization with the plasma-derived hepatitis B vaccine reduced the rate of infection even further[69,70]. Since rates of infection were similar in untreated infants born either in the United States or in highly endemic areas to $HBsAg^+/HBeAg^+$ mothers, medical practices had no apparent effect on the rate of perinatal transmission. Furthermore, inclusion of a placebo-controlled group would have been ethically questionable in the light of the availability of the licensed Heptavax B® product. Thus, in lieu of a placebo control group, it was considered appropriate to calculate the efficacy of the yeast-derived vaccine on the basis of historical control data.

Among infants receiving HBIG at birth plus 5-μg doses of the yeast-derived vaccine at 0, 1 and 6 months, only 5% became chronic carriers[66]. This rate of protection from chronic carriage (95%) was comparable to that in a group of infants in the same study[66] receiving HBIG and three doses of the Heptavax B®. This study demonstrated the effectiveness of anti-HBs elicited by either Recombivax HB® or Heptavax B® in preventing viral infection. This result is consistent with the immunological comparability of the two vaccines in terms of the qualitative properties of the antibodies elicited by each one. As a watershed for worldwide public health this study describes the means for preventing the most common mode of transmission of HBV in the world, i.e., the use of a vaccine which now can be reproduced in an essentially unlimited supply.

Future direction

The excellent immunogenicity and protective efficacy profile of the recombinant yeast-derived hepatitis B vaccine present a formidable challenge to the development of a third generation of hepatitis B vaccines. The preS domains, especially preS2, represent the major focus for further vaccine development in light of their surface disposition on virions and their ability to elicit virus-neutralizing antibodies. Yeast-derived vaccines containing either the preS2 + S or preS1 + preS2 + S polypeptides have been formulated and are being tested[61,71]. Nevertheless, beyond extensive preclinical testing of products made by these or other methods, only human clinical trials will establish whether such approaches warrant future vaccine development.

HEPATITIS A VACCINE

Epidemiology

Ecology

HAV is one of the most stable human pathogens, being resistant to many conventional inactivating conditions. This resistance, coupled with the excretion of HAV in copious amounts in the stools of infected individuals, is a major factor in the survival and spread of the virus. HAV is unusually resistant to heat-inactivation, especially in a non-purified state, and it also resists inactivation by low pH and organic solvents[72–75]. More recent studies have confirmed this resistance and have shown that infectious HAV persists for unusually long periods of time under a variety of natural environmental situations and conditions (water, soil, dried surfaces) and from which transmission to humans beings is possible[76,77].

HAV is excreted in the stools of infected individuals at concentrations as high as 10^9 infectious particles per gram[78]; excretion may occur over 2–3 weeks preceding the onset of disease symptoms. There is also significant viraemia associated with HAV infection in humans, with levels of infectivity in the order of 10^4–10^5/ml documented in blood[78]. Though less well documented, there also is evidence suggesting the presence of infectious HAV in saliva[78]. HAV infection of human beings generally is considered to be non-chronic in nature. However, there are recent reports indicating that relapses of hepatitis A do occur[79]. During relapse, HAV has been reported to be excreted in the stool[80] and to be present in the liver[81].

There is no known natural animal reservoir of HAV infection. However, it is clear that currently there is a high rate of infection in Old World monkeys housed in various facilities in the United States. Infection of these animals probably results from primary contact with human beings and rapid spread from animal to animal. Possible indications for natural HAV infection in monkeys are the demonstration of antibody positivity in freshly captured macaques in Malaysia[82] and the HAV-related agent described in Panamanian owl monkeys[83] which differs in nucleotide sequence from human HAV strains to such an extent that it might be an HAV strain indigenous to monkeys.

Disease transmission

HAV may infect humans either through ingestion or by percutaneous entry. The incubation period, and possibly the severity of the disease, are influenced by the dose of infecting virus[84]. In developed countries, HAV infection is usually associated with crowded living conditions, inadequate sanitation facilities and poor personal hygienic practices. This usually results in person-to-person transmission of infection or limited outbreaks of infection due to contamination of food or water. In less-developed countries the disease is endemic, and there is widespread contamination of food and water supplies[85]. These areas present a special risk to travellers from developed areas.

Circumstances facilitating HAV transmission in developed countries are being recognized increasingly. These include numerous outbreaks of hepatitis A traced to homosexual practices and to day-care centres where non-immune adults handle diapered children[85]. Faecal–oral transmission continues its predominant role, but transmission of blood-borne virus appears to play a role in some areas, particularly in intravenous drug abusers[86,87]. In this regard it is pertinent that transmission of hepatitis A infection by blood transfusion also has been documented[88].

Seroepidemiology

Seroepidemiologic studies have shown that hepatitis A is endemic in the less-developed areas of the world, resulting in a high rate of infection (usually clinically mild) in children and an adult population retaining immunity generated from childhood infection[84,85]. Whereas HAV infection once tended to be endemic in the United States and other more developed countries, this pattern has been changing due to improvements in sanitation, housing and general socioeconomic conditions[84,85]. Serosurveys show that 10–20% of 20-year-old Americans have been exposed to HAV. Thus, a large proportion of adults in developed countries is susceptible to hepatitis A. This is unfortunate, as hepatitis A in adults is characterized by greater clinical severity[84,85]. Since sporadic outbreaks of hepatitis A will inevitably continue to occur, it is desirable to develop appropriate vaccines for use in the more-developed and also in developing areas of the world[84,85].

Strategy for vaccine development

Two closely related marmoset species, *Saguinus mystax* and *S. labiatus*, were validated as suitable primate hosts for human HAV infection[74,89,90]. Subsequent studies in these animals led to several advances which provide the framework on which current vaccine strategies are based. A first significant observaton was that animals recovering from infection were solidly immune to reinfection[74]. Another was that HAV infectivity for these animals was neutralized by *in vitro* incubation with human convalescent sera or with pooled human immune globulin[74]. The discovery of high levels of HAV in the infected livers of these animals provided HAV antigen for the first practical serological assays for HAV antibody (complement fixation; immune adherence haemaglutination (IAHA))[18,91,92]. Most significantly, infected liver tissue from these animals provided a source of HAV antigen later used to demonstrate the feasibility of making a formalin-inactivated HAV vaccine The vaccine successfully induced antibodies which provided solid protection against HAV infection in the marmoset[93]. Furthermore, HAV derived from infected marmoset livers after 31 serial *in vivo* passages of the CR326 strain was of such quality and potency as an inoculum that it produced the first documented replication of HAV in cell culture[94]. The knowledge that formalin-inactivated HAV retained vaccinating capacity, coupled with the newly discovered ability to produce HAV *in vitro* in cell culture, suggested pursuit of an inactivated HAV vaccine. With the growth of HAV in cell culture it was established quickly that virulence of CR326 HAV for the marmoset was attenuated upon continued serial passaging of the agent in cell culture[95,96]. This observation suggested pursuit of the first strategy for HAV vaccine development, a live attenuated vaccine. Both marmosets and chimpanzees have served to guide this vaccine development programme[16,95,97,98].

Live, attenuated vaccine

Strain development

Following 31 serial *in vivo* passages in *S. labiatus*, the CR326 srain of HAV was grown for 34 serial *in vitro* passages at 35°C in fetal rhesus monkey kidney (FRhK6) cells[94], a low-passage, non-transformed cell preparation[99]. The passaged virus was tested after 5, 10, 15, 20, 25, 30 and 34 passages in FRhK6 by intravenous inoculation into *S. labiatus*. Through passage 20 the virus retained its virulence, inducing elevated levels of a liver enzyme (isocitric dehydrogenase, ICD) in all animals. At passages 25 and 30 some recipient animals showed virulent infection and others little or no evidence of enzyme elevation. At passage 34 all recipient marmosets showed non-virulent but antibody-inducing infection, *viz.*, an attenuated vaccine-like response[95,96]. These findings served as the first clear indication that production of an attenuated, live HAV vaccine was feasible. However, FRhK6 cells were not available in quantity, and primary adult monkey kidney cultures, in which HAV also could be propagated[94], contained endogenous contaminating agents. Thus, CR326 was adapted to growth in WI-38 and MRC-5 human diploid lung fibroblast cells[100]. This was accomplished by using virus already adapted to growth in FRhK6. Eventually, work with CR326 focused on growth in MRC-5 cells which were available in quantity and were judged acceptable for live vaccine development.

A number of variants purified by limit dilution were derived from CR326 by various regimens of serial passaging in FRhK6 cells at 35°C and in MRC-

5 cells at either 35°C or 32°C. The development and assessment of these many variants as live vaccines in marmosets and chimpanzees has been described[95–97]. Some variants retained virulence, some appeared appropriately attenuated, and some appeared inert in test animals. Three of these variants (A, B, D) were non-immunogenic upon subcutaneous injection into human volunteers (Table 2). This was expected with A, and to some extent with B, both of which had minimal activity in test animals. Most disappointing was the apparent lack of vaccinating activity of D, as it had shown appropriate vaccine properties in both marmosets and chimpanzees[95,97]. The inability of the CR326-derived variants to serve as vaccines for man remains unexplained. It may be related to the long passage history of the CR326 in the marmoset, a possibility strengthened by finding in studies of CR326F.

The CR326F strain of HAV was isolated from the frozen-stored stool of the same hepatitis A patient whose blood had yielded the CR326 strain isolated in marmosets some years earlier[15,101]. The isolation of CR326F was made in FRhK6 cells, with no intervening passaging *in vivo* in marmosets. A similar regimen of attenuation by passaging in FRhK6 and MRC-5 cells was carried out as had been done for CR326. Two variants derived from CR326F were formulated into vaccines for clinical trials. One of these variants (F) had some attributes of virulence in test animals and appeared to induce mild enzyme elevations in some of the human volunteers[102]. The second and more highly passaged variant (F′) appeared to be fully attenuated both in test animals and in man while eliciting vaccine-induced antibodies[102]. In contrast to findings with CR326 variants, it appeared that the behaviour of F and F′ in both marmosets and chimpanzees was an excellent predictor of behaviour in man (Table 2). Both F and F′ variants were shown to induce solid protection against virulent HAV challenge in inoculated marmosets (Table 3).

Variant F vaccine containing $10^{5.6}$ infectious units for tissue culture ($TCID_{50}$)/dose was given subcutaneously to nine adult volunteers[102]. All nine developed antibody to HAV using standard RIA testing. Mean time to

Table 2 Behaviour of live HAV vaccine candidates in marmosets, chimpanzees and man

HAV Strain	*Letter Designation*	*In Vitro Passages in* FRhK6	*MRC−5*[a]	*Behavior*[b] *in* Marmoset	*Chimpanzee*	*Man*
CR326	A	15	9,11(32°C)	ATT/IN	IN	IN
CR326	B	25	8,10(35°C)	ATT/IN	ATT	IN
CR326	D	16	8,10(35°C)	ATT	ATT	IN
CR326F	F	15	8,10(35°C)	VI/ATT	VI/ATT	VI/ATT
CR326F	F'	15	16,18(35°C)	ATT	ATT	ATT

[a]First digit is the number of passages to production of a master seed; second digit is the number of passages to producing a lot of vaccine; temperature of growth in cell culture is in parentheses
[b]IN = inert; no serological response following injection
ATT = attenuated no elevated level of enzymes, no liver pathology, modest antibody titres
VI = virulent; evidence of elevated enzymes and/or liver pathology, high antibody titres
ATT/IN = some with attenuated, some with inert responses
VI/ATT = some with virulent, some with attenuated responses

Table 3 Protective efficacy of live HAV vaccine candidates F and F' in the marmoset

Group	*Post- vaccination*[a]		*Post-challenge*[b]	
	Number of animals	*Antibody titre*[c]	*Number of protected animals*	*Antibody titre*[c]
F Vaccinees	4	80	4	240
Controls	4	<5	0	>2560
F' Vaccinees	6	27	6	67
Controls	3	<5	0	1280

[a]F vaccine group was challenged at 16 months post-vaccination, F' group at 24 months post-vaccination
[b]F vaccinees were challenged intravenously with 10^5 marmoset infectious doses (ID_{50}), F' vaccinees with 10^4 ID_{50}
[c]HAV antibody measured by IAHA and expressed as GMT
[d]Protection was based on no ICD enzyme elevations and no boost in antibody titre

seroconversion was 6.6 weeks, and the GMT of IAHA was 1:53, a value on the order of 1% of that seen following virulent infection. A negative aspect of this study was that mild, brief ALT elevations were detected in three out of nine recipients, consistent with the slight virulence seen in marmosets and chimpanzees given F vaccine.

Subsequently the more attenuated F' variant of CR326F HAV was inoculated subcutaneously into 11 adult volunteers[102]. The vaccine contained $10^{6.3}$ $TCID_{50}$/dose. None of the recipients exhibited serum enzyme elevations. However, the level of antibody produced in the volunteers was lower than that seen with variant F. Six of 11 vaccinees seroconverted in the standard RIA, while a modified version of this assay (providing about 10-fold greater sensitivity) detected seroconversion in 10/11 subjects. Antibody induction in these same individuals was confirmed by detection of neutralizing antibody activity in a radioimmunofocus assay (S. Lemon, personal communication). Another very positive finding in this study was that antibody persisted in bleedings obtained at 3 years post-vaccination from all nine of these individuals tested, and that antibody levels similar to those induced in these vaccinees routinely protected marmosets from HAV infection. Continuing development and clinical testing of these vaccine candidates is ongoing[96].

Another major programme of live HAV vaccine development has been carried out with the HM175 strain of HAV, serially passaged in primary African green monkey kidney cells[103]. This strain of HAV was tested in both marmosets and chimpanzees after 21 passages in cell culture; it retained virulence for the marmoset but appeared attenuated for chimpanzees. After 32 passages it remained attenuated for chimpanzees and showed a greater degree of attenuation for marmosets than had been found at passage 21. No clinical studies with this strain have been reported yet.

Other ongoing efforts at live HAV vaccine development have been reported. These include the demonstration that the MS-1 strain of HAV was attenuated for chimpanzees by 20 serial *in vivo* passages in marmosets[104], the reported attenuation of the MBB and L-A-1 strains of HAV for marmosets by *in vitro* passage of HAV in human fetal lung fibroblast cells[105], the attenuation of the GBM strain of HAV for chimpanzees by *in vitro* passaging of the virus in human fetal kidney and human diploid fibroblast cells[106], and the development of cell culture-adapted variants of HAV whose attenuation was demonstrated in Old World monkeys[107].

In addition to proving efficacy, ongoing and future studies of live HAV vaccines will have to address several areas of concern. First is the question of how much virus is excreted in the stools of vaccinees. Second is the question of what tissues other than liver may serve as sites of viral replication. Third is the issue of whether HAV may persist in liver or other tissues of vaccinees. Also of obvious concern is the question of what incidence of reversion to virulence may be encountered. Finally, it will be necessary to develop meaningful markers to identify the attenuated HAV strains. Currently, these consist strictly of behaviour in marmosets/chimpanzees and the capacity to grow in MRC-5 cells.

In view of the long records of safe and effective use of many existing live virus vaccines (yellow fever, smallpox, polio, measles, mumps, rubella), it is reasonable to anticipate ultimate success with a live HAV vaccine as well. The closest corollary vaccine to HAV would be poliovirus. Although there is concern about rates of reversion of Sabin polioviruses types 2 and 3, it should be noted that Sabin poliovirus type 1, the most extensively modified strain of the group[108], has been problem-free through many years and millions of doses of use[109].

Alternative live vaccine approaches

To the best of current understanding, HAV replicates primarily if not entirely in the liver. It has been suggested that a live vaccine replicating in the alimentary tract might be ideal for producing intestinal immunity and for avoiding potential damage to liver cells[110]. Evidence of a low level of infectious HAV in the saliva of acutely ill human hepattis A patients has been documented[78]. It may be possible that appropriate viral modification could produce a vaccine strain limited in its replication to the alimentary tract and not capable of infecting the liver. This would appear to be a long-range goal.

It has been demonstrated by the study of recombinant polioviruses made with cDNA clones of wild-type Mahoney parental virus and Sabin type 1 vaccine strain that the strong neurovirulence properties of wild-type poliovirus for cynomolgus monkeys reside in the 5′ non-coding region of the genome[109]. This finding suggested two strategies for producing attenuated picornavirus vaccines[109]. One is to use the recognized safe Sabin type 1 virus as a vector to carry foreign picornavirus antigens. The other approach is the *in vitro* construction of attenuated viruses by deliberate mutations in the 5′ non-coding region. Recombinant viruses were made by incorporating Sabin poliovirus types 2 or 3 coat proteins into Sabin type 1 genome[109]. The recombinants were tested satisfactorily in monkey neurovirulence and are undergoing further study. Alternatively, it might be possible to incorporate HAV coat protein into the Sabin type 1 genome[109]. This approach to an attenuated HAV vaccine would have to be pursued with great caution, since a potentially dangerous phenotype might result and a novel virus would be released into the environment, but it could conceivably accomplish vaccination against hepatitis A while avoiding liver infection.

It has also been shown that deliberate nucleotide deletions in the 5′ noncoding region of wild-type Mahoney and even of Sabin type 1 poliovirus resulted in reduced neurovirulence of each strain for cynomolgus monkeys[109]. It is possible that this approach could be applied to further attenuate or to stabilize the existing candidate live HAV vaccines. That these approaches are readily applicable to live HAV vaccine development is bolstered by the recent accomplishment of producing infectious RNA transcripts from cDNA of the HM175 attenuated strain of HAV[111].

A similar approach has been reported using Sabin type 1 poliovirus to incorporate critical antigens of types 2 and 3[112]. A 69-base oligonucleotide from antigen site 1 of VP1 of type 3 poliovirus was inserted into the full-length cDNA of Sabin poliovirus type 1. The chimeric virus induced neutralizing antibody to type 3 poliovirus in mice. It is possible that such an approach may be useful for HAV if an appropriate antigen can be identified. Evidence to date suggests that such a site does exist in HAV in the first 70 N-terminal amino acids of VP1[113,114].

Alternatives to the use of poliovirus as a vector for HAV coat protein antigens may lie in such vectors as vaccinia virus, varicella-zoster virus, adenovirus, and live *Salmonella* vaccines. No attempts to use as these vectors for HAV have been reported.

Inactivated HAV vaccine

Technical development

The feasibility of developing a formalin-inactivated HAV vaccine was demonstrated 10 years ago[93], prior to the era of successful growth of HAV *in vitro*, using strain CR326 HAV partially purified from the livers of acutely infected *S. labiatus* marmosets. Multiple doses of vaccine were administered to *S. labiatus*. Antibody to HAV was induced in all vaccinated animals, and they were solidly immune to viral challenge as a result.

Subsequently, following the growth of HAV in cell culture, a highly purified, formalin-inactivated HAV vaccine was prepared from strain CR326 grown in LLC-MK2 cell culture[115]. This cell is transformed in nature and thus not readily amenable to use in human vaccine development. Nevertheless, this prototype vaccine generated the key finding that nanogram (ng) doses of HAV vaccine had the capacity to induce immunity. In mice, a single 10 ng dose of HAV antigen was found to induce HAV antibody in 50% of the animals. Three subcutaneous doses of 1 ng each induced HAV antibody in 50% of marmosets, and three 10 ng doses induced antibody in 100% of the marmosets (Table 4). All animals with detectable antibody were protected against HAV infection when challenged with virulent virus.

Another successful prototype-inactivated vaccine was prepared from the HM175 strain of HAV grown in BSC-1 cells[116], also a transformed cell line. Although not a highly purified preparation of defined antigen content, this vaccine was used to demonstrate convincingly that both antibody induction

Table 4 Potency and protective efficacy in marmosets of formalin-inactivated, purified HAV vaccine of cell culture origin

Vaccine dose[a] (ng)	*Number*[b] *seroconverted* *Total*	*Number protected*[c] *vs. Challenge/total*
0	0/3	0/3
1	2/4	2/4
10	4/4	4/4
100	2/2	2/2

[a]Animals received three doses of 0, 1, 10 or 100 ng of vaccine formulated on alum
[b]Seroconversion based on detection of antibody in a RIA of enhanced sensitivity
[c]Protection was based on no serum enzyme elevations and no pronounced boost in antibody. Animals were challenged intravenously with 10^5 ID_{50}

and protection against challenge were achievable in the owl monkey. A similar HM175 vaccine now has been made in MRC-5 cells and has been tested in man.

The second major clinical study of HAV vaccine is the recently reported study of formalin-inactivated HM175 HAV in eight volunteers[117]. The vaccine, a clarified extract from MRC-5 cells[118], contained about 17 ng HAV antigen/ml. It was inoculated intramuscularly at days 0, 23, 56 and again at 6–8 months. No adverse effects were noted. Importantly, antibody induction was achieved in all volunteers after the fourth dose of vaccine. The remarkable capacity of such a small dose of HAV antigen (4 x 17 ng) to induce antibody in man is consistent with the earlier study in marmosets in which as little as three doses of 1 ng each induced antibody in 50% of marmosets[115]. These findings with inactivated vaccine in humans are most important and portend well for the eventual success of an inactivated HAV vaccine.

Major efforts to develop inactivated HAV vaccines are under way with both the CR326F and HM175 strains of HAV grown in MRC5 cells[96,117]. An inactivated HAV vaccine offers the potential for greater safety than a live, attenuated vaccine. Particularly desirable in this regard is the large-scale effort under way to use inactivated F′ attenuated HAV strain, purified from MRC5 cells, as a killed vaccine[96].

Alternative approaches to an inactivated vaccine

A low-level induction of neutralizing antibody was found in rabbits inoculated with disrupted HAV and in rats given purified HAV subunit proteins[119], but other workers were less successful in attempting to induce neutralizing antibodies in rabbits given either subunit proteins or synthetic peptides[120]. Thus it appears that native epitopes present on the intact virion are necessary for the efficient induction of neutralizing antibodies. Studies to date of synthetic peptides of HAV in rabbits and guinea pigs also have shown a very low order of induction of neutralizing antibodies against HAV[114,121]. Efficient vaccines made from virion subunits undoubtedly will be developed using advancing technology, but are not feasible at present.

Overall comparison of live and inactivated vaccines

Table 5 summarizes the advantages, disadvantages, and unknowns of the candidate live and inactivated HAV vaccines. Neither approach is convincingly superior to the other at present. Both vaccines have good chances for success, and both undoubtedly will be improved with advancing technology. Perhaps both will find a niche in the public health armamentarium, since the advantages of single-dose inoculation with the live attenuated vaccine may be essential to provide protection in developing countries where the health delivery infrastructure is minimal, while the multiple doses of inactivated vaccine may be an acceptable tradeoff in developed countries where live virus vaccines are viewed less favourably by some potential vaccinees.

Table 5 Comparison of live vs. inactivated HAV vaccines: advantages, disadvantages, unknowns

	Live vaccine	*Inactivated vaccine*
Advantages	1. More complete immune response 2. Longer duration antibody 3. Single dose 4. No adjuvant 5. Simpler manufacture 6. Less expensive 7. More widespread use 8. Heat-stable virus	1. No concern with reversion 2. Greater safety 3. Greater stability 4. Can use attenuated F' variant
Disadvantage	1. Potential reversion 2. Probable excretion 3. Interference by other infections	1. Lesser duration of antibody 2. Multiple doses required 3. Adjuvant probably required 4. More complex manufacture 5. More expensive 6. Less widespread use
Unknowns:	1. Optimal variant achieved? 2. Rate of reversion? 3. Optimal route? 4. Tissue tropism altered? 5. Virus persistence in liver? 6. Protection vs. oral infection?	1. Less complete and effective immunity? 2. Protection vs. oral infection? 3. Minimum number of doses?

REFERENCES

1. Gerety, R. J. (1984). Introduction. In Gerety, R. J. (ed.), *Hepatitis A*, pp. 1–8. (Orlando, Florida: Academic Press)
2. Bradley, D. W. and Maynard, J. E. (1986). Etiology and natural history of post-transfusion and enterically-transmitted non-A, non-B hepatitis. *Sem. Liver Dis.*, **6**, 56–66
3. Bradley, D., Andjaparidze, A., Cook, E. H., McCaustland, K., Balayan, M., Stetler, H., Velazquez, O., Robertson, B., Humphrey, C., Kane, M. and Weisfuse, I. (1988). Aetiological agent of enterically transmitted non-A, non-B hepatitis. *J. Gen. Virol.*, **69**, 731–8

4. Krugman, S., Ward, R. and Giles, J. P. (1962). The natural history of infectious hepatitis. *Am. J. Med.*, **32**, 717–28
5. Krugman, S., Giles, J. P. and Hammond, J. (1967). Infectious hepatitis: Evidence for two distinctive clinical, epidemiological, and immunological types of infection. *J. Am. Med. Assoc.*, **200**, 365–73
6. Blumberg, B. S., Alter, H. J. and Visnich, S. (1965). A new antigen in leukemia sera. *J. Am. Med. Assoc.*, **191**, 541–6
7. Blumberg, B. S., Gersley, B. J. and Hungerford, D. A. (1967). A serum antigen (Australia antigen) in Down's syndrome, leukemia, and hepatitis. *Ann. Intern. Med.*, **66**, 924–31
8. Prince, A. M. (1968). An antigen detected in the blood during the incubation period of serum hepatitis. *Proc. Natl. Acad. Sci. USA*, **60**, 814–21
9. Giles, J. P., McCollum, R. W., Berndtson, L. M. and Krugman, S. (1969). Viral hepatitis: relation of Australia-SH antigen to the Willowbrook MS-2 strain. *N. Engl. J. Med.*, **281**, 119–22
10. Bayer, M. E., Blumberg, B. S. and Werner, B. (1968). Particles associated with Australia antigen in the sera of patients with leukaemia, Down's syndrome and hepatitis. *Nature (Lond.)*, **218**, 1057–9
11. Dane, D. S., Cameron, C. H. and Briggs, M. (1970). Virus-like particles in serum of patients with Australia antigen-associated hepatitis. *Lancet*, **1**, 695–8
12. Tiollais, P., Pourcel, C. and Dejean, A. (1985). The hepatitis B virus. *Nature (Lond.)*, **317**, 489–95
13. Ganem, D. and Varmus, H. E. (1987). The molecular biology of the hepatitis B viruses. *Ann. Rev. Biochem.*, **56**, 651–93
14. Holmes, A. W., Wolfe, L., Rosenblatt, H. and Deinhardt, F. (1969). Hepatitis in marmosets. Induction of disease with coded specimens from a human volunteer study. *Science*, **165**, 816–17
15. Mascoli, C. C., Ittensohn, O. L., Villarejos, V. M., Arguedas, J. A., Provost, P. J. and Hilleman, M. R. (1973). Recovery of hepatitis agents in the marmoset from human cases occurring in Costa Rica. *Proc. Soc. Exp. Biol. Med.*, **142**, 276–82
16. Dienstag, J. L., Feinstone, S. M., Purcell, R. H., Hoofnagle, J. H., Barker, L. F., London, W. T., Popper, H., Peterson, J. M. and Kapikian, A. Z. (1975). Experimental infection of chimpanzees with hepatitis A virus. *J. Infect. Dis.*, **132**, 532–45
17. Feinstone, S. M., Kapikian, A. Z. and Purcell, R. H. (1973). Hepatitis A. Detection by immune electron microscopy of a virus-like antigen associated with acute illness. *Science*, **182**, 1026–8
18. Krugman, S., Friedman, H. and Lattimer, C. (1975). Viral hepatitis, type A. Identification by specific complement fixation and immune adherence tests. *New. Engl. J. Med.*, **292**, 1141–3
19. Melnick, J. L. (1982). Classification of hepatitis A virus as enterovirus type 72 and of hepatitis B virus as hepadnavirus type 1. *Intervirology*, **18**, 105–6
20. Feinstone, S. M., Moritsugu, Y., Shih, J. W. K., Gerin, J. L. and Purcell, R. H. (1979). Characterization of HAV. In Vyas, G. N., Cohen, S. N. and Schmid, E. R. (eds), *Viral Hepatitis*, pp. 41–8. (Philadelphia: Franklin Institute Press)
21. Szmuness, W., Harley, E. J., Ikram, H. and Stevens, C. E. (1981). Sociodemographic aspects of the epidemiology of hepatitis B. In Szmuness, W., Alter, H. J. and Maynard, J. E. (eds.) *Viral Hepatitis*, pp. 297–320. (Philadelphia: Franklin Institute Press)
22. Beasley, R. P. and Hwang, L.-Y. (1984). Epidemiology of hepatocellular carcinoma. In Vyas, G. N., Dienstag, J. H. and Hoofnagle, J. H. (eds), *Viral Hepatitis and Liver Disease*, pp. 204–9. (Orlando: Grune & Stratton)
23. Szmuness, W. (1978). Hepatocellular carcinoma and the hepatitis B virus: evidence for a causal association. *Prog. Med. Vir.*, **24**, 40–69
24. Krugman, S., Giles, J. P. and Hammond, J. (1970). Hepatitis virus: effect of heat on the infectivity and antigenicity of the MS-1 and MS-2 strains. *J. Infect. Dis.*, **122**, 432–6
25. Krugman, S., Giles, J. P. and Hammond, J. (1971). Viral hepatitis, type B (MS-2 strain). Studies on active immunization. *J. Am. Med. Assoc.*, **217**, 41–5
26. Seeff, L. B. (1988). Passive immunoprophylaxis. In Gerety, R. J. (ed.), *Hepatitis B*, pp. 353–84. (Orlando: Academic Press)
27. Hilleman, M. R., McAleer, W. J., Buynak, E. B. and McLean, A. A. (1983). The preparation and safety of hepatitis B vaccine. *J. Infect.*, **7**, 3–8

28. Barker, L. F., Maynard, J. E., Purcell, R. H., Hoofnagle, J. H., Berquist, K. R., London, W. T., Gerety, R. J. and Krushak, D. H. (1975). Hepatitis B virus infection in chimpanzees: titration of subtypes. *J. Infect. Dis.*, **132**, 451–8
29. Tabor, E., Purcell, R. H., London, W. T. and Gerety, R. J. (1983). Use of and interpretation of results using inocula of hepatitis B virus with known infectivity titers. *J. Infect. Dis.*, **147**, 531–4
30. Seidl, S. and Trautman, L. (1981). Detection of hepatitis B surface antigen in blood donors a comparative study using radio-immunoassay and enzyme immunoassay reverse passive hemagglutination and latex test. *Blood Transfus. Immunohaematol.*, **24**, 319–35
31. LeBouvier, G. L. and Williams, A. (1975). Serotypes of hepatitis B antigen (HBsAg): the problem of 'new' determinants, as exemplified by 't'. *Am J. Med. Sci.*, **270**, 165–71
32. Holland, P. V. (1975). Hepatitis B antigen subtypes - history, significance and immunogenicity. *Am. J. Med. Sci.*, **270**, 161–4
33. Tabor, E., Buynak, E. B., Smallwood, L. A., Snoy, P., Hilleman, M. R. and Gerety, R. J. (1983). Inactivation of hepatitis B virus by three methods: treatment with pepsin, urea, or formalin. *J. Med. Virol.*, **11**, 1–9
34. Francis, D. P., Feorino, P. M., McDougal, S., Warfield, D., Getchell, J., Cabradilla, C., Tong, M., Miller, W. J., Schultz, L. D., Bailey, F. J., McAleer, W. J., Scolnick, E. M. and Ellis, R. W. (1986). The safety of the hepatitis B vaccine. *J. Am. Med. Assoc.*, **256**, 869–72
35. Gerety, R. J., Tabor, E., Purcell, R. H. and Tyeryar, F. (1979). Summary of an international workshop on hepatitis B vaccines. *J. Infect. Dis.*, **140**, 642–8
36. Tabor, E., Barker, L. F. and Gerety, R. J. (1980). Failure to detect infectious hepatitis B virus using high dose safety test for hepatitis B vaccine. *J. Med. Virol.*, **6**, 279–84
37. Hilleman, M. R., Bertland, A. V., Buynak, E. B., Lampson, G. P., McAleer, W. J., Rochin, R. R. and Tyrell, A. A. (1978). Clinical laboratory studies of HBsAg vaccine. In Vyas, G. N., Cohen, S. N. and Schmid, R. (eds), *Viral Hepatitis*, pp. 525–42. (Philadelphia: Franklin Institute Press)
38. Waters, J. A., O'Rourke, S. M., Richardson, S. C., Papaevangelou, G. and Thomas, H. C. (1987). Qualitative analysis of the humoral immune response to the 'a' determinant of HBs antigen after inoculation with plasma-derived or recombinant vaccine. *J. Med. Virol.*, **21**, 155–60
39. Iwarson, S., Tabor, E., Thomas, H. C., Godall, A., Waters, J., Snoy, P., Shih, J. W.-K. and Gerety, R. J. (1985). Neutralization of hepatitis B virus infectivity by a murine monoclonal antibody: an experimental study in the chimpanzee. *J. Med. Virol.*, **16** 89–96
40. Krugman, S., Holley, P., Davidson, M., Simberkoff, M. S. and Matsaniotis, N. (1981). Immunogenic effect of inactivated hepatitis B vaccine: comparison of 20-microgram and 40-microgram doses. *J. Med. Virol.*, **8**, 119–21
41. Szmuness, W., Stevens, C. E., Harley, E. J., Zang, E. A., Taylor, P. E., Alter, H. J. and the Dialysis Vaccine Trial Group (1981). The immune response of healthy adults to a reduced dose of hepatitis B vaccine. *J. Med. Virol.*, **8**, 123–9
42. Szmuness, W., Stevens, C. E., Zang, E. A., Harley, E. J. and Kellner, A. A. (1981). Controlled clinical trial of the efficacy of the hepatitis B vaccine (Heptavax B): A final report. *Hepatology*, **1**, 377–85
43. Francis, D. P., Hadler, S. C., Thompson, S. E., Maynard, J. E., Ostrow, D. G., Altman, N., Braff, E. H., O'Malley, P., Hawkins, D., Judson, F. N., Penley, K., Nylund, T., Christie, G., Mayers, F., Moore, J. N., Gardner, A., Doto, I. L., Miller, J. H., Reynolds, G. H., Murphy, B. L., Schable, C. A., Clark, B. T., Curran, J. W. and Redeker, A. G. (1982). The prevention of hepatitis B with vaccine. *Ann. Intern. Med.*, **97**, 362–6
44. Stevens, C. E., Alter, H. J., Taylor, P. E., Zaug, E. A., Harley, E. J. and Szmuness, W. (1984). Hepatitis B vaccine in patients receiving hemodialysis: immunogenicity and efficacy. *N. Engl. J. Med.*, **311**, 496–501
45. Centers for Disease Control (1987). Update on hepatitis B prevention. *Morb. Mort. Weekly Rep.*, **36**, 353–66
46. Galibert, F., Mandart, E., Fitoussi, F., Tiollais, P. and Charnay, P. (1979). Nucleotide sequence of the hepatitis B virus genome (subtype *ayw*) cloned in *E. coli*. *Nature (Lond.)*, **281**, 646–50
47. Pasek, M., Goto, T., Gilbert, W., Zink, B., Schaller, H., MacKay, P., Leadbetter, G. and Murray, K. (1979). Hepatitis B virus genes and their expression. *Nature (Lond.)*, **282**, 575–9

48. Valenzuela, P., Gray, P., Quiroga, N., Zaldivar, J., Goodman, H. M. and Rutter, W. J. (1979). Nucleotide sequence of the gene coding for the major protein of hepatitis B virus surface antigen. *Nature (Lond.)*, **280**, 815-19
49. Peterson, D. L., Roberts, I. M. and Vyas, G. N. (1977). Partial amino acid sequence of two major component polypeptides of hepatitis B surface antigen. *Proc. Natl. Acad. Sci. USA*, **74**, 1530–40
50. Valenzuela, P., Medina, A., Rutter, W. J., Ammerer, G. and Hall, B. D. (1982). Synthesis and assembly of hepatitis B virus surface antigen particles in yeast. *Nature (Lond.)*, **298**, 347–50
51. Heerman, K. H., Goldman, V., Schwartz, W., Seyffarth, T., Baumgarten, H. and Gerlich, W. H. (1984). Large surface proteins of hepatitis B virus containing the pre-S sequence. *J. Virol.*, **52** 396–402
52. Peterson, D. L. (1981). Isolation and characterization of the major protein and glycoprotein of hepatitis B surface antigen. *J. Biol. Chem.*, **256**, 6975–82
53. Hilleman, M. R. and Ellis, R. W. (1986). Vaccines made from recombinant yeast cells. *Vaccine*, **4** 75–6
54. Ellis, R. W. (1989). Vaccines, diagnostic proteins and hormones. In Rehm, H. J. and Reed, G. (eds), *Biotechnology, A Comprehensive Treatise*, Vol. 7b *Gene Technology*. pp. 167–194. (Weinham: Verlag Chenne)
55. Holland, J. P. and Holland, M. J. (1980). Structural expression of two nontandemly repeated yeast glyceraldehyde-3-phosphate dehydrogenase genes. *J. Biol. Chem.*, **255**, 2596–605
56. Bennetzen, J. L. and Hall, B. D. (1982). The primary structure of the *Saccharomyces cerevisiae* gene for alcohol dehydrogenase I. *J. Biol. Chem.*, **257**, 3018–25
57. Jayaram, M., Li, Y.-Y. and Broach, J. R. (1983). The yeast plasmid in 2μ circle encodes components required for its high copy propagation. *Cell*, **34** 95–104
58. Ellis, R. W. (1989). Recombinant-derived hepatitis B vaccine - A paradigm for other subunit vaccines. In Putney, S. and Bolognesi, D. (eds), *AIDS Vaccine, Basic Research and Clinical Trials*. (New York: Marcel Dekker). (In press)
59. Emini, E. A., Ellis, R. W., Miller, W. J., McAleer, W. J., Scolnick, E. M. and Gerety, R. J. (1986). Production and immunological analysis of recombinant hepatitis B vaccine. *J. Infect.*, **13(A)**, 3–9
60. Hauser, P., Voet, P., Simoen, E., Thomas, H. C., Petre, J., DeWilde, M. and Stephenne, J. (1987). Immunological properties of recombinant HBsAg produced in yeast. *Postgrad. Med. J.*, **63**(2), 83–91
61. Ellis, R. W., Kniskern, P. J., Hagopian, A., Schultz, L. D., Montgomery, D. L., Maigetter, R. Z., Wampler, D. E., Emini, E. A., Wolanski, B., McAleer, W. J., Hurni, W. M. and Miller, W. J. (1988). Preparation and testing of a recombinant-derived hepatitis B vaccine consisting of pre-S2 + S polypeptides. In Zuckerman, A. (ed.), *Viral Hepatitis and Liver Disease*, pp. 1079–85. (New York: Alan Liss)
62. Zajac, B. A., West, D. J., McAleer, W. J. and Scolnick, E. M. (1986). Overview of clinical studies with hepatitis B vaccine made by recombinant DNA. *J. Infect.*, **13**(A), 39–45
63. West, D. J., Zajac, B. A., Ellis, R. W. and Gerety, R. J. (1988). Improved immunogenicity of a yeast-derived hepatitis B vaccine. *Infektionsklinik.*
64. Hollinger, F. B., Troisi, C. L. and Pepe, P. E. (1986). Anti-HBs responses to vaccination with a human hepatitis B vaccine made by recombinant DNA technology in yeast. *J. Infect. Dis.*, **153**, 156–9
65. Morton, D. and Krugman, S. (1986). Recombinant yeast hepatitis B vaccine compared with plasma-derived vaccine: Immunogenicity and effect of a booster dose. *J. Infect.*, **13**(A), 31–8
66. Stevens, C. E., Taylor, P. E., Tong, M. J., Toy, P. T., Vyas, G. N. and Krugman, S. (1987). Yeast-recombinant hepatitis B vaccine: efficacy with hepatitis B immunoglobulin in prevention of perinatal hepatitis B virus transmission. *J. Am. Med. Assoc.*, **257**, 2612–16
67. Okada, K., Kamiyama, I., Inomata, M., Imai, M., Miyakura, Y. and Mayumi, M. (1976). E antigen and anti-e in the serum of asymptomatic carrier mothers as indicators of positive and negative transmission of hepatitis B virus to their infants. *N. Engl. J. Med.*, **294**, 746–9
68. Beasley, R. P., Hwang, L.-Y., Stevens, C. E., Lin, C.-C., Hsieh, F.-J., Wang, K.-Y., Sun, T.-

S. and Szmuness, W. (1983). Efficacy of hepatitis B immune globulin for prevention of perinatal transmission of the hepatitis B virus carrier state: final report of a randomized double-blind, placebo-controlled trial. *Hepatology*, **3**, 135–41

69. Beasley, R. P., Hwang, L. Y., Lee, G. C.-Y., Lau, C. C., Roan, C. H., Huang, F. and Chen, C. L. (1983). Prevention of perinatally transmitted hepatitis B virus infections with hepatitis B immune globulin and hepatitis B vaccine. *Lancet*, **2**, 1099–102
70. Stevens, C. E., Toy, P. T., Tong, M. J., Taylor, P. E., Vyas, G. N., Nair, P. V., Guadavalo, M. and Krugman, S. (1985). Perinatal hepatitis B virus transmission in the United States: prevention by passive-active immunization. *J. Am. Med. Assoc.*, **253**, 1740–5
71. Kniskern, P. J., Hagopian, A., Burke, P., Dunn, N., Emini, E. A., Miller, W. J., Yamazaki, S. and Ellis, R. W. (1988). A candidate vaccine for hepatitis B containing the complete viral surface protein. *Hepatology*, **8**, 82–7
72. Havens, W. P. (1945). Properties of the etiologic agent of infectious hepatitis. *Proc. Soc. Exp. Biol. Med.*, **58**, 203–4
73. MacCallum, F. O. (1972). Early studies of viral hepatitis. *Br. Med. Bull.*, **28**, 105–8
74. Provost, P. J., Ittensohn, O. L., Villarejos, V. M., Arguedas, J. A. and Hilleman, M. R. (1973). Etiologic relationship of marmoset-propagated CR326 hepatitis A virus to hepatitis in man. *Proc. Soc. Exp. Biol. Med.*, **142**, 1257–67
75. Provost, P. J., Wolanski, B. S., Miller, W. J., Ittensohn, O. L., McAleer, W. J. and Hilleman, M. R. (1975). Physical, chemical and morphologic dimensions of human hepatitis A virus strain CR326 (38578). *Proc. Soc. Exp. Biol. Med.*, **148**, 532–9
76. Coulepis, A. G., Anderson, B. N. and Gust, I. D. (1987). Hepatitis A. *Adv. Virus Res.*, **32**, 129–69
77. Sobsey, M. D., Shields, P. A., Hauchman, F. S., Davis, A. L., Rullman, V. A. and Bosch, A. (1988). Survival and persistence of hepatitis A virus in environmental samples. In Zuckerman, A. J. (ed.), *Viral Hepatitis and Liver Disease*, pp. 121–4. (New York: Alan Liss)
78. Purcell, R. H., Feinstone, S. M., Ticehurst, J. R., Daemer, R. J. and Baroudy, B. M. (1984). Hepatitis A virus. In Vyas, G. N., Dienstag, J. L. and Hoofnagle, J. H. (eds), *Viral Hepatitis and Liver Disease*. pp. 1–22. (Orlando: Grune & Stratton)
79. Jacobson, I. M., Nath, B. J. and Dienstag, J. L. (1985). Relapsing viral hepatitis type A. *J. Med. Virol.*, **16**, 163–9
80. Sjögren, M. H., Tanno, H., Fay, O., Sileoni, S., Cohen, B., Burke, D. S. and Feighny, R. J. (1987). Hepatitis A virus in stool during clinical relapse. *Ann. Intern. Med.*, **106**, 221–6
81. Van den Anker, J. N., Sukhai, R. N. and Dumas, A. M. (1988). Relapsing hepatitis in a child, associated with isolation of hepatitis A antigen from the liver. *Eur. J. Pediatr.*, **147**, 333–42
82. Burke, D. S. and Heisey, G. B. (1984). Wild Malaysian cynomolgus monkeys are exposed to hepatitis A virus. *Am. J. Trop. Med. Hyg.*, **33**, 940–4
83. Lemon, S. M., Chao, S.-F., Jansen, R. W., Binn, L. N. and LeDuc, J. W. (1987). Genomic heterogeneity among human and nonhuman strains of hepatitis A virus. *J. Virol.*, **61**, 735–42
84. Lemon, S. M. (1985). Type A viral hepatitis. New developments in an old disease. *N. Engl. J. Med.*, **313**, 1059–67
85. Papaevangelou, G. J. (1987). Epidemiology of hepatitis A and B. *Infection*, **15**, 221–7
86. Widell, A., Hansson, B. G., Moestrup, T., Serleus, Z., Mathiesen, L. R. and Johnsson, T. (1982). Acute hepatitis A, B and non-A, non-B in a Swedish community studied over a ten-year period. *Scand. J. Infect. Dis.*, **14**, 253–9
87. Centers for Disease control (1988). Hepatitis A among drug abusers. *Morb. Mort. Weekly Rep.*, **37**, 299–305
88. Sherertz, R. J., Russel, B. A. and Reumann, P. D. (1984). Transmission of hepatitis A by transfusion of blood products. *Arch. Intern. Med.*, **144**, 1579–80
89. Lorenz, D., Barker, L., Stevens, D., Peterson, M. and Kirschstein, R. (1970). Hepatitis in the marmoset. *Saguinus mystax. Proc. Soc. Exp. Biol. Med.*, **135**, 348–54
90. Provost, P. J., Villarejos, V. M. and Hilleman, M. R. (1977). Suitabiity of the rufiventer marmoset as a host animal for human hepatitis A virus. *Proc. Soc. Exp. Biol. Med.*, **155**, 283–6
91. Provost, P. J., Ittensohn, O. L., Villarejos, V. M. and Hilleman, M. R. (1975). A specific complement-fixation test for human hepatitis A employing CR326 virus antigen. Diagnosis and epidemiology. *Proc. Soc. Exp. Biol. Med.*, **148**, 962–9

92. Miller, W. J., Provost, P. J., McAleer, W. J., Ittensohn, O. L., Villarejos, V. M. and Hilleman, M. R. (1975). Specific immune adherence assay for human hepatitis A antibody. Application to diagnostic and epidemiologic investigations. *Proc. Soc. Exp. Biol. Med.*, **149**, 254–61
93. Provost, P. J. and Hilleman, M. R. (1975). An inactivated hepatitis A virus vaccine prepared from infected marmoset liver. *Proc. Soc. Exp. Biol. Med.*, **159**, 201–3
94. Provost, P. J. and Hilleman, M. R. (1979). Propagation of human hepatitis A virus in cell culture *in vitro*. *Proc. Soc. Exp. Biol. Med.*, **160**, 213–21
95. Provost, P. J., Banker, F. S., Giesa, P. A., McAleer, W. J., Buynak, E. B. and Hilleman, M. R. (1982). Progress toward a live attenuated human hepatitis A vaccine. *Proc. Soc. Exp. Biol. Med.*, **170**, 8–14
96. Provost, P. J., Emini, E. A., Lewis, J. A. and Gerety, R. J. (1988). Progress toward the development of a hepatitis A vaccine. In Zuckerman, A. J. (ed.), *Viral Hepatitis and Liver Disease*, pp. 83–6. (New York: Alan Liss)
97. Provost, P. J., Conti, P. A., Giesa, P. A., Banker, F. S., Buynak, E. B., McAleer, W. J. and Hilleman, M. R. (1983). Studies in chimpanzees of live, attenuated hepatitis A vaccine candidates. *Proc. Soc. Exp. Biol. Med.*, **172**, 357–63
98. Karron, R. A., Daemer, R., Ticehurst, J., D'Hondt, E., Popper, H., Mihalik, K., Phillips, J., Feinstone, S. and Purcell, R. H. (1988). Studies of prototype live hepatitis A virus vaccines in primate models. *J. Infect. Dis.*, **157**, 338–45
99. Wallace, R. E., Vasington, P. J., Petricciani, J. C., Hopps, H. E., Lorenz, D. E. and Kadanka, Z. (1973). Development and characterization of cell lines from subhuman primates. *In Vitro*, **8**, 333–41
100. Provost, P. J., McAleer, W. J. and Hilleman, M. R. (1981). *In vitro* cultivation of hepatitis A virus. In Szmuness, W., Alter, H. and Maynard, J. (eds), *Viral Hepatitis*, pp. 21–30. (Philadelphia: Franklin Institute Press)
101. Provost, P. J., Giesa, P. A., McAleer, W. J. and Hilleman, M. R. (1981). Isolation of hepatitis A virus *in vitro* in cell culture directly from human specimens. *Proc. Soc. Exp. Biol. Med.*, **167**, 201–6
102. Provost, P. J., Bishop, R. P., Gerety, R. J., Hilleman, M. R., McAleer, W. J., Scolnick, E. M. and Stevens, C. E. (1986). New findings in live attenuated hepatitis A vaccine development. *J. Med. Virol.*, **20**, 165–75
103. Gust, I. D., Lehmann, N. I., Crowe, S., McCrorie, M., Locarnini, S. A. and Lucas, C. R. (1985). The origin of the HM175 strain of hepatitis A virus. *J. Infect. Dis.*, **151**, 365–7
104. Bradley, D. W., Schable, C. A., McCaustland, K. A., Cook, E. H., Murphy, B. L., Fields, H. A., Ebert, J. W., Wheeler, C. and Maynard, J. E. (1984). Hepatitis A virus: growth characteristics of *in vivo* and *in vitro* propagated wild and attenuated virus strains. *J. Med. Virol.*, **14**, 373–86
105. Hu, M., Scheid, R., Deinhardt, F., Gauss-Muller, V., Sun, B. and Zhou, Y. (1988). Attenuated hepatitis A virus for vaccine development: attenuation and virulence for marmosets. In Zuckerman, A. J. (ed.), *Viral Hepatitis and Liver Disease*, pp. 81–2. (New York: Alan Liss)
106. Flehmig, B., Mauler, R., Noll, G., Weinmann, E. and Gregersen, J. P. (1988). Progress in the development of an attenuated live hepatitis A vaccine. In Zuckerman, A. J. (ed.), *Viral Hepatitis and Liver Disease*, pp. 87–90. (New York: Alan Liss)
107. Mao, J., Xie, R., Huang, H., Chai, S., Chen, N., Yu, P., Wan, X., Liu, C., Cao, Y., Dong, D., Lian, Y., Zou, Y., Liang, W., Li, H. and Chen, T. (1988). Studies in monkeys of attenuated hepatitis A variants. *Scientia Sinica*, **31**, 338–43
108. Sabin, A. B. and Boulger, L. R. (1973). History of Sabin attenuated poliovirus oral live vaccine strains. *J. Biol. Stand.*, **1**, 115–18
109. Nomoto, A., Iizuka, N., Kohara, M. and Arita, M. (1988). Strategy for construction of live picornavirus vaccines. *Vaccine*, **6**, 134–7
110. Feinstone, S. M. (1986). Hepatitis A. *Prog. Liver Dis.*, **8**, 199–310
111. Cohen, J. I., Ticehurst, J. R., Feinstone, S. M., Rosenblum, B. and Purcell, R. H. (1988). Hepatitis A virus cDNA and its RNA transcripts are infectious in cell culture. *J. Virol.*, **61**, 3035–9
112. Burke, K. L., Dunn, G., Ferguson, M., Minor, P. D. and Almond, J. W. (1988). Antigenic chimaeras of polovirus as potential new vaccines. *Nature* (*Lond.*), **332**, 81–2

113. Ostermayr, R., von der Helm, K., Gauss-Muller, V., Winnacker, E. L. and Deinhardt, F. (1987). Expression of hepatitis A virus cDNA in *Escherichia coli*: Antigenic VP1 recombinant protein. *J. Virol.*, **61**, 3645–7
114. Emini, E. A., Hughes, J. V., Perlow, D. S. and Boger, J. (1985). Induction of hepatitis A virus-neutralizing antibody by a virus-specific synthetic peptide. *J. Virol.*, **55**, 836–9
115. Provost, P. J., Hughes, J. V., Miller, W. J., Giesa, P. A., Banker, F. S. and Emini, E. A. (1986). An inactivated hepatitis A viral vaccine of cell culture origin. *J. Med. Virol.*, **19**, 23–31
116. Binn, L. N., Bancroft, W. H., Lemon, S. M., Marchwicki, R. H., LeDuc, J. W., Trahan, C. J., Staley, E. C. and Keenan, C. M. (1986). Preparation of a prototype inactivated hepatitis A virus vaccine. *J. Infect. Dis.*, **153**, 749–56
117. Sjogren, M. H., Eckels, K. H., Binn, L. N., Dubois, D. R., Hoke, C. H., Burke, D. S. and Bancroft, W. H. (1988). Safety and immunogenicity of an inactivated hepatitis A vaccine. In Zuckerman, A. J. (ed.), *Viral Hepatitis and Liver Disease*, pp. 94–6. (New York: Alan Liss)
118. Binn, L. N., Bancroft, W. H., Eckels, K. H., Marchwicki, R. H., Dubois, D. R., Asher, L. V. S., LeDuc, J. W., Trahan, C. J. and Burke, D. S. (1988). Inactivated hepatitis A virus vaccine produced in human diploid MRC-5 cells. In Zuckerman, A. J. (ed.), *Viral Hepatitis and Liver Disease*, pp. 91–3. (New York: Alan Liss)
119. Hughes, J. V. and Stanton, L. W. (1985). Isolation and immunizations with hepatitis A viral structural proteins: induction of antiprotein, antiviral, and neutralizing responses. *J. Virol.*, **55**, 395–401
120. Gauss-Müller, V. and Deinhardt, F. (1988). Immunoreactivity of human and rabbit antisera to hepatitis A virus. *J. Med. Virol.*, **24**, 219–28
121. Wheeler, C. M., Roberston, B. H., Van Nest, G., Dina, D., Bradley, D. W. and Fields, H. A. (1986). Structure of the hepatitis A virion: Peptide mapping of the capsid region. *J. Virol.*, **58**, 307–18

11
Chemical synthesis of hepatitis B vaccine

A. R. NEURATH

INTRODUCTION

Hepatitis B is a common disease representing a serious worldwide health problem. An estimated 20 million new infections occur annually which in 5–10% of infected people lead to a chronic carrier state. The number of chronic carriers of the virus throughout the world is considered to be 280 million (Figure 1). The hepatitis B carrier state leads at high frequency to primary hepatocellular carcinoma (~1 million new cases per year) representing a major cause of death in countries with a high prevalence of hepatitis B. The disease is transmitted both horizontally and perinatally. The prevention, and possble eradication, of this disease can be accomplished by active immunoprophylaxis.

Hepatitis B virus (HBV) contains a lipoprotein envelope surrounding the hepatitis B core antigen (HBcAg) containing the hepatitis B virus genome. In addition to the virion, there are subviral particles which circulate in the blood of infected individuals. These are tubular and 20 nm spherical forms (Figure 2). These two forms are antigenically very similar but not completely identical to the envelope (env) of HBV. Discovery of these differences contributed to the understanding of protective immunity to HBV.

In 1974 it was shown by electron microscopy that sera from some HBV-infected individuals contain immune complexes consisting exclusively of virus particles but lacking the other two forms[2]. The most reasonable way to explain this was by assuming that antibodies in the immune complexes were directed against epitopes of the HBV envelope which were absent, or at least present at lower levels, in the two subviral forms. This hypothesis was later confirmed[3]. Rabbits were immunized with preparations enriched in virus particles. The resulting antisera were adsorbed on 20 nm spherical particles. This led to removal of all antibodies recognizing these particles as measured by radioimmunoassays (RIA). They adsorbed serum agglutinated virus particles. This was a direct proof for additional specificities on the surface

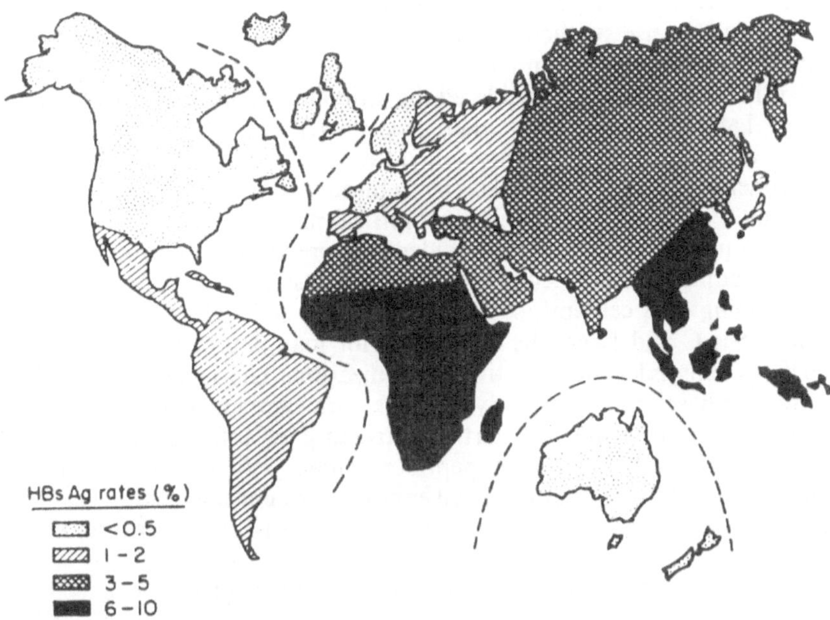

Figure 1 Schematic map of the worldwide distribution of HBsAg carriers (reprinted with permission from ref. 1)

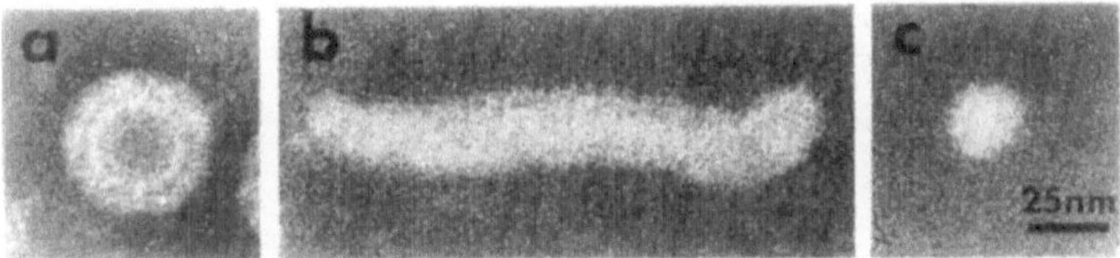

Figure 2 The HBV particle (**a**), and subviral particles: the tubular form (filament) (**b**) and the ~20 nm spherical particle (**c**)

of the virus. This conclusion was supported by findings of Alberti *et al.*[4], who demonstrated the presence of anti-HBV-specific antibodies in sera of humans early during the recovery phase from HBV infection. However, the nature and importance of these antibodies remained unclear until after the cloning and sequencing of HBV DNA and the delineation of HBV envelope (env) protein epitopes using synthetic peptides.

The first hepatitis B vaccines were prepared from plasma of infected individuals using purified 20 nm spherical HBsAg particles. In the production of one of these vaccines these particles were treated with pepsin, urea and formaldehyde to eliminate all other contaminating viruses which might have been present in the blood of infected people[5]. This procedure, resulting in proteolytic cleavage of HBV env proteins, was not used in the preparation of other serum-derived vaccines. All these vaccines proved to be quite efficient in preventing hepatitis B[6]. However, since the source of the vaccines was not uniform, and extensive purification procedures were required, new vaccines based on recombinant DNA technology were developed. Another possibility is to use synthetic peptides for vaccination. To accomplish this it is necessary to define B- and T-cell epitopes on the HBV env protein.

Synthetic peptides are considered the ultimate step in vaccine development (D, E, Table 1). Unlike the other vaccines (A–C, Table 1), the design of synthetic vaccines depends on detailed knowledge concerning immunogenic components of viral proteins, i.e. their amino acid sequence, the localization of B and T cell epitopes (based on empirical mapping of epitopes along the entire sequence of the protein aided by predictive algorithms[8-10]) and understanding of their secondary and tertiary structure. Approaches useful for mapping of B cell epitopes are summarized in Table 2. At present only approaches C and D can be considered for mapping of B cell epitopes on HBV proteins relevant to active immunization. The localization of B cell epitopes is based predominantly on work with synthetic peptides until more information concerning the tertiary structure of HBV proteins becomes available. However, synthetic peptides mimic only continuous, but not topographical (discontinuous) B cell epitopes. For consideration as candidate components of synthetic vaccines, peptides have to satisfy criteria listed in Table 3.

As with viruses in general, those HBV proteins which are exposed either on the surface of virions or on the membrane of infected cells (i.e. HBV env proteins and HBcAg, respectively) play a role in protective immunity. HBV env proteins exposed on the surface of the virus elicit virus-neutralizing

Table 1 The pattern of progress in vaccine production*

Vaccine	*Relies on*
A. Conventional vaccines	Empirical knowledge; living attentuated and crude killed vaccines
B. Improved vaccines	Large-scale culture including mammalian cell culture; purification of antigens; genetic basis for virulence; immunological understanding
C. Single protein vaccines	Monoclonal antibodies; pure antigens; gene cloning and sequencing; improved adjuvants
D. Simpler synthetic peptide vaccines	Immunochemistry; computer chemistry understanding of basis of adjuvanticity
E. Simpler synthetic peptide vaccines active orally	Medicinal chemistry

*Reprinted with permission from Vane and Cuatrecasas[7]

Table 2 Approaches for B-cell epitope mapping

A.	Understanding of the three-dimensional structure of antigens (viruses) or of antigen–antibody complexes
B.	Effect of site-directed mutagenesis (deletion and point mutations) on antibody binding
C.	Synthetic peptides binding anti-protein antibodies
D.	Knowledge concerning amino acid variability between related antigens (antigenic subtypes of viruses)

Table 3 Criteria for peptide components of synthetic hepatitis B vaccines

1. Optimally designed peptides should be recognized by antibodies to the native env protein, and the affinity constant (K) for the reaction between these antibodies and the peptides should be of the same order of magnitude as K for the reaction between the same antibodies and the native env protein
2. Antipeptide antisera should recognize the native env protein well. That is, the anti-peptide antisera should correspond as closely as possible to the anti-native protein antisera
3. The synthetic peptides should be highly immunogenic, i.e. able to elicit high levels of antibodies reacting with the native protein in the absence of any carrier. This can also be stated as requiring that peptides should contain not only B cell but also T cell epitopes
4. T cell epitopes on the synthetic peptides should mimic the corresponding T cell epitopes on the native protein, and immunization with synthetic peptides should prime the immunized animals for a response to the native env protein
5. The synthetic peptides should correspond to functionally important segments of the env protein, and anti-peptide antibodies should have inhibitory activity on the corresponding biological functions
6. The synthetic peptides should elicit virus-neutralizing antibodies and should be protective in man and animals suceptible to hepadnavirus infection

protective antibodies. HBcAg, which is not exposed on the surface of intact virions, is accessible on the surface of infected cells[11]. Epitopes on HBcAg may elicit protection by two distinct mechanisms: (a) a specific cytotoxic response against infected hepatocytes[12–14] and (b) generation of anti-HBc-specific T helper cells for antibody response to HBV env proteins[13–16]. For this reason it is necessary to consider synthetic peptides derived from both the HBV env protein and from the HBcAg sequence as potential components of synthetic vaccines.

Proteins of the HBV envelope, although representing translational products of a single gene, consist of several species differing in the extent of glycosylation and having a common C-terminus but differing in their N-termini (Figure 3). The most abundant protein in the 20 nm subviral particles is S protein in its unglycosylated and glycosylated forms (P25 and GP29). The content of M-protein, and especially of L-protein, is higher in virus particles than in subviral particles. Due to the presence of multiple protein species in the HBV envelope, the antigenicity and immunogenicity of peptides corresponding to different segments (S, pres2 and preS1) of the HBV envelope will be discussed separately.

SYNTHETIC PEPTIDES DERIVED FROM THE SEQUENCE OF S PROTEIN

S protein is the major component of 20 nm spherical HBsAg particles, each of which contains about 100 copies of S protein[18]. Four major antigenic subtypes of HBsAg can be discerned by serological reactions using human or animal anti-HBs. These can be further subdivided (as indicated in parentheses) into the following subtypes: *adw* (*adw2*, *adw4*); *adr* ($adrq^-$,

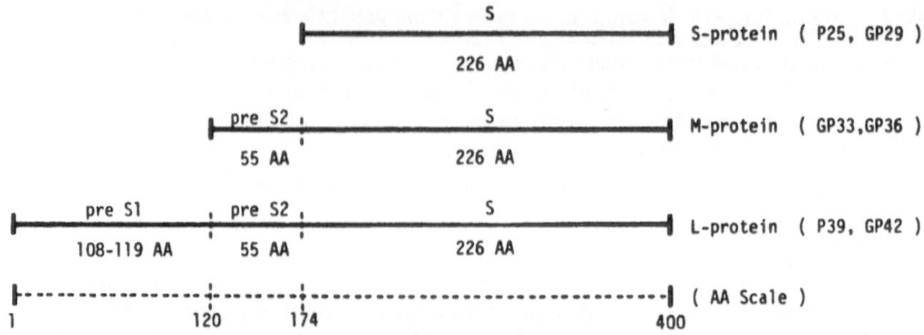

Figure 3 Schematic representation of HBV env proteins and their relatedness. The open reading frame on HBV DNA coding for HBV env proteins has the capacity to code for a protein consisting of 389–400 amino acids (AA) depending on the antigenic subtype of HBV. The earliest identified HBV env component was the 25 kd S-protein derived from the C-terminal half of this open reading frame and consisting of 226 AA. It exists in a non-glycosylated (P25) and a glycosylated (GP29) form. The middle (M) protein (281 AA) contains the sequences of the S-protein with 55 additional N-terminal AA encoded by the preS2 region of HBV DNA, and occurs in two distinct glycosylated forms, GP33 and GP36. The large (L) protein (389 or 400 AA) contains the sequence of M-protein with 108 or 119 additional N-terminal AA encoded by the preS1 region of HBV DNA, and exists in a non-glycosylated (P39) and a glycosylated (GP42) form[17]

adrq$^+$); *ayw* (*ayw1*, *ayw2*, *ayw3*, *ayw4*) and *ayr*. The letter *a* denotes antigenic specificities common to all HBV subtypes; the letters *d*/*y* and *w*/*r*, respectively, denote pairs of mutually exclusive specificities: numbers 1–4 further subdivide the *w* specificity and the presence or absence of *q* determinants subdivides the *adr* subtypes[19]. The *a* specificity, common to all HBV subtypes, appears to consist of a group of distinct antigenic determinants. Antibodies to some of these *a* determinants provide protection against infection by any of the HBV subtypes. Failure to respond to *a* determinants after infection (immunization) by one HBV subtype may later result in reinfection by another HBV subtype[19].

Dominant B-cell epitopes are localized within the sequence S(105–161) of S protein. The corresponding amino acid sequence for subtype *adw*2 is evident from Table 4. There are eight cysteine residues in this sequence, all of which are conserved among the distinct HBV subtypes. Residues 110, 113, 114, 120, 122, 125–127, 131, 133, 134, 143 and 159–161 are not conserved among the distinct HBV subtypes[19]. Substitution of arginine (R) for lysine

Table 4 Amino acid sequence of peptides derived from the S(105–161) region of HBsAg S-protein (subtype *adw*2)

Peptide	Sequence
Peptide 1 S(105–120)	PV<u>C</u>PLIPGSTTTSTGP
Peptide 2 S(121–136)	<u>C</u>KT<u>C</u>TTPAQGNSMFPS
Peptide 3 S(137–146)	<u>CCC</u>TKPTDGN
Peptide 4 S(147–161)	<u>C</u>T<u>C</u>IPIPSSWAFAKY

(K) corresponding to amino acid residue 122 is the single essential difference between S protein subtypes *d* and *y*[20]. A single point mutation changing the codon for amino acid 160 from K to R converts the subtype determinant *w* into *r*[21]. The significance of other amino acid replacements within the S(105–161) sequence remains unclear.

The dominant B cell epitopes on S protein appear to be topographical (discontinuous), since reduction of disulphide bonds within S protein results in a drastic reduction of binding of antibodies specific for the native protein (anti-HBs) and in increased binding of antibodies generated by immunization with the altered reduced–alkylated protein (Figure 4). Since the dominant B cell epitopes of S protein are discontinuous, it proved difficult to mimic them by linear synthetic peptides. This problem was partially overcome by using cyclic peptides generated by intramolecular disulphide bond formation between two (four) cysteine residues present in the peptides[19,23] (Figure 5).

The role of disulphide bonds between particular cysteine residues within the S protein sequence in the recognition of peptides by anti-HBs and in eliciting antibodies recognizing native S protein is demonstrated by results from two sets of experiments. In one set of experiments, four distinct peptides,

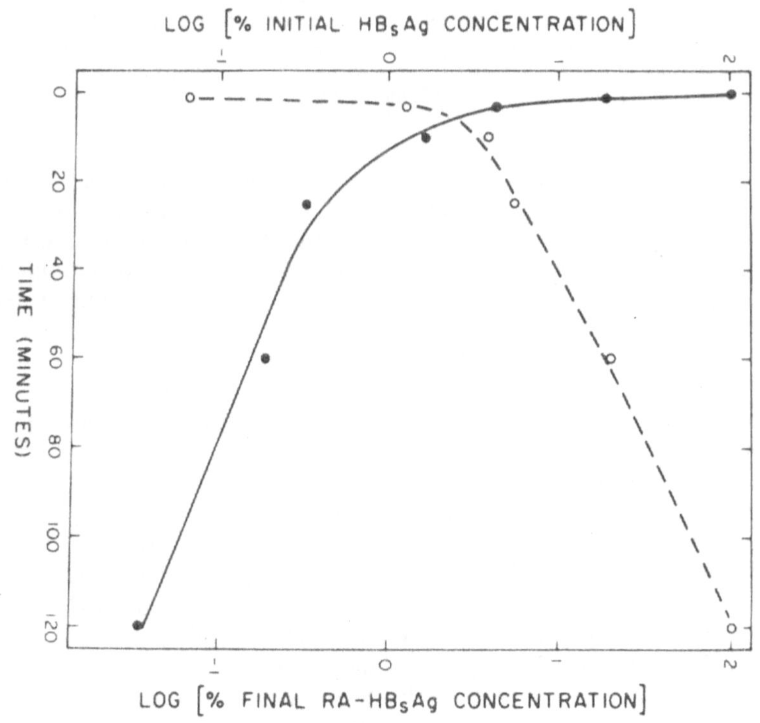

Figure 4 Kinetics of conversion of native HBsAg by reduction and alkylation into an antigenically distinct form detectable by antibodies to reduced and alkylated HBsAg (RA-HBsAg) (reprinted with permission from ref. 22)

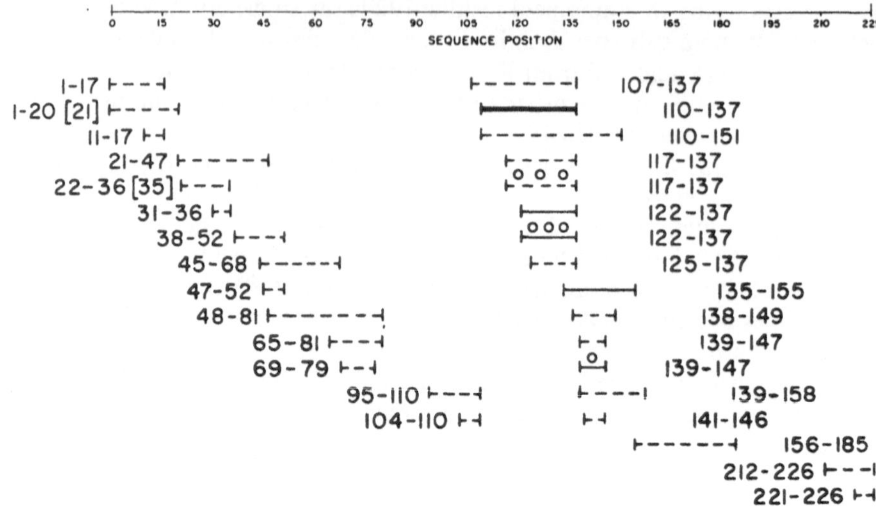

Figure 5 Schematic representation of results of studies on synthetic analogues of the HBV S protein. Synthetic peptides eliciting anti-S antibodies are represented by dashed bars; peptides which, in addition, were reported to react with antibodies to native protein (anti-HBs) are represented by solid bars. The thicker solid bar indicates the peptide reported to elicit protective antibodies in chimpanzees. Numbers to the left or right of the bars indicate N- and C-termini of the peptides. Circles on top of the bars indicate cyclic peptides. All peptides listed were immunogenic when bound to protein carriers and administered with complete and incomplete Freund's adjuvant. Immungenicity without protein carriers and Freund's adjuvant was reported only for S(122–137) (cyclic) and S(135–155) (derived from results presented in ref. 23)

each containing at least one cysteine residue, were synthesized (Table 4). Antigenicity (ability to be recognized by anti-HBs) and immunogenicity (elicitation of antibodies to native S protein) of the individual peptides, as well as of di- and tripeptides, generated by intermolecular disulphide bond formation between the individual peptides, was measured. The tripeptide $2 + 3 + 4$ was optimally recognized by anti-HBs (Table 5). The same tripeptide also elicited the highest level of anti-HBs (Table 6). In a complementary set of experiments, peptides derived from the sequence S(121–151) were synthesized, each peptide having five out of seven cysteine residues replaced by serine at distinct positions. Each of the peptides, having two cysteine residues, was oxidized to form intramolecular disulphide bonds and tested for immunogenicity. The results (Figure 6) demonstrate the importance of disulphide bonds between particular cysteine residues within the S protein sequence. The best results were obtained with peptides expected to have disulphide bonds between residues 121–138, 124–138 and 139–147. The corresponding antipeptide antibodies recognized both native HBsAg and denatured P25 and GP29 (Figure 7, lanes D–F).

Since all cysteine residues in the S protein sequence are involved in disulphide bonds, synthetic peptides with multiple pairs of cysteine residues at defined locations will have to be synthesized in order to optimally mimic native S protein. The synthesis of the peptide [(S119–159)] with four cysteines and two disulphide loops between residues 124–137 and 139–147,

Table 5 Antigenicity of peptides 1, 2, 3, 4 and of di- and tripeptides generated by disulphide bond formation between the distinct peptides

Peptide	*Dilution endpoints with*	
	Human anti-HBs	*Rabbit anti-HBs*
1	<1:40	<1:40
2	<1:40	<1:40
3	<1:40	<1:40
4	<1:40	<1:40
1 + 2	<1:40	<1:40
1 + 3	<1:40	1:40
1 + 4	<1:40	1:80
2 + 3	<1:40	<1:40
2 + 4	<1:40	<1:40
3 + 4	<1:40	1:100
1 + 2 + 3	1:500	<1:40
1 + 3 + 4	1:500	1:100
2 + 3 + 4	1:2500	1:500

Table 6 Elicitation of anti-HBs by tripeptides generated by disulphide bond formation between peptides 1, 2, 3, 4

Peptide	*Dilution endpoints of anti-HBs antibodies measured by double-antibody RIA*
1 + 2 + 3	1:300*
1 + 3 + 4	1:335*
2 + 3 + 4	1:7200*

*Geometric mean dilution endpoints corresponding to two rabbit antisera per peptide

respectively, was reported[24]. The bi-cyclic peptide elicited anti-HBs while the linear form was unable to do so. However, the level of elicited antibodies was much lower than the level of antibodies elicited by intact HBsAg. A peptide [(S122–148)] with three cysteine residues at positions 124, 139 and 147 was better recognized by anti-HBs, and was able to elicit considerably higher levels of anti-HBs than shorter peptides S(122–137) and S(139–148) each having only two cysteine residues[25]. A cyclic peptide S(139–147) having a C-terminal tyrosine residue, added for labelling with ^{125}I, bound anti-HBs with an affinity similar to that determined for the reaction between HBsAg and anti-HBs[26–28]. The same peptide, when polymerized with glutaraldehyde, elicited antibodies reacting with native HBsAg with affinity values similar to those found for antibodies from individuals immune to hepatitis B[29].

LOCATION OF T CELL EPITOPES IN THE SEQUENCE OF S PROTEIN

Unlike the topographical B cell epitopes, T cell epitopes on S protein are sequential. Reduced and alkylated HBsAg[30], HBsAg denatured by formic acid[31], denatured S protein (P25) isolated from HBsAg and tryptic fragments

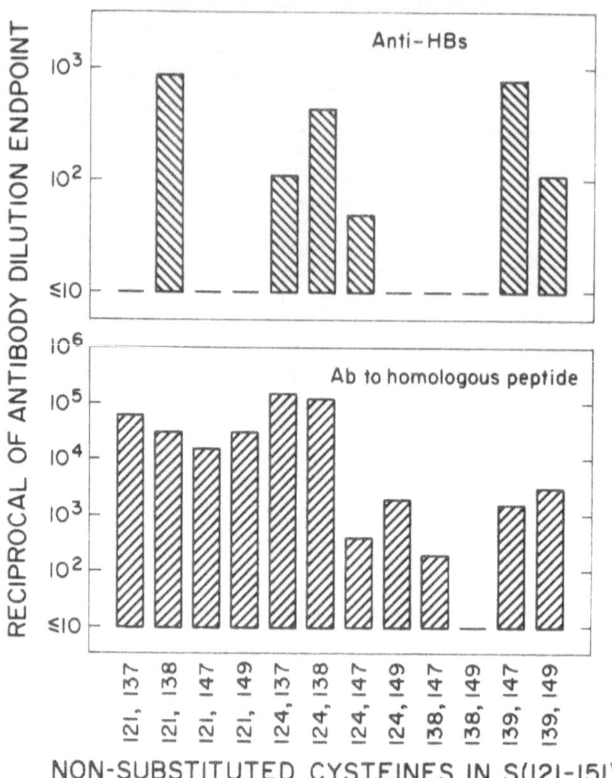

Figure 6 Immunogenicity of a series of peptides corresponding to the S protein sequence S(121–151), having five out of seven cysteine residues replaced by serines. Free peptides and subsequently peptides linked to bovine serum albumin were used to immunize rabbits. The antisera were tested for antibodies recognizing the homologous peptide (bottom) and HBsAg (top)

of P25[32] were all recognized by HBsAg-specific T cells and, when used for immunization, elicited an HBsAg-specific T cell response. In attempts to identify the sequences recognized by HBsAg-primed T cells from congenic strains of mice, several synthetic peptide analogues were screened for their ability to induce proliferation of these cells. The active peptides were distinct for different congenic strains of mice. Some of the peptides overlapped B cell epitopes while others did not. The following peptides were found to elicit T cell proliferation: S(38–52), S(95–109), S(110–137) and S(140–154)[32,33]. These peptides were much less efficient in eliciting T cell proliferation than equimolar quantities of HBsAg. It was also reported that peptides S(110–137) and S(38–52) stimulated T cells isolated from some recipients of a hepatitis B vaccine.

Detailed studies[34] in which T cell lines of the helper/inducer class, isolated from recipients of a hepatitis B vaccine, were used, indicated that the

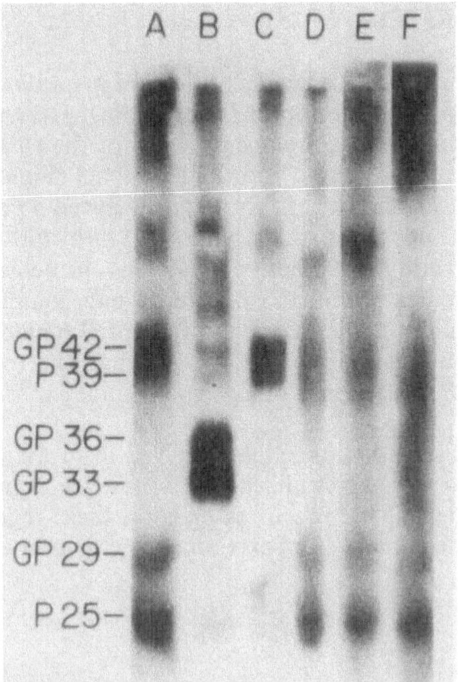

Figure 7 Western immunoblots of HBsAg containing S, preS and preS1 sequences with distinct antisera to synthetic peptides derived from the S-protein sequence. The peptides were: S(122–148)GGY (lane A); hybrid preS(120–153)–S(122–148)GGY (lane B); hybrid preS(12–47)–S(122–148)GGY (lane C); and S(121–151) with non-substituted cysteines at positions 121,138 (lane D) 124,138 (lane E) and 139,147 (lane F)

dominant T cell epitope is localized near the N-terminus of the S protein sequence. A single peptide [S(4–33)] contained a dominant T cell epitope and was highly efficient in eliciting T cell proliferation to the same extent as equimolar concentrations of formic acid-denatured HBsAg. Shorter peptides S(14–33), S(19–33), and S(19–28) were equally efficient in eliciting proliferative T cell responses. Cytotoxic human T lymphocytes were able to kill autologous target cells coated with these peptides. Thus, the shortest peptide carrying a dominant epitope recognized by both helper and cytotoxic T cells is S(19–28) having the sequence FFLLTRLTI, common to all HBV subtypes[19]. These results suggest that the T cell epitopes for two species, mice and humans, are distinct. Furthermore, the dominant epitope recognized by human T lymphocytes is distant in the primary sequence from dominant B cell epitopes. Therefore, synthetic S protein immunogens will have to be derived from distinct regions of the S protein sequence in order to fulfil criteria listed in Table 3. These requirements, and the need to mimic dominant topographic B cell epitopes, makes the task of developing a synthetic vaccine based on S protein challenging, and the design of vaccines based on other regions of the HBV envelope protein, more attractive.

SYNTHETIC PEPTIDES DERIVED FROM THE preS REGION OF THE HBV env PROTEIN

When electrophoretically separated denatured polypeptide components from HBV were reacted with an antiserum raised against HBV (anti-HBV), only the larger M- and L-protein components, but not the smaller components P25 and GP29, corresponding to S protein, reacted (Figure 8). This result is in agreement with the finding that native and reduced S protein are distinct antigens (Figure 4) and shows that antibodies with anti-preS specificities elicited by immunization with native HBV env proteins recognized the corresponding sequences within the denatured env components separated by electrophoresis. Thus, the antigenicity of the preS region of the HBV env proteins is affected by denaturation much less than that of S protein. This is in agreement with the absence of cysteine residues in the preS sequence (Figure 9).

Initial studies with synthetic peptides derived from the preS2 and preS1 regions of HBV env proteins established the presence of immunodominant disulphide bond-independent B cell epitopes on these regions of the HBV env protein[35,36]. Based on results of experiments with mouse congenic strains

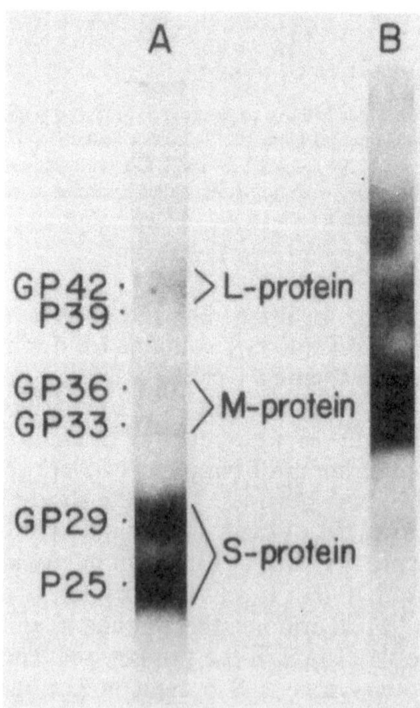

Figure 8 Western immunoblot of HBV env protein components separated by polyacrylamide gel electrophoresis. An antiserum to native HBV env proteins was used for immunoblotting. Separated HBV env proteins stained with silver (lane A); HBV env components detected with anti-HBV (lane B)

```
                                          1                   2                   3                   4
          1 2 3 4 5 6 7 8 9 0 1 2 3 4 5 6 7 8 9 0 1 2 3 4 5 6 7 8 9 0 1 2 3 4 5 6 7 8 9 0

1 adw2    M G G W S S K P R K G M G T N L S V P N P L G F F P D H Q L D P A F G A N S N N
2 adw                           M G T N L S V P N P L G F L P D H Q L D P A F G A N S T N
3 adyw                          M G Q N L S T S N P L G F F P D H Q L D P A F R A N T N N
4 ayw                           M G Q N L S T S N P L G F F P D H Q L D P A F R A N T A N
5 ayw                           M G Q N L S T S N P L G F F P D H Q L D P A F R A N T A N
6 adr     M G G W S S K P R Q G M G T N L S V P N P L G F F P D H Q L D P A F G A N S N N
7 adr     M G G W S S K P R Q G M G T N L S V P N P L G F F P D H Q L D P A F G A N S N N
8 adr     M G G W S S K P R Q G M G T N L S V P N P L G F F P D H Q L D P A F G A N S H N

                                M G   N L S     N P L G F   P D H Q L D P A F   A N     N

                                          5                   6                   7                   8
          1 2 3 4 5 6 7 8 9 0 1 2 3 4 5 6 7 8 9 0 1 2 3 4 5 6 7 8 9 0 1 2 3 4 5 6 7 8 9 0

1 adw2    P D W D F N P V K D D W P A A N Q V G V G A F G P R L T P P H G G I L G W S P Q
2 adw     P D W D F N P I K D H W P A A N Q V G V G A F G P G L T P P H G G I L G W S P Q
3 adyw    P D W D F N P N K D T W P D A N K V G A G A F G L G F T P P H G G L L G W S P Q
4 ayw     P D W D F N P N K D T W P D A N K V G A G A F G L G F T P P H G G L L G W S P Q
5 ayw     P D W D F N P N K D T W P D A N K V G A G A F G L G F T P P H G G L L G W S P Q
6 adr     P D W D F N P N K D Q W P E A N Q V G A G A F G P G F T P P H G G L L G W S P Q
7 adr     P D W D F N P N K D H W P E A I K V G A G D F G P G F T P P H G G L L G W S P Q
8 adr     P D W D F N P N K D H W P E A N Q V G A G A F G P G F T P P H G G L L G W S P Q

          P D W D F N P   K D   W P   A     V G   G   F G       T P P H G G   L G W S P Q

                                          9                  10                  11                  12
          1 2 3 4 5 6 7 8 9 0 1 2 3 4 5 6 7 8 9 0 1 2 3 4 5 6 7 8 9 0 1 2 3 4 5 6 7 8 9 0

1 adw2    A Q G I L T T V S T I P P P A S T N R Q S G R Q P T P I S P P L R D S H P Q A M
2 adw     A Q G I L T T V S T I P P P A S T N R Q S G R Q P T P I S P P L R D S H P Q A M
3 adyw    A Q G I M Q T L P A N P P P A S T N R Q S G R Q P T P L S P P L R T T H P Q A M
4 ayw     A Q G I L Q T L P A N P P P A S T N R Q S G R Q P T P L S P P L R N T H P Q A M
5 ayw     A Q G I L E T L P A N P P P A S T N R Q S G R Q P T P L S P P L R N T H P Q A M
6 adr     A Q G I L T T V P A A P P P A S T N R Q S G R Q P T P I S P P L R D S H P Q A M
7 adr     A Q G I L T T V P A A P P P V S T N R Q S G R Q P T P I S P P L R D S H P Q A M
8 adr     A Q G V L T T V P V A P P P A S T N R Q S G R Q P T P I S P P L R D S H P Q A M

          A Q G       T         P P P   S T N R Q S G R Q P T P   S P P L R     H P Q A M

                                         13                  14                  15                  16
          1 2 3 4 5 6 7 8 9 0 1 2 3 4 5 6 7 8 9 0 1 2 3 4 5 6 7 8 9 0 1 2 3 4 5 6 7 8 9 0

1 adw2    Q W N S T A F H Q T L Q D P R V R G L Y L P A G G S S S G T V N P A P N I A S H
2 adw     Q W N S T A L H Q A L Q D P R V R G L Y L P A G G S S S G T V N P A P N I A S H
3 adyw    H W N S T T F H Q T L Q D P R V R G L Y F P A G G S S S G T V N P V P T T T S P
4 ayw     Q W N S T T F H Q T L Q D P R V R G L Y F P A G G S S S G T V N P V L T T A S P
5 ayw     Q W N S T T F H Q T L Q D P R V R G L Y F P A G G S S S G T V N P V P T T V S P
6 adr     Q W N S T T F H Q A L L D P R V R G L Y F P A G G S S S G T V N P V P T T A S P
7 adr     Q W N S T T F H Q A L L D P R V R G L Y F P A G G S S S G T V N P V P T T V S P
8 adr     Q W N S T T F H Q A L L D P R V R G L Y F P A G G S S S G T V N P V P T T A S P

            W N S T     H Q   L   D P R V R G L Y   P A G G S S S G T V N P           S

                                         17
          1 2 3 4 5 6 7 8 9 0 1 2 3 4

1 adw2    I S S I S A R T G D P V T N
2 adw     I S S I S A R T G D P V T I
3 adyw    I S S I F S R I G D P A L N
4 ayw     L S S I F S R I G D P A L N
5 ayw     I S S I F S R I G D P A L N
6 adr     I S S I F S R T G D P A P N
7 adr     I S S I F S R T G D P A P N
8 adr     I S S I S S R T G D P A P N

            S S I     R   G D P
```

Figure 9 Amino acid sequences of the preS (preS1 and preS2) region of HBV env protein derived from HBV DNA sequencing data. The preS1 and preS2 sequences correspond to residues 1–119 (12–119) and 120–174, respectively. Sequences for several HBV subtypes, indicated at the left of the sequences, are shown. Bottom line shows common sequences (derived from ref. 17). (Single-letter abbreciations for the amino acid residues are A, alanine; R, arginine; N, asparagine; D, aspartic acid; C, cysteine; Q, glutamine; E, glutamic acid; G, glycine; H, histidine; I, isoleucine; L, leucine; K, lysine; F, phenylalanine; M, methionine; P, proline; S, serine; T, threonine; W, tryptophan; Y, tyrosine; V, valine

primed with HBsAg containing the preS2 region, it was suggested that the native preS2 sequence is more immunogenic at both the B- and T-cell level than native S protein[33,37]. Other experiments confirmed that anti-pre-S2-specific antibodies appear in serum of immunized animals earlier than anti-S-specific antibodies. However, after boosting, the differences in anti-S and anti-preS2-specific antibody levels disappear[38]. There are no inherent differences in the imunogenicities of preS1, preS2, and S regions. The relative proportions of antibodies against these distinct regions reflect approximately the molar ratios of these three domains in the native immunogen used[39]. The conclusion that the preS2 region is significantly more immunogenic than the S region at the T-cell level[40] may apply mostly to the experimental conditions used, i.e. congenic strains of mice primed with one dose of HBsAg as a stimulating antigen to measure proliferation of T cells. Results of other experiments in which human helper T-cell clones specific for S-protein were utilized, indicated that formic acid-denatured HBsAg induces T-cell proliferation at doses more than one order of magnitude lower than native HBsAg[31]. Comparisons between concentrations of preS-specific peptides[41,42] and an appropriately selected peptide from the S protein sequence[34] suggest that S protein peptides are not inherently inferior as compared with preS peptides in stimulating the proliferation of T cells with appropriate specificities. Taking into account the above findings, as well as the documented efficacy of vaccines based on HBsAg containing S protein only[6,15], the prevailing reason for attempting to design a synthetic vaccine based on preS sequences is the demonstrated success in mimicking native preS sequences by synthetic peptides[15,17,33,35,36] and the limited success in designing synthetic immunogens mimicking with high enough fidelity B-cell epitopes on S protein.

The inclusion of preS immunogens into hepatitis B vaccines in addition to S protein would broaden the repertoire of anti-HBV-specific antibodies elicited by active immunization, and make it qualitatively similar to the repertoire of antibodies elicited as a result of recovery from natural infection[15]. A more rapid immune response to preS as compared with S epitopes could be of great importance for post-exposure prophylaxis of HBV infections, eliminating the need for simultaneous administration of anti-HBs antibodies. Furthermore, the inclusion of preS epitopes into hepatitis B vaccines is expected to contribute to the overcoming of immunological non-responsiveness to S protein in a portion of vaccine recipients: (1) by providing preS-specific T-cell help for an immune response to S protein, in analogy with results in congenic strains of mice[33] and (2) by eliciting anti-preS-specific antibody responses which are sufficient for protection (see below)[43–47].

Synthetic peptides derived from the preS region of the HBV env protein, in order to be considered as components of a synthetic vaccine, have to fulfil criteria listed in Table 3. To demonstrate that these requirements are indeed met required extensive research. It was necessary in initial studies to eliminate those regions of the preS sequence which are not recognized by anti-HBV antibodies. Non-overlapping peptides from the preS sequence were synthesized and screened for reactivity with rabbit anti-HBV. The only peptides which failed to react were preS(53–73) and preS(153–171)[43].

Therefore, only peptides from the N-terminal half of the preS2 region (residues 120–153) and peptides from both the N-terminal and the C-terminal half of the preS1 sequence had to be considered for further studies[45]. A few peptides, at least 19 amino acids in length[43], from both the preS1 and preS2 region were selected for more detailed studies. These peptides were preS(12–32), and related peptides from the preS1 region containing the receptor binding site for hepatocytes[44,48] preS(94–117), preS(120–145) and a longer peptide, preS(120–153), which is better recognized by some anti-preS2-specific monoclonal antibodies (McAb)[49]. The properties of these peptides conform with the requirements listed in Table 3.

1. The peptides are recognized by polyclonal human and animal anti-HBV[36,50] and by some McAb specific for the native preS2 sequence[49,51]. However, these peptides, as well as other peptides derived from the preS sequence, are not recognized by other preS1 and preS2-specific McAb which are probably directed against topographic epitopes[39,52]. The reaction of anti-HBV with a fusion protein containing the entire preS2 sequence linked to β-galactosidase was completely inhibited by preS(120–145) (Figure 10). These results show that anti-preS2-specific antibodies present in anti-HBV were predominantly if not exclusively directed towards epitopes within the preS(120–145) region in agreement with results that anti-HBV did not recognize the preS(153–174) sequence[43]. Molar concentrations of the peptide and of the native preS2 sequence within HBV required for equal degrees of inhibition were approximately identical, indicating that epitopes on the synthetic peptide and on the corresponding segment of the native preS2 sequence are identical or closely related.

McAb specific for the native preS2 sequence may preferentially recognize synthetic peptides derived from the pres2 sequence corresponding to the HBV subtype used for raising the McAb[49]. The affinity constant (K) for the

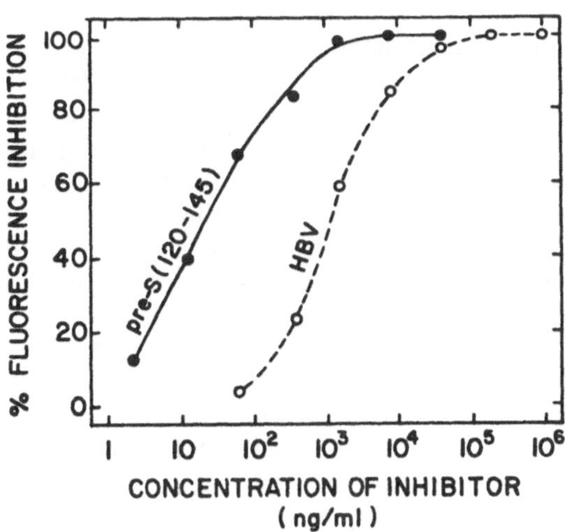

Figure 10 Inhibition by peptide preS(120–145) or by HBV of the reaction of anti-HBV with a preS(120–174)–4β-galactosidase fusion protein (reprinted with permission from ref. 53)

reaction between these McAb and the subtype-matched peptide (3.2×10^7 l/mol) was of the same order of magnitude as K for the reaction between these McAb and the native preS2 sequences (5.2×10^7)[49].

Recognition of peptides derived from the preS1 sequence by anti-HBV was also studied in detail. Humans who recovered from HBV infection, or who received appropriate hepatitis B vaccines, developed antibodies to peptides preS(12–32) and preS(94–117)[43,54]. The detection of antibodies to peptides preS(1–21), preS(32–53) and preS(53–74) was also reported[41]. The only synthetic peptide binding antibodies from sera of all strains of congenic mice immunized with HBV env proteins containing the preS1 region was peptide preS(94–117)[41]. Sera from some of the congenic mouse strains also recognized preS(53–73). Among inbred strains of mice only SJL/J (haplotype S) mice recognized the peptide preS(12–32)[55,41]. The sequence preS(1–11) is present only in some of the HBV subtypes (Figure 9). Little attention was given to synthetic peptides containing this region. Most of the research was concerned with the preS(12–47) and preS(94–117) regions of the preS1 sequence.

Peptides derived from the N-terminal half of the preS1 sequence, preS(12–32), preS(13–47), preS(15–47), preS(17–47), preS(19–47), preS(21–47), preS(26–32), preS(29–47) and preS(32–47), all reacted with polyclonal rabbit anti-HBV and no preferential binding of antibodies by any of the peptides was evident. Since the peptide preS(1–21) was recognized about ten times less efficiently than preS(12–32) by anti-HBV, the immunodominant B cell epitope within the preS(12–47) region is likely to be localized C-terminally from residue 21[56]. In agreement with this conclusion is the finding that preS(21–47) elicited antibodies recognizing HBV and inhibiting its attachment to receptors on hepatoma cells[48].

Based on studies with congenic strains of mice immunized with HBsAg containing the preS1 sequence, B cell epitopes were localized within sequences preS(32–53), preS(41–53), preS(94–105) and preS(106–117)[57].

2. Antisera to the selected peptides mentioned above recognized well the native HBV env proteins, and were applied to the detection of preS2 and preS1 sequences in HBV (HBsAg)[17,35,36,48,58]. Antibodies to synthetic peptides from the preS1 and preS2 regions [preS(15–47) and preS(120–153)] derived from one subtype of HBV recognized preS sequences corresponding to all HBV subtypes[58], unlike some McAb, the specificity of which is subtype-restricted. This suggests that synthetic peptides derived from the preS region of one or two HBV subtypes can lead to immunity to the whole range of HBV subtypes.

Quantitative aspects of immunological cross-reactivities between native preS1 and preS2 sequences exposed on HBV (HBsAg) and the synthetic peptide analogues were studied in detail. HBV completely inhibited the reaction between anti-preS(120–145) and preS(120–145) linked to β-galactosidase used as an enzyme marker (Figure 11A). This indicates that there is no significant population of anti-peptide antibodies which would recognize only the synthetic peptide but not the native preS2 sequence. The approximately molar concentrations of the synthetic peptide and the native preS2 sequence

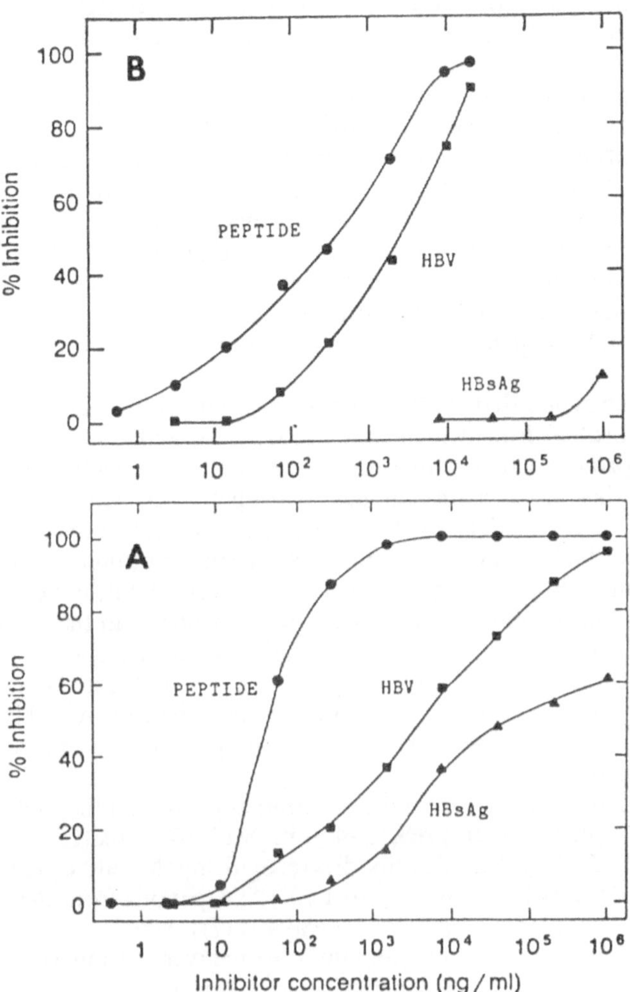

Figure 11 A: Inhibition of the reaction of anti-preS(120–145) with the peptide preS(120–145) (conjugated to β-galactosidase) by free unconjugated homologous peptide (●), HBV (■), and HBsAg particles (▲) (derived from ref. 36). **B**: Inhibition of the reaction of anti-preS(15–47) with the peptide preS(15–47) (conjugated to β-galactosidase). Similar results were obtained with preS(12–32)

in HBV required for 50% inhibition of the reaction were about equal, indicating that the synthetic peptide mimics epitopes on the preS2 sequence with considerable fidelity[36]. The 22 nm HBsAg particles were much less inhibitory, in agreement with their much lower content of preS2 sequences as compared with HBV. Similar results were obtained with antisera to synthetic peptides derived from the preS1 sequence, preS(12–32) or preS(15–47) (Figure 11B).

The K value for the reaction between anti-preS(120-153) and the homologous peptide was of the same order of magnitude as (K) for the reaction between these antibodies and preS2 sequences on native HBsAg (approximately 10^7 l/mol)[49]. K values for the reaction between antibodies to peptides derived from the preS1 sequence and the homologous peptides and the native preS1 sequence, respectively, are not yet available.

Among inbred strains of mice only the SJL/J mice responded to the peptide preS(12–32)[55], and the corresponding antisera were reported to recognize preferentially the sequence preS(16–27), while peptides (12–21) and (22–32) were not recognized[57]. It was also reported that anti-preS(12–32) antisera from SJL/J mice do not recognize the native preS1 sequence[57]. This appears to be contrary to the findings that rabbit antisera to preS(12–32) recognize the native preS1 sequence[35,56] (Figures 11B and 13).

3. It is often stated that synthetic peptides are much less immunogenic than the native protein from which they are derived, and that they have to be linked to protein carriers in order to become sufficiently immunogenic. Neither of these two claims applies to properly selected peptides derived from the preS region. The synthetic peptides preS(120–145) and preS(120–153) elicited higher levels of anti-preS2-specific antibodies than HBsAg particles containing the preS2 sequence. The levels of antibodies recognizing the homologous peptide and the native preS2 sequence in the corresponding anti-peptide antisera were very similar, indicating the absence of a subpopulation of antibodies recognizing the peptide alone, but not the native preS2 sequence, in agreement with results presented in Figure 11A[56]. The endpoint dilutions of the respective antibodies in the antipeptide antisera were between $1{:}10^6$ and $1{:}10^7$.

Several peptide derived from the N-terminal portion of the preS1 sequence [preS(1–21), preS(12–32), preS(12–47), preS(13–47), preS(15–47), preS(17–47) and preS(19–47)] elicited antibodies recognizing the native preS1 sequence (dilution endpoints between $1{:}10^3$ to $1{:}10^5$)[56]. A peptide from the C-terminal portion of the preS1 sequence [preS(94–117)] which is recognized by antibodies from sera of some humans who recovered from HBV infection, and which represents the only peptide partly homologous to preS sequences of other hepadnaviruses[54], also elicited antibodies recognizing HBV (endpoint dilution 1:2000).

The middle portion of the preS(120–145) sequence [residues preS(132–137/139)] appears to be most prominently involved in the binding of antibodies with anti-preS2 specificity[56]. However, the N-terminal and C-terminal thirds of the preS(120–145) sequence [preS(120–134) and preS(134–145)] were also recognized by anti-HBV antibodies[53,59] indicating that the entire preS(120–145) sequence is exposed on the surface of HBV and is accessible to antibodies. Furthermore, residues located C-terminally from preS(145) can improve the binding of antibodies, probably due to conformational effects[56]. However, the N-terminal residues preS(120–123) do not seem to contribute to the binding of anti-HBV and may be dispensable in the design of synthetic preS2-antigens (but not immunogens, as shown below)[56]. In conclusion, peptides optimally mimicking B cell epitopes on the preS2 region should encompass residues preS(124) at the N-terminus and

153 ⩾ preS > 145 at the C-terminus.

Since the dominant B-cell epitope on the preS(120–145) [153] sequence is localized in its middle portion and can be influenced by residues at the C-terminus, the possibility was investigated that shorter peptides truncated on the N-termini might serve as synthetic hepatitis B immunogens. Shorter peptides, preS(128–153) and preS(124–153), were synthesized and tested for immunogenicity. They were much less immunogenic than the full-length peptide preS(120–153) (Figure 12). Consequently, residues preS(120–127) are essential for the immunogenicity of preS2 peptides, indicting that T-cell epitopes are localized on this part of the preS2 sequence.

Cysteine residues were added to most of the peptides used in the author's work to allow their linking to carriers and enzymes. These residues were separated from the peptide sequence by a Gly–Gly spacer. Surprisingly ,the addition of cysteine residues enhanced about ten-fold the immunogenicity of peptides preS(120–145) and preS(120–153) (the Gly–Gly spacer was not used

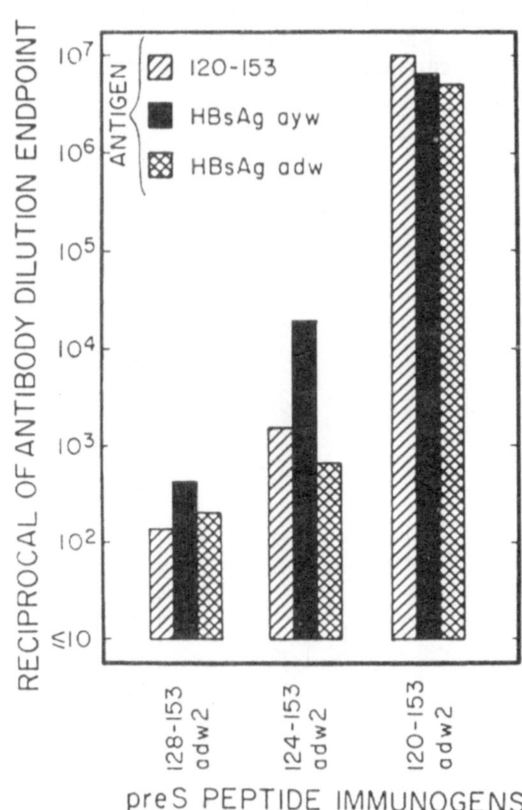

Figure 12 Evidence for the essential role of residues preS(120–127) for the immunogenicity of synthetic peptides from the preS2 region of the HBV env protein. All peptides had Gly–Gly–Cys–NH_2 residues at their C-termini. The antigens indicated in the insert were used for the coating of polystyrene 96-well plates. Dilutions of anti-peptide antisera were tested in double-antibody RIA tests (adapted from ref. 56)

for the preS(120–145) peptide which contains Gly residues at positions 144 and 145; Figure 9)[59].

When preS2 responder strains of mice were immunized with preS(120–145) and subsequently the *in vitro* proliferative T cell responses elicited by the homologous peptide and by shorter peptides preS(120–132), preS(128–138) and preS(133–145) were determined, the highest T cell proliferation was observed with the full-length peptide and by the N-terminal peptide preS(120–132), indicating the localization of a T cell epitope within the 13 N-terminal amino acids of the preS2 sequence. Single subtype-dependent amino acid substitutions at position 126 (Figure 9) eliminated the T cell proliferative response, indicating the subtype specificity of the T cell epitope and the essential role of residue 126. Additional studies indicated that residue preS(120–126) are essential for T cell recognition, in agreement with results shown in Figure 7[33,42].

The peptides preS(1–21) and preS(12–32) (in unconjugated form) elicited high levels of antibodies recognizing the homologous peptide and preS1 sequences in native HBV env proteins (column 1 and 2, Figure 13). However, the peptide preS(21–47) was poorly immunogenic (column 3, Figure 13) and had to be linked to carriers to elicit high levels of anti-preS1 specific

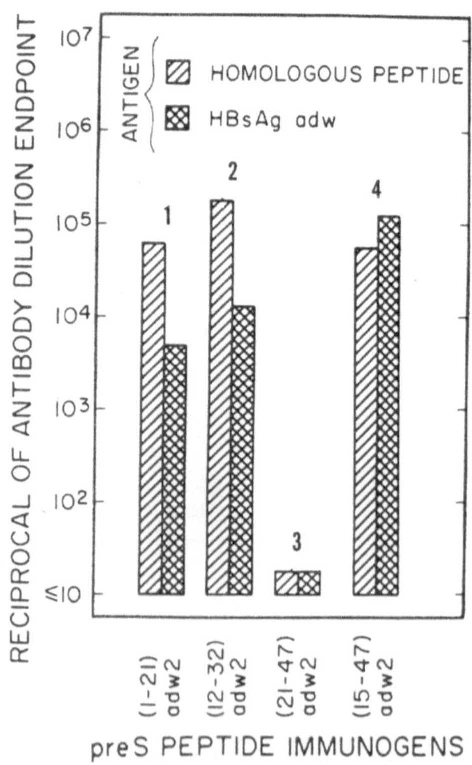

Figure 13 Immunogenicity of selected peptides from the preS1 region of the HBV env protein. For further details see text to Figure 12 (results are derived from ref. 56)

antibodies[48]. Therefore, longer synthetic peptides with preS(47) C-termini were synthesized (12–47, 13–47, 15–47, 17–47 and 19–47). All these peptides were about equally immunogenic in rabbits. Results obtained with the peptide preS(15–47) are shown in Figure 13 (column 4). The results indicate the importance of residues (12–20) for the immunogenicity of peptides derived from the N-terminal portion of the preS1 sequence and suggest a critical role for Val, Pro and Asn residues at positions 18–20 of the *adw*2, *adw* and *adr* subtypes (Figure 9) for T cell recognition. Experiments with SJL/J mice indicated the localization of immunodominant T cell epitopes within the preS(12–21) and preS(94–117) regions[57]. There is only minimal cross-reactivity between T cell epitopes, located within the preS(12–21) sequence, corresponding to subtypes *adw*2 and *ayw*, suggesting the importance of residues 14, 18, and/or 19 (see Figure 9) for T cell recognition. Further experiments indicated that residues 18 and 19 are the most critical[57].

4. The high immunogenicity in experimental animals of selected synthetic peptides from the preS region, the presence of immunodominant B and T cell epitopes on these peptides and the high cross-reactivity between B cell epitopes on the peptides and on native HBV env proteins has justified further evaluation of these peptides for protective efficacy against HBV infection. However, preS-specific immunity elicited by the synthetic peptides would still be qualitatively different from that elicited during recovery from HBV infection or by immunization with HBV env proteins. The synthetic peptides would not prime immunized individuals for an effective immune response against HBV, unless T cell epitopes on the synthetic peptides were strongly cross-reactive with the corresponding T cell epitopes on the native preS2 and preS1 sequences. Studies related to this problem were carried out exclusively in the murine model system. It was shown that T cell determined H2 restriction of the immune response to the preS(120–145) sequence within the synthetic peptides and the HBV env protein was distinct. Thus, some mouse strains were good responders to the synthetic peptide but did not respond to the native preS2 sequence while other strains failed to respond to the synthetic peptide but responded to preS2 sequences within HBsAg particles[42,55]. These results indicated that T cell recognition sites on the native preS2 region are not identical to those on the synthetic peptide preS(120–145). The reported failure of preS(120–145)-primed T cells to proliferate when exposed *in vitro* to HBsAg particles containing the preS2 sequence and the failure of the synthetic peptide to prime mice for an antibody response to the native preS2 sequence supported this conclusion[42]. On the other hand, it was shown that immunization of S-non-responder strains of mice with three doses of preS(120–145) primed them for a subsequent response to HBsAg containing S protein and the preS2 region. These results indicate that the non-responsiveness to S protein can be circumvented more effectively in mice preimmunized with the synthetic peptide[55].

Several synthetic peptides from the preS1 region [preS(1–21), preS(12–32), preS(32–53), preS(53–74) and preS(94–117)] elicited the proliferation of T cells from mice primed with HBsAg containing preS1 sequences. The highest proliferation was elicited by the peptide preS(12–32)[41]. In reciprocal experiments, T cells from mice primed with preS(12–32) were induced to proliferate by both the homologous peptide and HBsAg containing preS1 sequences, the latter being about six times more efficient on a molar basis. Lymphocytes primed with preS(94–117) proliferated when challenged with HBsAg containing preS1 sequences[57]. This indicates that T cell epitopes on the synthetic peptides preS(12–32) and preS(94–117), respectively, were cross-reactive with the corresponding epitopes on the native preS1 sequence. In accordance with this finding, priming of S non-responder strains of mice with peptides preS(12–32), preS(12–21) and preS(94–117), respectively, led, after challenge with a suboptimal dose of HBsAg containing preS1 and preS2 sequences, to *in vivo* antibody production specific for several epitopes on the preS1, preS2 and S regions of the HBV env protein[33,57].

Since the N-terminal half of the preS(12–32) sequence contains immunodominant Tcell epitopes[56,57] mimicking epitopes on the native preS1 sequence, hybrid immunogens containing a T cell epitope derived from the preS1 sequence and a B cell epitope derived from the preS2 sequence were synthesized. Their ability to elicit an anti-preS2-specific antibody response in mice[57] and rabbits[60] was evaluated. Addition of the T cell epitope from the preS1 sequence significantly enhanced the antibody response to the preS2 portion of the hybrid peptide. However, hybrid peptides were less immunogenic than peptides preS(120–145) or preS(120–153) containing both B and T cell epitopes derived from the preS2 sequence. Hybrid peptides from the preS1 and preS2 sequence, respectively, linked to a peptide from the S-protein sequence were also prepared. The immunogenicity of the S peptide was not enhanced by the addition of either preS1 or preS2 peptides containing both T and B cell epitopes[60]. The hybrid peptides elicited higher antibody responses to preS1 and preS2 sequences than to the S sequence, since the anti-peptide antisera reacted stronger with M-protein (lane B, Figure 7) or with L protein (lane C, Figure 7) than with S protein. These results suggest that synthetic peptides containing B and T cell epitopes which are adjacent (overlapping) in the native sequence are preferable to hybrid peptides containing B and T cell epitopes from non-adjacent portions of the HBV env protein sequence.

Proliferative effects of distinct peptides from the preS1 and preS2 sequence on preS-specific lymphocytes from humans recovered from HBV infection or immunized with appropriate serum-derived or recombinant hepatitis B vaccines will have to be studied to define more precisely preS-specific T cell epitopes playing an immunodominant role in human anti-HBV responses.

5. Group-specific *a* determinants on S protein elicit protective antibodies against HBV infection[19]. McAb with anti-*a* specificity are virus-neutralizing[61]. Ironically, the functional role of S protein, and specifically of those determinants which are involved in the process of virus-neutralization, remains unknown. It was reported that HBsAg consisting exclusively of S protein attached to cell lines derived from African green monkey kidneys but not to human liver cells or hepatoma cells lines[62]. The biological significance of this binding reaction, as well as the region of S protein

involved in the attachment of HBsAg, remain to be defined.

The preS2 region is involved in the binding of HBV env proteins to human serum albumin (HSA). Residues preS(146–153) appear to play an important role in the binding process, since the peptide preS(120–145) did not bind to HSA, while peptides preS(120–153) from both the *adw*2 and *ayw* subtypes did[60]. Other synthetic peptides from the preS1 and preS2 region failed to react with HSA. It has not been established whether the interaction between HBV env proteins and HSA plays any role in the replication of HBV.

The preS1 region is involved in the attachment of HBV to human hepatoma cell lines. This attachment can be inhibited by the synthetic peptide preS(21–47) and by the corresponding anti-peptide antiserum. The synthetic peptide itself reacted with the cells[48]. The shortest peptide inhibiting the HBV–hepatoma cell interaction was preS(32–47). Other longer peptides extended toward the N-terminus and containing the preS(32–47) sequence also inhibited the reaction[44,56]. Since one of several virus-neutralization pathways involves virus attachment blockade by antibodies, it was expected that synthetic peptides including the preS(21–47) sequence would elicit virus-neutralizing and protective antibodies.

6. Evidence that synthetic peptides can elicit virus-neutralizing and protective antibodies is crucial for their potential application as components of hepatitis B vaccines. The virus-neutralizing acitivity of antisera and the protective efficacy of vaccines can be demonstrated in chimpanzees, the only model for HBV infection in humans. Therefore, the immunochemical properties of synthetic HBV analogues and their corresponding antisera had to be defined in detail before embarking on difficult and expensive chimpanzee experiments. Excessive concern about the use of oil-containing adjuvants in chimpanzees, some of which have even been approved for use in humans[63], has led to suboptimal designs of tests for protective efficacy of synthetic peptides and to attempts to ascertain the potential of synthetic immunogens by virus-neutralization assays rather than by direct protective efficacy tests.

Synthetic peptides derived from S protein, S(110–137) (both in linear and cyclic forms) and S(125–137) were linked to keyhole limpet haemocyanin (KLH) and mixed either with incomplete Freund's adjuvant (for one chimpanzee) or with alum (for eight chimpanzees) (alum is an unsuitable adjuvant for synthetic peptides[64]). After immunized chimpanzees were challenged with subtype-matched HBV, complete protection was observed in 2/9 animals and partial protection in 4/9 animals[65]. Similar results were obtained with analogous peptides in the woodchuck model for HBV-like infection. These results indicate that the S(110–137) region contains a protective epitope of HBV and HBV-like viruses. Considering the fact that the described immunogens probably did not contain the major S-specific T cell epitopes for primates, and were combined with suboptimal carriers and adjuvants, these results should encourage the design of better immunogens derived from the S protein region.

To avoid dealing with the issue of selection of an appropriate adjuvant, locally approved for usage in chimpanzees, the potential of synthetic analogues of the preS region as protective immunogens was evaluated by virus-neutralization assays with high-titred rabbit anti-peptide antisera instead of directly studying the protective efficacy of synthetic peptides. In the neutralization tests the anti-peptide antisera were mixed with HBV and the mixtures were injected into chimpanzees subsequently followed for markers of HBV infection. The virus-neutralizing activity of anti-preS(120–145) was demonstrated in 2/2 chimpanzees[43]. In similar experiments with anti-preS(21–47), one chimpanzee remained uninfected and another developed an attenuated HBV infection probably due to residual infectious HBV in the antiserum–HBV mixture[44] (Figure 14). The quantity of infectious HBV used for virus-neutralization assays was 2×10^3 and 1.6×10^4 CID_{50}, respectively. It must be appreciated that 99.9% neutralization of virus infectivity would still result in a positive score in this type of assay. These results provide evidence that the two peptides from the preS2 and preS1 regions, respectively, should be protective when used for immunization in combination with appropriate adjuvants.

Using a suboptimal carrier (= KLH)–adjuvant(= alum) combination, two chimpanzees were immunized with preS(120–145). They developed anti-peptide antibodies as well as antibodies to the native preS2 sequence. The antibody dilution endpoints of the corresponding antisera were approximately three orders of magnitude lower in comparison with sera from rabbits immunized with peptides in combination with Freund's adjuvant (Figure 12). After challenge with HBV, one chimpanzee was protected while the other one developed signs of attenuated disease[47]. Immunization with preS(123–151) lacking the three N-terminal amino acids of the preS2 sequence, possibly contributing to the T-cell epitope (Figure 12), linked to KLH and combined with incomplete Freund's adjuvant protected two chimpanzees against subsequent challenge with 10^6 CID_{50}[46]. These results indicate the important role of an oil-containing adjuvant and/or the contributory role of residues preS(146–151) for protection against HBV infection.

To investigate the protective role of epitopes on the preS1 sequence, the peptide preS(12–47) (myristylated at the N-terminus) was used in free form to immunize two chimpanzees in combination with an adjuvant from Ribi Immunochem Research Inc. without any oil to comply with local restrictions concerning work with chimpanzees. Because of an inadequate antibody response the chimpanzees were hyperimmunized with the same peptide linked to bovine serum albumin (BSA). The chimpanzees developed antibodies recognizing the peptide and the native preS1 sequence. After challenge with HBV, one of the chimpanzees developed attenuated inapparent, anicteric hepatitis B while the other one was protected completely[45] (Figure 15).

Cumulatively, these results indicate that synthetic peptides derived from either the preS1 or the preS2 region can individually elicit protetion against HBV infection. However, for application as components of synthetic vaccines it will be necessary to combine these peptides with appropriate adjuvants. Considering potential problems arising from the genetic restriction of the immune response, and the advantage of having multiple rather than a single protective epitope present in a vaccine, it is preferable to include several distinct peptides into future synthetic hepatitis B vaccines.

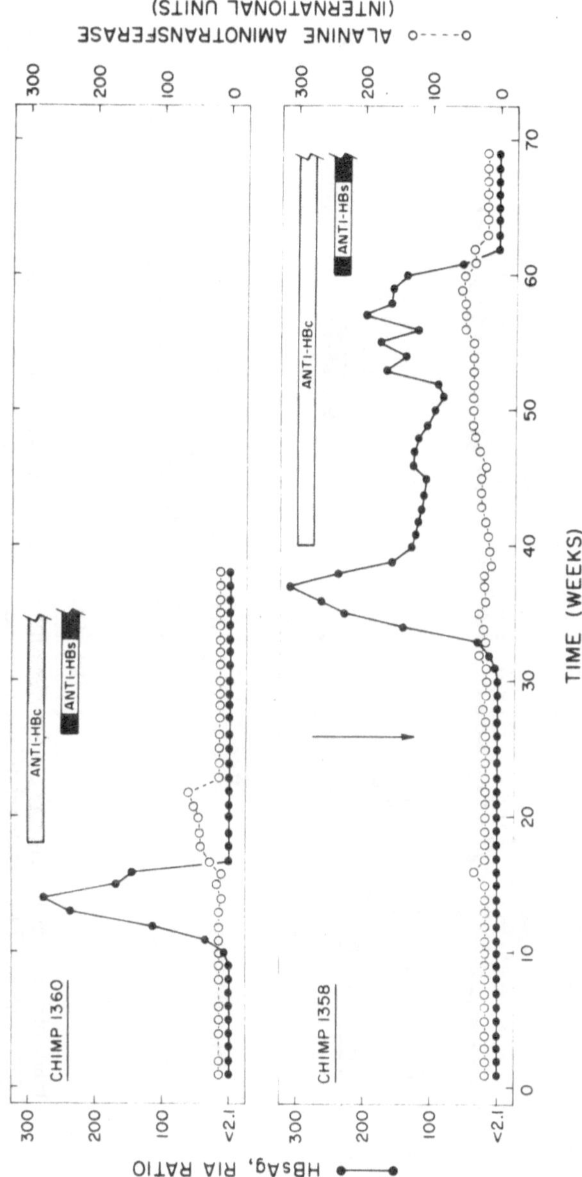

Figure 14 Results of virus-neutralization tests with anti-preS(21–47). Chimpanzees were injected with antiserum-HBV mixtures at time 0. Chimpanzee 1360 developed attenuated disease with short HBsAg antigenaemia and alanine amino transferase (ALT) elevations. Chimpanzee 1358 remained uninfected. To prove susceptibility to HBV infection he was infected at week 26 (arrow) with HBV. Long-lasting HBsAg antigenaemia and ALT elevations developed

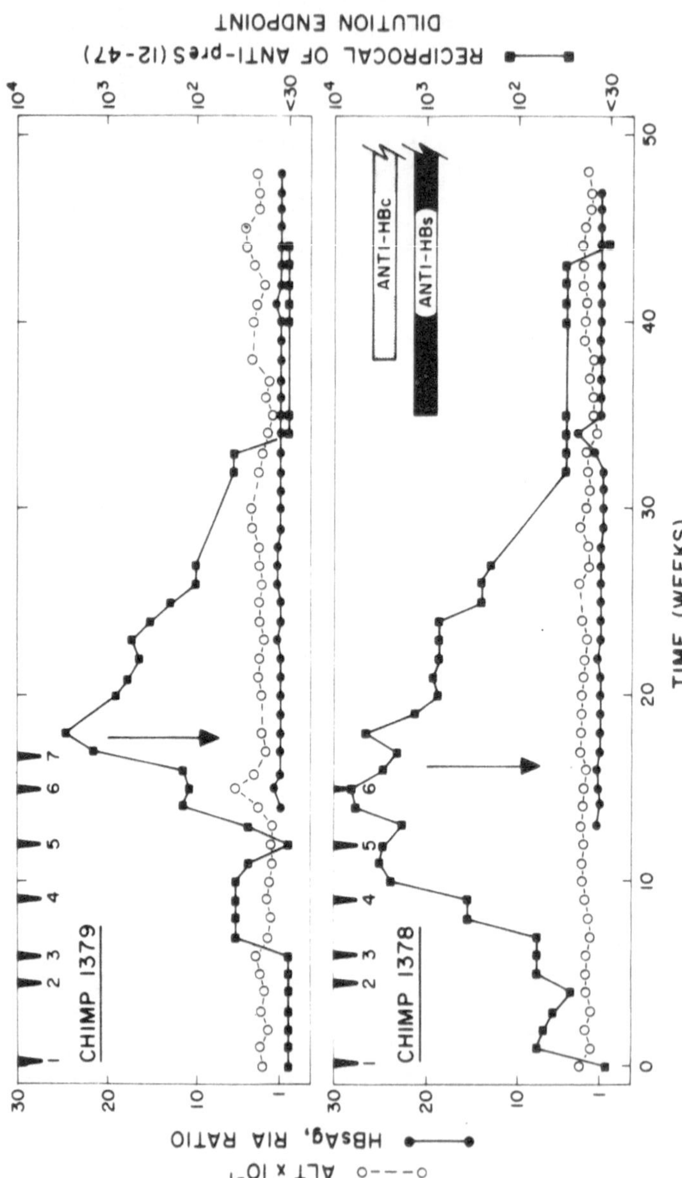

Figure 15 Results of active immunization of chimpanzees with myristylated preS(12–47). Chimpanzees were vaccinated with the unconjugated immunogen (400 μg peptide per dose) at times indicated by short arrows 1–4, followed by booster doses of peptide conjugated to BSA (short arrows 5-7). At times indicated by long arrows, chimpanzees 1378 and 1379 were challenged intravenously with $10^{4.5}$ and $10^{3.5}$ CID_{50}, respectively, of HBV subtype adw. Chimpanzee 1378 developed, low, short-lasting (~1 week, at the 34th week) HBsAg antigenaemia immediately followed by production of anti-HBs and later of anti-HBc chapter 7

SYNTHETIC PEPTIDES DERIVED FROM HBcAg

There is no evidence for a role in virus clearance and recovery of antibodies to HBcAg (anti-HBc) which develop early during the course of HBV infection. However, immunization of chimpanzees with HBcAg protects them against subsequent challenge with live virus[66-68]. The protective immunity may be explained by elicitation of HBcAg-specific cytotoxic T lymphocytes contibuting to the elimination of HBV-infected cells[13,69] and by intermolecular/intrastructural help provided by anti-HBc-specific helper T lymphocytes[14] for anti-HBV env protein-specific B lymphocytes[15,16]. Since the HBcAg-specific protective immunity is T cell-mediated, synthetic immunogens with a potential for vaccination against HBV should mimic T cell epitopes on the highly immunogenic HBcAg[70]. Several synthetic peptides derived from the HBcAg sequence induced proliferation of HBcAg-primed T lymphocytes from several congenic mouse strains. The distinct mouse strains recognized multiple but distinct sites within the HBcAg sequence. HBcAg was more efficient in eliciting proliferation of HBcAg-specific T lymphocytes than were the synthetic peptides. Immunization of mice with the synthetic peptides elicited T cells which recognized native HBcAg. The dominant T cell epitopes were localized within the region C(120–140) (for H2 haplotypes s and b); C(100–120) (haplotypes f and q) and C(85–100) (haplotype d)[71]. *In vivo* priming of helper T cells with appropriate synthetic peptides induced B cells to produce antibodies recognizing HBcAg and multiple epitopes on the HBV env protein. Priming with these synthetic peptides can overcome anti-protein S non-responsiveness in S non-responder strains of mice[16,33]. Synthetic hybrid immunogens composed of HBcAg-specific T cell epitopes and of preS2-specific B cell epitopes were synthesized and shown to elicit antibodies which recognize the native preS2 sequence within the HBV env M-protein[72]. However, the level of these antibodies was lower than the level of antibodies elicited by preS2 specific peptides containing both B and T cell epitopes. Taking into consideration that dominant T cell epitopes for S protein are distinct for humans and mice, as described before, HBcAg-specific epitopes for human T cells will have to be defined in order to design complex synthetic immunogens containing peptides derived from the HBcAg sequence.

AUGMENTATION OF THE IMMUNOGENICITY OF PEPTIDES DERIVED FROM THE HBV env SEQUENCE

Selected peptides from the preS region described above were highly immunogenic when combined with Freund's adjuvant. Protein carriers enhancing the immunogenicity of the peptides are not required since they contain both B and T cell epitopes. To replace Freund's adjuvant the synthetic peptides will have to be combined with other oil-based adjuvants, some of which have already been approved for clinical trials of synthetic vaccines[63]. The description of adjuvants applicable for synthetic immunogens is beyond the scope of this chapter.

Alternative approaches for increasing the immunogenicity of peptides are based on the use of liposomes, iscoms[73-75], polysaccharide carriers[60] and proteosomes[76].

MULTIVALENT FULLY SYNTHETIC HEPATITIS B IMMUNOGENS

Results of the virus-neutralization tests and of direct efficacy trials of synthetic peptides from the preS region show the presence of protective epitopes on each of the preS1 and preS2 portions of the HBV env protein. Synthetic peptides from each of these regions are sufficient to elicit protection against HBV infection. It is possible that single peptides derived from either the preS2 or the preS1 region will elicit protective immunity against HBV to the same extent as do current vaccines based on HBsAg containing mostly or exclusively S protein. This possibility will have to be assessed in large-scale clinical trials. However, the combination of peptides from both the preS1 and the preS2 regions is likely to be more efficacious. Incorporation of additional components corresponding to B and T cell epitopes of S protein and to T cell epitopes of HBcAg may increase the efficacy of a fully synthetic vaccine. Such vaccine will be feasible in the future after synthetic peptides corresponding to the latter three epitopes have been designed and technical aspects of developing a vaccine consisting of several synthetic peptides have been solved. The presentation of epitopes from several synthetic peptides on the surface of high molecular weight polysaccharides[60], liposomes[73], iscoms[74,75], and proteosomes[76] may offer advantages in preparing multimeric polyvalent synthetic hepatitis B vaccines. The presentation of such multimeric synthetic antigens to the immune system, and thereby their immunogenicity, could potentially be enhanced by addition of human anti-HBV antibodies of the IgG subclass[31,77-81].

SEMI-SYNTHETIC HEPATITIS B VACCINES

Hepatitis B vaccines consisting exclusively of S protein prepared by recombinant DNA techniques, or serum-derived vaccines containing HBsAg consisting predominantly of S protein, elicit a repertoire of antibodies which is narrower than the repertoire of antibodies elicited by natural infection. This limitation can potentially be overcome by linking peptides derived from the preS region to HBsAg particles. The peptide preS(133–151) was covalently linked to HBsAg particles and the resulting complex immunogen elicited antibodies to both S protein and the preS2 region[82]. However, chemical linkage of the synthetic peptide to HBsAg diminished the immunogenicity of S protein. To overcome this problem a new approach for linking of synthetic peptides to HBsAg particles was developed. Synthetic peptides were extended with a hydrophobic tail which mediated their attachment to hydrophobic domains exposed on the surface of S protein. The peptide preS(12–47) was linked by this method to recombinant HBsAg particles containing S protein and the preS2 sequene[38]. The resulting immunogen elicited antibodies to S protein, preS2 and preS1 sequences. The addition of the peptide derived from the preS1 region significantly enhanced the antibody response to S protein. Linking of synthetic peptides derived from the sequence of the HBV env protein to HBcAg is also expected to result in immunogens which may elicit a broad spectrum of protective antibodies against HBV, considering the successful results obtained with recombinant HBcAg containing an epitope of an unrelated virus[83].

SAFETY OF HEPATITIS B VACCINES CONTAINING EPITOPES DERIVED FROM THE preS REGION

Concern has been expressed that anti-idiotypic antibodies elicited during an immune response to epitopes on the preS2 and preS1 region, known to react with HSA and with hepatocyte receptors, respectively, would be directed against host components and cause autoimmunity deleterious to the liver[84]. Results of laboratory[60,85] and clinical[86] studies indicate that these concerns are unwarranted. There is no evidence that the native preS2 sequence or unconjugated peptides derived from that sequence elicit anti-HSA antibodies in experimental animals. Antibodies to synthetic peptides derived from the preS1 or preS2 sequence do not recognize proteins exposed on liver cells having the receptor for HBV. An antibody response to preS2 epitopes elicited in humans, either by HBV infection or by vaccines containing the preS2 region, leads neither to an anti-HSA response nor to liver damage. In the course of HBV infection, a response to the preS2 sequence is a marker of HBV clearance and has no role in the pathogenesis of HBV-related liver damage.

ACKNOWLEDGEMENTS

Help in preparation of this manuscript was provided by L. Greene, T. Huima and M. Zucker. Synthetic peptides for the described studies were provided by Dr S. B. H. Kent, Neosystem Laboratories, Strasbourg, France and Cambridge Research Biochemicals Ltd, Cambridge, England. The studies were supported in part by a grant from the American Cancer Society. Virus-neutralization and protective efficacy assays were carried out at the Bureau of Biologics, FDA under the guidance of Dr B. Seto.

NOTE ADDED AT PROOF

A human T cell line cloned from blood of a recipient of a serum-derived hepatitis B vaccine was induced to proliferate by preS1 peptides 1–28, 12–32 and 21–47 in association with MHC class I antigens. This suggested the location of a T cell epitope in the overlapping sequence preS(21–28)[87].

REFERENCES

1. Szmuness, W., Harley, E. J., Ikram, H. and Stevens, C. E. (1978). Sociodemographic aspects of the epidemiology of hepatitis B. In Vyas, G. N., Cohen, S. N. and Schmid, R. (eds), *Viral Hepatitis: Etiology, Epidemiology, Pathogenesis and Prevention*, pp. 297–320. (Philadelphia: Franklin Institute Press)
2. Moodie, J., Stannard, L. M. and Kipps, A. (1974). Dane complexes in hepatitis B antigen. *J. Gen. Virol.*, **24**, 375–9
3. Neurath, A. R., Trepo, C., Chen, M. and Prince, A. M. (1976). Identification of additional antigenic sites on Dane particles and the tubular forms of hepatitis B surface antigen. *J. Gen. Virol.*, **30**, 277–85
4. Alberti, A., Diana, S., Sculard, G. H., Eddleston, W. F. A. and Williams, R. (1978). Detection of a new antibody system reacting with Dane particles in hepatitis B virus infection. *Br. Med. J.*, **2**, 1056–8
5. Hilleman, M. R., Bertland, U. A., Buynak, E. G., Lampson, G. P., McAleer, W. J., McLean, A. A., Roehm, R. R. and Tytell, A. A. (1978). Clinical and laboratory studies of HBsAg vaccine. In Vyas, G. N., Cohen, S. N. and Schmid, R. (eds), *Viral Hepatitis: Etiology, Epidemiology, Pathogenesis and Prevention*, pp. 525–537. (Philadelphia: Franklin Institute Press)
6. Stevens, C. E., Taylor, P. E., Tong, M. J., Toy, P. T. and Vyas, G. N. (1984). Hepatitis B vaccine: an overview. In Vyas, G. N., Dienstag, J. L. and Hoofnagle, J. H. (eds), *Viral Hepatitis and Liver Disease*, pp. 275–291. (Orlando: Grune & Stratton)
7. Vane, J. and Cuatrecasas, P. (1984). Genetic engineering and pharmaceuticals. *Nature*, **312**, 303–5
8. Van Regenmortel, M. H. V. and de Marcillac, D. (1988). An assessment of prediction methods for locating continuous epitopes in proteins. *Immunol. Lett.*, **17**, 95-108
9. Berzofsky, J. A., Cease, K. B., Cornette, J. L., Spouge, J. L., Margalit, H., Berkower, I. J., Good, M. F., Miller, L. H. and DeLisi, C. (1987). Protein antigenic structures recognized by T cells: Potential applications to vaccine design. *Immunol. Rev.*, **98**, 9–52
10. Rothbard, S.-N. and Taylor, W.R. (1988). A sequence pattern common to T cell epitopes. *EMBO J.*, **7**, 93–100
11. Huang, S-N. and Neurath, A. R. (1979). Immunohistologic demonstration of hepatitis B viral antigens in liver with reference to its significance in liver injury. *Lab. Invest.*, **40**, 1–17
12. Mondelli, M., Vergani, G. M., Alberti, A., Vergani, D., Portmann, B., Eddleston, A. L. W. F. and Williams, R. (1982). Specificity of T lymphocyte cytotoxicity to autologous hepatocytes in chronic hepatitis B virus infection: evidence that T cells are directed against HBV core antigen expressed on hepatocytes. *J. Immunol.*, **129**, 2773–8
13. Ferrari, C., Penna, A., Giuberti, T., Tong, M. J., Ribera, E., Fiaccadori, F. and Chisari, F. V. (1987). Intrahepatic, nucleocapsid antigen-specific T cells in chronic active hepatitis B. *J. Immunol.*, **139**, 2050–8
14. Ferrari, C., Mondelli, M. U., Penna, M., Fiaccadori, F. and Chisari, F. V. (1987). Functional characterization of cloned intrahepatic, hepatitis B virus nucleoprotein-specific helper T cell lines. *J. Immunol.*, **139**, 539–44
15. Neurath, A. R., Jameson, B. A. and Huima, T. (1987). Hepatitis B virus proteins eliciting protective immunity. *Microbiol. Sci.*, **4**, 45–51
16. Milich, D. R., McLachlan, A., Thornton, G. B.and Hughes, J. L. (1987). Antibody production to the nucleocapsid and envelope of the hepatitis B virus primed by a single synthetic T cell site. *Nature*, **329**, 547–9
17. Neurath, A. R. and Kent, S. B. H. (1988). The preS region of hepadnavirus envelope proteins. In Maramorosh, K., Murphy, F. A. and Shatkin, A. J. (eds), *Advances in Virus Research*, Vol. 34, pp. 65–142. (Orlando: Academic Press)
18. Peterson, D. L., Gavilanes, F., Paul, D. A. and Achord, D. T. (1984). Hepatitis B surface antigen: Protein structure and the development of alternative hepatitis B virus vaccines. In Chisari, F. V. (ed.), *Advances in Hepatitis Research*, pp. 30–39. (New York: Masson)
19. Neurath, A. R. and Kent, S. B. H. (1985). Antigenic structure of human hepatitis viruses. In Van Regenmortel, M. H. V. and Neurath, A. R. (eds), *Immunochemistry of Viruses: The Basis for Serodiagnosis and Vaccines*, pp. 325–366. (New York: Elsevier)
20. Okamoto, H., Imai, M., Tsuda, F., Tanaka, T., Miyakwa, Y. and Mayumi, M. (1987). Point

mutation in the S gene of hepatitis B virus for a d/y or w/r subtypic change in two blood donors carrying a surface antigen of compound subtype adyr or adwr. *J. Viriol.*, **61**, 3030–4

21. Okamoto, H., Imai, M., Miyakawa, Y. and Mayumi, M. (1987). Site-directed mutagenesis of hepatitis B surface antigen sequence at codon 160 from arginine to lysine for conversion of subtypic determinant from r to w. *Biochem. Biophys. Res. Commun.*, **148**, 500–4
22. Neurath, A. R. and Strick, N. (1980). Antibodies as immunological probes for studying the denaturation of HBsAg. *J. Med. Virol.*, **6**, 309–22
23. Neurath, A. R., Kent, S. B. H., Strick, N. and Parker, K. (1988). Vaccination with synthetic hepatitis B virus peptides. In Kurstak, E., Marusyk, R. G., Murphy, F. A. and Van Regenmortel, M. H. V. (eds), *Applied Virology Research: New Vaccines and Chemotherapy*, pp. 107–128 (New York: Plenum)
24. Kanda, P., Kennedy, R. C. and Sparrow, J. T. (1986). Immunization studies using resin-bound synthetic peptides. In Peeters, H. (ed.), *Protides of the Biological Fluids: Proceedings of the Thirty-fourth Colloquium*, 1986, pp. 125–8. (New York: Pergamon Press)
25. Zheng, J., Hu, P.-S., Xu, L.-G., Liu, Z.-P. and Huang, W.-T. (1986). Serotypic antigenic structure and immunological activity of synthetic peptide vaccine for hepatitis-B. *Biopolymers*, **25**, S201–S208
26. Brown, S. E., Zuckerman, A. J., Howard, C. R. and Stewart, M. W. (1984). Affinity of antibody responses in man to hepatitis B vaccine determined with synthetic peptides. *Lancet*, **2**, 184–7
27. Brown, S. E., Howard, C. R., Zuckerman, A. J. and Steward, M. W. (1984). Determination of the affinity of antibodies to hepatitis B surface antigen in human sera. *J. Immunol. Methods*, **72**, 41–8
28. Thanavala, Y. M., Brown, S. E., Howard, C. R., Roitt, I. M. and Steward, M. W. (1986). A surrogate hepatitis B virus antigenic epitope represented by a synthetic peptide and an internal image antiidiotype antibody. *J. Exp. Med.*, **164**, 227-36
29. Howard, C. R., Allan, J., Chen, S.-H., Brown, S. E. and Steward, M. H. (1986). Progress toward a synthetic hepatitis B vaccine. In Peeters, H. (ed.), *Protides of the Biological Fluids: Proceedings of the Thirty-fourth Colloquium*, 1986, pp. 133–136. (New York: Pergamon Press)
30. Roberts, I. M., Bernard, C. C., Vyas, G. N. and MacKay, I. R. (1975). T-cell dependence of immune response to hepatitis B surface antigen in mice. *Nature*, **254**, 606-7
31. Celis, E., Kato, I., Miller, R. W. and Chang, T.-E. (1985). Regulation of the human immune response to HBsAg: effects of antibodies and antigen conformation in the stimulation of helper T cells by HBsAg. *Hepatology*, **5**, 744–51
32. Milich, D. R., Peterson, D. L., Leroux-Roels, G. G., Lerner, R. A. and Chisari, F. V. (1985). Genetic regulation of the immune response to hepatitis B surface antigen (HBsAg). *J. Immunol.*, **134** 4203–11
33. Milich, D. R. (1987). Genetic and molecular basis for T- and B-cell recognition of hepatitis B viral antigens. *Immunol. Rev.*, **99**, 71–103
34. Celis, E., Ou, D. and Otvos, L., Jr (1988). Recognition of hepatitis B surface surface antigen by human T lymphocytes: Proliferative and cytotoxic responses to a major antigenic determinant defined by synthetic peptides. *J. Immunol.*, **140**, 1808–15
35. Neurath, A. R., Kent, S. B. H. and Strick, N. (1984). Location and chemical synthesis of a pre-S gene coded immunodominant epitope of hepatitis B virus. *Science*, **224**, 392–5
36. Neurath, A. R., Kent, S. B. H., Strick, N., Taylor, P. and Stevens, C. E. (1985). Hepatitis B virus contains pre-S gene-encoded domains. *Nature*, **315**, 154-6
37. Milich, D. R., Thornton, G. B., Neurath, A. R., Kent, S. B. H., Michel, M.-L. and Tiollais, P. (1985). Enhanced immunogenicity of the pre-S region of hepatitis B surface antigen. *Science*, **228**, 1195–9
38. Neurath, A. R., Strick, N. and Girard, M. (1989). Hepatitis B virus surface antigen (HBsAg) as carrier for synthetic peptides having an attached hydrophobic tail. *Mol. Immunol.*, **26**, 53–62
39. Heermann, K.-H., Kruse, F., Seifer, M. and Gerlich, W. H. (1987). Immunogenicity of the gene S and pre-S domains in hepatitis B virions and HBsAg filaments. *Intervirology*, **28**, 14–25
40. Milich, D. R., McNamara, M. K., McLachlan, A., Thornton, G. B. and Chisari, F. V. (1985).

Distinct H-2-linked regulation of T-cell responses to the pre-S and S regions of the same hepatitis B surface antigen polypeptide allows circumvention of nonresponsiveness to the S region. *Proc. Natl. Acad. Sci. USA*, **82**, 8168–72

41. Milich, D. R., McLachlan, A., Chisari, F. V., Kent, S. B. H. and Thornton, G. B. (1986). Immune response to the pre-S(1) region of the hepatitis B surface antigen (HBsAg): A pre-S(1)-specific T cell response can bypass nonresponsiveness to the pre-S(2) and S regions of HBsAg. *J. Immunol.*, **137**, 315–22
42. Milich, D. R., McLachlan, A., Chisari, F. V. and Thornton, G. B. (1986). Nonoverlapping T and B cell determinants on an hepatitis B surface antigen pre-S(2) region synthetic peptide. *J. Exp. Med.*, **164**, 532–47
43. Neurath, A. R., Kent, S B. H., Parker, K., Prince, A. M., Strick, N., Brotman, B. and Sproul, P. (1986). Antibodies to a synthetic peptide from the preS 120–145 region of the hepatitis B virus envelope are virus-neutralizing. *Vaccine*, **4**, 35–7
44. Neurath, A. R., Strick, N., Kent, S. B. H., Parker, K., Seto, B. and Girard, M. (1988). Design of synthetic peptides mimicking the immunologic and biologic functions of the pre-S1 sequence of the hepatitis-B virus envelope strain. In Ginsberg, H., Brown, F., Lerner, R. A. and Chanock, R. M. (eds), *Vaccines*, Vol. 88, pp. 229–34. (New York: Cold Spring Harbor Laboratory)
45. Neurath, A. R., Seto, B., Strick, N. and Girard, M. (1989). Peptides from the preS1 region of the hepatitis B virus (HBV) envelope (env) protein as components of polyvalent (hybrid) vaccines. In Ginsberg, H., Brown, F., Lerner, R. A. and Chanock, R. M. (eds), *Vaccines*, Vol. 89. (New York: Cold Spring Harbor Laboratory) (In press)
46. Itoh, Y., Takai, E., Ohnuma, H., Kitajima, K., Tsuda, F., Machida, A., Mishiro, S., Nakamura, T., Miyakawa, Y. and Mayumi, M. (1986). A synthetic peptide vaccine involving the product of the pre-S(2) region of hepatitis B virus DNA: Protective efficacy in chimpanzees. *Proc. Natl. Acad. Sci. USA*, **83**, 9174–8
47. Thornton, G. B., Milich, D., Chisari, F., Mitamura, K., Kent, S. B. H., Neurath, R., Purcell, R. and Gerin, J. (1987). Immune response in primates to the pre-S2 region of hepatitis-B surface antigen: Identification of a protective determinant. In Chanock, R. M., Lerner, R. A., Brown, F. and Ginsberg, H. (eds), *Vaccines*, Vol. 87, pp. 77–80. (New York: Cold Spring Harbor Laboratory)
48. Neurath, A. R., Kent, S. B. H., Strick, N. and Parker, K. (1986). Identification and chemical synthesis of a host cell receptor binding site on hepatitis B virus. *Cell*, **46**, 429–36
49. Neurath, A. R., Kent, S. B. H., Adamowicz, P., Riottot, M. M., Price, P., Strick, N., Parker, K., Petit, M. A., Budkowska, A., Girard, M. and Pillot, J. (1987). Immunological cross-reactivity between preS2 sequences of the hepatitis B virus envelope proteins corresponding to serological subtypes adw2 and ayw. *Mol. Immunol.*, **24** 561–8
50. Neurath, A. R., Kent, S. B. H. and Strick, N. (1986). Detection of antiviral antibodies with predetermined specificity using synthetic peptide-β-lactamase conjugates: application to antibodies specific for the preS region of the hepatitis B virus envelope proteins. *J. Gen. Virol.*, **67**, 453–61
51. Neurath, A. R., Adamowicz, P., Kent, S. B. H., Riottot, M. M., Strick, N., Parker, K., Offensperger, W., Petit, M. A., Wahl, S., Budkowska, A., Girard, M. and Pillot, J. (1986). Characterization of monoclonal antibodies specific for the pre-S2 region of the hepatitis B virus envelope protein. *Mol. Immunol.*, **23**, 991–7
52. Heermann, K. H., Goldmann, U., Schwartz, W., Seyffarth, T., Baumgarten, H. and Gerlich, W. H. (1984). Large surface proteins of hepatitis B virus containing the pre-S sequence. *J. Virol.*, **52**, 396–402
53. Neurath, A. R., Kent, S. B. H. and Strick, N. (1985). Synthetic peptides in immunoprophylaxis and diagnosis of hepatitis B. In Alitalo, K., Partanen, P. and Vaheri, A. (eds), *Synthetic Peptides in Biology and Medicine*, pp. 113–31 (New York: Elsevier)
54. Neurath, A. R., Strick, N. and Kent, S. B. H. (1986). Human antibody responses to pre-S-gene-coded sequences of the hepatitis-B virus envelope protein. In Brown, F., Chanock, R. M. and Lerner, R. A. (eds), *Vaccines*, Vol. 86, pp. 371–75. (New York: Cold Spring Harbor Laboratory)
55. Neurath, A. R., Kent, S. B. H., Strick, N., Stark, D. and Sproul, P. (1985). Genetic restriction of immune responsiveness to synthetic peptides corresponding to sequences in the pre-S region of the hepatitis B virus (HBV) envelope gene. *J. Med. Virol.*, **17**, 119–25

56. Neurath, A. R., Kent, S. B. H., Strick, N. and Parker, K. (1988). Delineation of contiguous determinants essential for biological functions of the pre-S sequence of the hepatitis B virus envelope protein: its antigenicity, immunogenicity and cell receptor recognition. *Ann. Inst. Pasteur. Virol.*, **139**, 13–38
57. Milich, D. R., McLachlan, A., Moriarity, A. and Thornton, G. B. (1987). A single 10-residue pre-S(1) peptide can prime T cell help for antibody production to multiple epitopes within the pre-S(1), pre-S(2), and S regions of HBsAg. *J. Immunol.*, **138**, 4457–65
58. Neurath, A. R., Kent, S. B. H., Strick, N., Parker, K., Curouce, A.-M., Riottot, M. M., Petit, M. A., Budkowska, A., Girard, M. and Pillot, J. (1987). Antibodies to synthetic peptides from the pre-S1 and pre-S2 regions of one subtype of the hepatitis B virus (HBV) envelope protein recognize all HBV subtypes. *Mol. Immunol.*, **24**, 975–80
59. Milich, D. R., McLachlan, A., Chisari, F. V., Nakamura, T. and Thornton, G. B. (1986). Two distinct but overlapping antibody binding sites in the pre-S(2) region of HBsAg localized within 11 continuous residues. *J. Immunol.*, **137**, 2703–10
60. Neurath, A. R., Strick, N., Kent, S. B. H., Parker, K., Kim, C. S., Girard, M., Ralph, H. E. and Valinsky, J. (1988). Biolgical role of preS sequences of the hepatitis B virus (HBV) envelope protein. In Tam, J. P. and Kaiser, E. T. (eds), *Synthetic Peptides: Approaches to Biological Problems* (New York: Alan R. Liss) (In press)
61. Iwarson, S., Tabor, E., Thomas, H. C., Goodall, A., Waters, J., Snoy, P., Shih, J. W.-K. and Gerety, R. J. (1985). Neutralization of hepatitis B virus infectivity by a murine monoclonal antibody: an experimental study in the chimpanzee. *J. Med. Virol.*, **16**, 89–96
62. Peeples, M. E., Komai, K., Radek, R. and Bankowski, M. J. (1987). A cultured cell receptor for the small S protein of hepatitis B virus. *Virology*, **160**, 135–42
63. Jones, W. R., Judd, S. J., Ing, R. M. Y., Powell, J., Bradley, J., Denholm, E. H., Mueller, U. W., Griffin, P. D. and Stevens, V. C. (1988). Phase I clinical trial of a World Health Organisation birth control vaccine. *Lancet*, **1**, 1295–8
64. Neurath, A. R., Strick, N. and Kent, S. B. H. (1985). Immune response to hepatitis-B virus determinants coded by the pre-S gene. In Lerner, R. A., Chanock, R. M. and Brown, F. (eds), *Vaccines*, Vol. 85, pp. 185–9. (New York: Cold Spring Harbor Laboratory)
65. Gerin, J. L., Purcell, R. H. and Lerner, R. A. (1985). Use of synthetic peptides to identify protective epitopes of the hepatitis-B surface antigen. In Lerner, R. A., Chanock, R. M. and Brown, F. (eds), *Vaccines*, Vol. 85, pp. 235–9. (New York: Cold Spring Harbor Laboratory)
66. Iwarson, S., Tabor, E., Thomas, H. C., Snoy, P. and Gerety, R. J. (1985). Protection against hepatitis B virus infection by immunization with hepatitis B core antigen. *Gastroenterology*, **88**, 763–7
67. Murray, K., Bruce, S. A., Hinnen, A., Wingfield, P., van Erd, P. M. C. A., de Reus, A. and Schellekens, H. (1984). Hepatitis B virus antigens made in microbial cells immunise against infection. *EMBO J.*, **3**, 645–60
68. Murray, K., Bruce, S. A., Wingfield, P., van Erd, P., de Reus, A. and Schellekens, H. (1987). Protective immunisation against hepatitis B with an internal antigen of the virus. *J. Med. Virol.*, **23**, 101–7
69. Mondelli, M., Vergani, G. M., Alberti, A., Vergani, D., Portmann, B., Eddleston, A. L. W. F. and Williams, R. (1982). Specificity of T lymphocyte cytotoxicity to autologous hepatocytes in chronic hepatitis B virus infection: Evidence that T cells are directed against HBV core antigen expressed on hepatocytes. *J. Immunol.*, **129**, 2773–8
70. Milich, D. R. and McLachlan, A. (1986). The nucleocapsid of hepatitis B virus is both a T-cell-independent and a T-cell-dependent antigen. *Science*, **234**, 1398–401
71. Milich, D. R., McLachlan, A., Moriarty, A. and Thornton, G. B (1987). Immune response to hepatitis B virus core antigen (HBcAg): Localization of T cell recognition sites within HBcAg/HBeAg. *J. Immunol.*, **139**, 1223–31
72. Milich, D. R., Hughes, J. L., McLachlan, A., Thornton, G. B. and Moriarty, A. (1988). Hepatitis B synthetic immunogen comprised of nucleocapsid T-cell sites and an envelope B-cell epitope. *Proc. Natl. Acad. Sci. USA*, **85**, 1610–14
73. Neurath, A. R., Kent, S. B. H. and Strick, N. (1984). Antibodies to hepatitis B surface antigen (HBsAg) elicited by immunization with a synthetic peptide covalently linked to liposomes. *J. Gen. Virol.*, **64**, 1009–14
74. Neurath, A. R. and Strick, N. (1987). Multimeric immunogens containing several synthetic peptide analogs of the hepatitis-B virus envelope protein. In Chanock, R. M., Lerner, R.

A., Brown, F. and Ginsberg, H. (eds), *Vaccines*, Vol. 87, pp. 33–37. (New York: Cold Spring Harbor Laboratory)

75. Howard, C. R., Sundquist, B., Allan, J., Brown, S. E. and Chen, S.-E. (1988). Immune-stimulating complexes (iscoms') as a novel hepatitis B vaccine. In Tam, J. P. and Kaiser, E. T. (eds), *Synthetic Peptides: Approaches to Biological Problems* (New York: Alan R. Liss) (In press)
76. Lowell, G. H., Ballou, W. R., Smith, L. F., Wirtz, R. A., Zollinger, W. D. and Hockmeyer, W. T. (1988). Proteosome–lipopeptide vaccines: enhancement of immunogenicity for malaria CS peptides. *Science*, **240**, 800–2
77. Celis, E., Zurawski, R., Jr. and Chang, T.-W. (1984). Regulation of T-cell function by antibodies: enhancement of the response of human T-cell clones to hepatitis B surface antigen by antigen-specific monoclonal antibodies. *Proc. Natl. Acad. Sci. USA*, **81**, 6846–50
78. Celis, E. and Chang, T.-W. (1984). Antibodies to hepatitis B surface antigen potentiate the response of human T lymphocyte clones to the same antigen. *Science*, **224**, 297–9
79. Ozaki, S. and Berzofsky, J. A. (1987). Antibody conjugates mimic specific B cell presentation of antigen: relationship between T and B cell specificity. *J. Immunol.*, **138**, 4133–42
80. Kennedy, R. C., Sparrow, J. T., Sanchez, Y., Melnick, J. L. and Dreesman, G. R. (1984). Enhancement of viral hepatitis B antibody (anti-HBs) response to a synthetic cyclic peptide by priming and anti-idiotype antibodies. *Virology*, **136**, 247–52
81. Steward, M. W., Brown, S. E. and Howard, C. R. (1988). Potentiation of antibody responses to synthetic hepatitis B peptide. In Tam, J. P. and Kaiser, E. T. (eds), *Synthetic Peptides, Approaches to Biological Problems* (New York: Alan R. Liss) (In press)
82. Machida, A., Ohnuma, H., Takai, E., Tanaka, T., Itoh, Y., Tsuda, F., Akahane, Y., Usuda, S., Nakamura, T., Miyakawa, Y. and Mayumi, M. (1987). A synthetic peptide coded for by the preS2 region of hepatitis B virus for adding immunogenicity to small spherical particles of the product of the S-gene. *Mol. Immunol.*, **24**, 523–9
83. Clarke, B. E., Newton, S. E., Carroll, A. R., Francis, M. J., Appleyard, G., Syred, A. D., Highfield, P. E., Rowlands, D. J. and Brown, F. (1987). Improved immunogenicity of a peptide epitope after fusion to hepatitis B core protein. *Nature*, **330**, 381–4
84. Hilleman, M. R. (1988). Perspectives in the quest for a vaccine against AIDS. In Gallo, R. C., Haseltine, W., Klein, G. and zur Hausen, H. (eds), *Human Retroviruses, Cancer and AIDS: Approaches to Prevention and Therapy*, p. 291. (New York: Alan R. Liss)
85. Neurath, A. R., Strick, N., Parker, K. and Kent, S. B. H. (1988). Antibodies recognizing human serum albumin are not elicited by immunization with preS2 sequences of the hepatitis B virus envelope protein. *J. Med. Virol.*, **24**, 137–51
86. Alberti, A., Pontisso, P., Tagariello, G., Cavalletto, D., Chemello, L. and Belussi, F. (1988). Antibody response to pre-S2 and hepatitis B virus induced liver damage. *Lancet*, **1** 1421–4
87. Jin, Y. J., Shih, W.-K. and Berkower, R. (1988). Human T cell response to the surface antigen of hepatitis B virus (HBsAg). *J. Exp. Med.*, **168**, 293–306

12
Prospects of immunization against EB virus

A. J. MORGAN and M. A. EPSTEIN

BACKGROUND

The EB virus

Epstein–Barr (EB) virus is one of the six human herpesviruses, a group made up of herpes simplex virus types I and II, cytomegalovirus, varicella-zoster virus, and the recently discovered human herpesvirus 6. As with all the viruses in this group the structure of EB virus is relatively complex. It consists of an outer, cell-derived, lipid membrane carrying several virus-coded glycoproteins of 340, 220 and 85 kd (gp340, gp220, gp85)[1], surrounding an icosahedral capsid of 162 capsomeres which encloses a 172 kb double-stranded DNA genome; the nucleotide sequence of the entire genome has been determined for the B95-8 laboratory strain of the virus[2].

The cellular host range of EB virus is strictly limited to those primate lymphocytes which carry the C3d complement component receptor CR2[3], and it is now clear that attachment of the virus to the target cell is mediated by the gp340/220 in the viral envelope[4,5]. Evidence has also been obtained indicating that the virus can bind to epithelial cells expressing the C3d receptor, and can replicate in oral and pharyngeal epithelium *in vivo*[6,7].

Biological behaviour of EB virus

Natural primary infection usually occurs in early childhood, is unaccompanied by obvious clinical manifestations, and leads only to the generation of antibodies to the viral antigens[8] and the development of specific cell-mediated immune responses[9]. A lifelong carrier-state ensues whereby the virus persists as a latent infection of circulating B cells[10] and continues to replicate in the region of the oropharynx, whence it is shed into the buccal fluid in considerable amounts in about 20% of those infected[11,12] and in small amounts in almost all the remainder[13]. This salivary virus provides the source for transmission of the infection in human populations.

When primary infection is delayed until early adult life, or later, there is then a 50% chance that it will be accompanied by the symptoms of infectious mononucleosis (IM)[14]. Although this disease is debilitating, and often unpleasant, it almost always resolves as immunological responses develop and a normal persisting virus carrier-state ensues[15]. Individuals with minor immunological defects may suffer prolonged chronic IM and where there is the rare, X-linked genetically predetermined major failure in EB virus-specific T cell function of Duncan syndrome, primary infection results in death[16].

EB virus and cancer

A highly significant aspect of EB virus is its association with certain human cancers. The role of this agent in the causation of endemic Burkitt's lymphoma (BL) has been extensively reviewed over the years, and it now appears that the virus, in conjunction with certain cofactors, is an essential link in a chain of events leading to excessive B cell proliferation in immunodepressed individuals, with a consequential increased chance of generating a malignant B cell clone whose c-myc gene is deregulated[17-19]. EB virus is also associated with undifferentiated nasopharyngeal carcinoma (NPC) and a role for the virus in the aetiology of this tumour appears even more compelling, perhaps with racial and genetic cofactors playing a more important part than environmental influences[20]. In this connection it is interesting to note that the mass screening of high-risk populations for NPC-specific antibody responses to EB virus infection has provided the first example of the use of viral seroepidemiology for the early detection of a human cancer[21].

In addition, it has become evident in recent years that patients receiving prolonged immunosuppressive therapy following organ grafting have an unusually high risk of developing malignant lymphomas[22,23] and these assumed special importance when it was found that all the tumour cells carried the EB virus genome[24,25].

In the context of oncogenesis, two attributes of EB virus in experimental systems are of relevance to its behaviour in man. First, its ability on infecting B lymphocytes *in vitro* to transform these cells into continuously growing lymphoblastoid cell lines[26], and second, its capacity on injection into cottontop tamarins (*Saguinus oedipus oedipus*) regularly and rapidly to induce multiple tumours[27] which the most stringent current criteria have characterized as malignant lymphomas[28].

VACCINES AGAINST EB VIRUS

Rationale for an antiviral vaccine to prevent EB virus-associated cancers

By the mid-1970s the links between EB virus and both BL and NPC were sufficiently strong for it to be deemed essential to explore the possibilities of an antiviral vaccine[29]. Although the exact mechanisms whereby the virus might contribute to the causation of the cancers were not known, an essential role was clear, so that removal of the virus by vaccine prevention of primary infection should lead to a decrease in the incidence of the tumours in populations at risk; the comparison with abstention from, or giving up, cigarette smoking in relation to bronchogenic carcinoma[30] seemed obvious.

Although endemic BL is not of much significance in total world cancer terms, undifferentiated NPC certainly is, since it is the most common cancer of men and the second most common of women in all populations of southern Chinese origin[31], and it also has a medium–high incidence across North Africa, in the Sudan, and in Kenya[32,33]. Efforts to control NPC would thus be well worth while.

As for a precedent for successful prevention of a naturally occurring cancer by antiviral vaccination, this was provided by the case of Marek's disease of chickens[34]. With this herpesvirus-induced condition huge numbers of commercial chickens were regularly lost from malignant lymphomas[35], until the introduction of efficient antiviral vaccines[36,37]. Although live apathogenic virus vaccines are currently used, experimental vaccines based on purified antigens from the membranes of cells infected with Marek's disease herpesvirus have also given excellent protection[38]. It was for this reason that, for an analogous vaccine against EB virus, the EB virus-determined membrane antigen (MA) was chosen from the outset as immunogen, and because antibodies to it were known to be virus neutralizing. Early work from several laboratories demonstrated that MA consists of two antigenically related, large glycoprotein molecules of 340 and 270 kd (MA gp340 and gp270) (reviewed in ref. 39) and the larger of these was selected for study. Over the years a prototype MA gp340-based vaccine was developed.

Validation of a prototype MA gp340-based subunit vaccine

In the first experiments MA gp340 was purified by a molecular weight-based procedure[40], ensuring optimum yields at each step by monitoring with a quantitative radioimmunoassay[41]. The product was rendered immunogenic by incorporation in artificial liposomes and the antibodies induced in banal laboratory animals were assessed by means of a highly sensitive ELISA[42] and standard virus-neutralization tests[43,44].

The only animal known to respond with lesions to experimental EB virus infection is the cottontop tamarin in which, as mentioned above, the virus rapidly induces multiple malignant lymphomas[27]. In order to provide enough individuals of this rare, and at the time little-known, species for testing protection by the vaccine, a successful breeding colony had to be established[45,46]. It was also necessary to determine the dose of virus for use as challenge after vaccination which would cause lymphomas in all unprotected animals of this outbred population[47]. Material prepared as outlined above was used as a prototype vaccine in cottontop tamarins and it was shown that the immunized animals were protected against tumour induction when challenged with the 100% lymphomagenic dose of virus, thus demonstrating the efficacy of MA gp340 as a protective immunogen[47].

Assessment of candidate vaccines for use in man

Production of MA gp340 in genetically engineered cells

The region of the EB virus genome carrying the gene coding for MA has been identified[48] and the nucleotide sequence of this gene is known[49]. For production of MA gp340 in genetically engineered cultured cells the gene has been cloned and expressed in *E. coli*[50], yeast[51], and several types of mammalian cells[52,53]. However, it has proved difficult to maintain cultures with a significant proportion of cells continuing to express MA gp340, and purification of the product in tractable amounts has not been successful. Little progress has been made with any of these systems up to the present, but further refinements of appropriate molecular techniques may in the future provide second-generation vaccine material suitable for use in man.

Recombinant viral vectors to express MA gp340

1. Two vaccinia virus recombinants have been prepared which express the MA gp340 gene under the control of a vaccinia virus promoter during replication[54]. The recombinants were derived, respectively, from the relatively virulent WR laboratory strain of vaccinia and the attenuated New York Board of Health Wyeth vaccine strain. Vaccination of tamarins intradermally with the WR recombinant caused skin lesions 4 or 5 cm in diameter in these small animals (of about 500 g) with a further crop of satellite pustules 1 week later. Antibodies to vaccinia ranged in titre from 1:5000 to 1:10 000, a second intradermal vaccination did not increase this response, and no antibodies to MA gp340 could be detected; yet when challenged with the 100% lymphomagenic dose of EB virus, three out of four animals were protected, suggesting that some form of cell-mediated immunity had been successfully elicited. The WR vaccinia virus is, of course, far too virulent for use in man, a point not usually stressed in reported work on recombinant vaccinia virus vaccines. Disappointingly, the Wyeth vaccine strain recombinant only induced minimal skin lesions in vaccinated tamarins, and gave much lower titres of antibody to vaccinia, presumably because of the rather restricted level of virus replication, and the vaccinated animals proved quite unresistant to challenge with EB virus[55]. Although it is possible to conceive of theoretically feasible strategies to overcome these difficulties with vaccinia recombinants, their realization lies well into the future.
2. A recombinant varicella virus has also been made using analogous genetic engineering techniques to insert the MA gp340 gene[56] and starting from the outset with the Oka vaccine strain[57]. This strain has been employed extensively over the years to vaccinate young children, and no adverse reactions have been reported[58]. It has been shown recently that the common marmoset (*Callithrix jacchus*) can be infected experimentally with the Oka strain of varicella virus[59], and although this species does not respond with disease manifestations when given EB virus[60] it is closely related phylogenetically to the cottontop tamarin, which does. There is reason to expect, therefore, that it may be possible to explore the protective effects of the recombinant Oka varicella against tumour induction by EB virus using tamarins, and this hope has been strengthened by current experiments indicating that the recombinant will grow in cottontop tamarin fibroblast cultures (Morgan *et al.*, unpublished); however, much preliminary work remains to be done.

Elaboration of a first-generation MA gp340 vaccine immunogen for human trials

Although the approaches discussed above are likely to give valuable second-generation vaccines in the long term, it was considered imperative to establish the efficacy and harmlessness of MA gp340 in humans before embarking on the major effort required to exploit them. Accordingly, other methods have been sought to elaborate a first-generation MA gp340-based vaccine immunogen suitable for human trials.

During a preliminary analysis of the structure of MA gp340 it was observed that the carbohydrate component was heavily sialylated[61]. On reviewing this finding it became clear that the molecule should remain negatively charged at a relatively low pH, and a purification procedure was accordingly developed using anion exchange chromatography on an automated fast protein liquid chromatography (FPLC) system[62]. With this method the membrane fraction of EB virus-infected cells (expressing therefore MA gp340) is solubilized in a synthetic non-ionic detergent (MEGA-9[63]) and passed down an ion exchange matrix (Mono-Q) under conditions of low ionic strength at pH 5.0. In these circumstances MA gp340 binds to the anion exchanger very efficiently, and can be readily eluted with a salt gradient. Although virtual purity is achieved with this single step, a final gel filtration guarantees the homogeneity of the product[62]. This new method has several important advantages, including the isolation of all MA gp340 molecules, avoidance of denaturing conditions, automation, reproducibility, and the potential for easy scale-up.

With FPLC-purified MA gp340 readily available, its efficacy in conjunction with two powerful new adjuvants has been investigated.

FPLC-purified MA gp340 and iscoms

Immunostimulating complexes (iscoms) based on the glycoside Quil A provide a novel method for enhancing immunogenic presentation[64,65]. If the antigen to be used is amphipathic and has a hydrophobic membrane anchor sequence, such as that of MA gp340, then under appropriate conditions supramolecular structures of the same order of size as small viruses (about 40 nm in diameter) can form as complexes between it and Quil A. These iscom structures are highly immunogenic, probably because the antigen is presented in an 'array' with which the Quil A adjuvant molecule is intimately associated multimerically, and induce both humoral and cell-mediated responses. Cottontop tamarins vaccinated with FPLC-purified MA gp340 incorporated into iscoms have subsequently been challenged with the 100% oncogenic dose of EB virus and were found to be completely protected[66]. Furthermore, the dose of antigen required was no more than three injections of 5 μg each. Preliminary tests have recently shown that iscoms are free from obvious short-term adverse effects[67] but a full-range toxicological study remains to be carried out, and will take a considerable time.

FPLC-purified MA gp340 and a synthetic MDP analogue

Muramyl dipeptide (MDP) has long been known to have important adjuvant activity, but it is also pyrogenic and induces such serious side-effects as arthritis, anterior uveitis, and central nervous system pathology. In an important advance the immunopotentiating activity has been separated from the functions causing side-effects with the introduction of a synthetic threonyl derivative of MDP which, when emulsified in squalane with a pluronic polymer, gives a powerful adjuvant formulation[68,69]. The formulation consists of microspherules that retain antigen on their surfaces and activate complement, and both humoral and cellular immunity have been induced when the formulation was given with a variety of inactivated viruses and viral subunits[69]. Extensive toxicological studies have failed to reveal harmful properties, and it is expected that the formulation will shortly be approved by the US FDA.

FPLC-purified MA gp340 and the MDP formulation have been used together as immunogen to vaccinate cottontop tamarins, and the immunized animals were found to be protected against the 100% oncogenic challenge dose of EB virus. A great advantage of this immunogen lies in the fact that the antigen and the adjuvant can simply be mixed together before injection without the need for any complicated coupling, and further studies have shown that, as with iscoms, the MDP formulation is so effective an adjuvant that three doses of 5 μg gp340 each are sufficient to induce complete immunity (Morgan *et al.*, in preparation).

Comment

It is clear from the foregoing that MA gp340 can now be easily prepared in tractable amounts by the FPLC purification procedure[62], and that the MDP formulation[68,69] provides a safe, easy-to-use, highly effective adjuvant giving excellent results with extraordinarily low doses of antigen. A first-generation subunit vaccine against EB virus is thus now available for use in humans, and planning for human trials is already under way.

Programme for human trials

The phase I trial

FPLC-purified MA gp340 is being prepared on contract in the commercial sector under conditions of good manufacturing practice which conform to the requirements of licensing authorities for products to be used in human subjects. The batch produced will be used, after appropriate testing for immunogenicity, sterility, and safety *in vitro* and in laboratory animals, for a phase I human trial. The objectives of the trial are:

1. to determine the immunogenicity in man of FPLC-purified EB virus MA gp340 administered with the MDP adjuvant formulation by injection;
2. to make a preliminary estimate of its tolerability, in particular if given to seropositive individuals.

The protocol for the phase I trial involves the following ethically approved steps:

1. serological screening for antibodies to EB virus of 100 young, informed, consenting human volunteers;

2. selection of 12 seronegative individuals and 12 seropositive individuals with low levels of antibody to MA gp340;
3. full clinical and laboratory screening of those chosen;
4. full investigation of EB virus status of those chosen (serology, salivary virus shedding, cytotoxic T-cell function, establishment of B-cell lines as subsequent targets for cell-mediated immunity);
5. administration of vaccine;
6. post-immunization clinical monitoring and scrutiny of daily diary of symptoms;
7. immunological assessment of antibody and cell-mediated responses to EB virus.

The analysis of the results will concentrate on the search for local or systemic reactions to the vaccine, and the detection in seronegative individuals of induced antibody and cellular reactivity to gp340 and in seropositive individuals of a boost in these measures of immunity.

Future double-blind confirmatory trial

It is intended that a double-blind placebo trial should be undertaken as soon as FPLC-purified MA gp340 with the MDP formulation has been shown to be safe and immunogenic for humans. The double-blind studies will have to be undertaken in the context of delayed primary infection and EB virus-induced infectious mononucleosis (IM) in young adults. Prevention of IM was never envisaged as the primary reason for developing a vaccine against EB virus but, as has frequently been pointed out, IM provides an excellent experimental testing ground for such a vaccine[29,39]. Young adults who have escaped the usual silent primary infection with EB virus in childhood can be routinely detected by serological screening, and in Western-style societies such people constitute a significant minority, especially in the upper socio-economic classes. As a group they are at risk for delayed primary infection which, as already mentioned, is accompanied by the symptoms of IM in 50% of cases[14].

There are thus good grounds for applying screening to a cohort of university or college students and undertaking the double-blind trial among volunteers who have never been infected by the virus. Monitoring would rather quickly determine the ability of the vaccine to prevent primary infection, and there would be the added advantage that those who were successfully protected would not have to face the disruption and discomfort of an attack of IM. At the same time there are strong ethical reasons for providing a vaccine programme for individuals with Duncan syndrome in which EB virus infection is life-threatening[16], even before a double-blind trial has been completed in healthy volunteers.

Future field trials

Once vaccine prevention of primary EB virus infection has been demonstrated with coincidental prevention of IM and the grave effects of Duncan syndrome, the way would be open for a phase of field trials to prevent EB virus-associated cancers. In the first place, the vaccine would have to be deployed in areas where endemic BL has a high incidence, by definition in a developing country, so that special considerations arise. Primary EB virus infection occurs in all children at a very early age in the social conditions and standards of hygiene of the Third World[70,71] and vaccinations would have to be carried out in the first few months of life.

However, such a schedule is exactly comparable to that required for vaccination against hepatitis B (HBV)[72,73] and the-logistics for an EB virus vaccine trial against BL in the tropics are less complicated than those already being implemented for a WHO 30-year prospective study of HBV vaccination to prevent primary liver cell cancer[74]. Incidentally, since the latter tumour is one of adult life, and the peak incidence for BL is at about age 7, the influence of EB virus vaccination would be apparent considerably sooner than that of HBV vaccination.

Field trials of EB virus vaccination to prevent NPC will require a greater and much longer-term effort. NPC is a tumour of later life, and immunity would have to be maintained for many decades, longer even than the HBV vaccine protection against liver cancer. Nevertheless, progress with a vaccine against EB virus continues steadily, and success at each step in demonstrating the efficacy of the MA gp340-based vaccine will generate acceleration in the rate of advance.

CONCLUDING REMARKS

It is sometimes argued that to attempt to use vaccines in humans to prevent infection with cancer-associated viruses, in order to decrease the incidence of the tumours themselves, cannot be justified in the absence of a clear understanding of the mechanisms by which the viruses cause the cancers, or even certain knowledge that they do so. The successful control of a human cancer by vaccination against its tumour virus, analogous to the antiviral vaccine control of Marek's disease lymphomas[35,36], is in fact the only way in which causality can be proven in the human context. As for councils of delay until mechanisms are understood, they can best be compared to the toleration of heavy smoking until the exact details of the role of cigarettes in the induction of lung cancer have been worked out.

Subunit antiviral vaccines have been highly effective both in human and animal diseases[75,76], and although it is hoped that the present first-generation MA gp340-based vaccine will soon be superseded by more sophisticated second-generation products, it is good that the protective immunogenicity of MA gp340 can be assessed in man in the meantime. The start of human trials in 1989 will take place 25 years after EB virus was originally discovered[77], and 13 years since a vaccine against it was first proposed[29]. The long-term goals have appeared dauntingly distant for many years, but it now seems likely that they will at least be explored sooner rather than later.

ACKNOWLEDGEMENTS

The early work discussed here was supported jointly by the Medical Research Council, London, and the Cancer Research Campaign, London; the more recent studies were funded by the Cancer Research Campaign alone.

REFERENCES

1. North, J. R., Morgan, A. and Epstein, M. A. (1980). Observations on the EB virus envelope and virus-determined membrane antigen (MA) polypeptides. *Int. J. Cancer*, **26**, 231–40
2. Baer, R., Bankier, A. T., Biggin, M. D., Deininger, P. L., Farrell, P. J., Gibson, T. J., Hatfull, G., Hudson, G. S., Satchwell, S. C., Sequin, C., Tuffnell, P. S. and Barrell, B. G. (1984). DNA sequence and expression of the B95-8 Epstein–Barr virus genome. *Nature*, **310**, 207–11
3. Fingeroth, J. D., Weiss, J. J., Tedder, T. F., Strominger, J. L., Biro, P. A. and Fearon, D. T. (1984). Epstein–Barr virus receptor of human B lymphocytes is the C3d receptor CR2. *Proc. Natl. Acad. Sci. USA*, **81**, 4510–14
4. Tanner, J., Weiss, J., Fearon, D., Whang, W. and Kieff, E. (1987). Epstein–Barr virus gp350/220 binding to the B lymphocyte C3d receptor mediates absorption, capping and endocytosis. *Cell*, **50**, 203–13
5. Nemerow, G. R., Mold, C., Schwend, V. K., Tollefson, V. and Cooper, N. (1987). Identification of gp350 as the viral glycoprotein mediating attachment of Epstein–Barr virus (EBV) to the EBV/C3d receptor of B cells: sequence homology of gp350 and C3 complement fragment C3d. *J. Virol.*, **61**, 1416–20
6. Sixbey, J. W., Davis, D. S., Young, L. S., Hutt-Fletcher, L., Tedder, L. F. and Rickinson, A. B. (1987). Human epithelial cell expression of an Epstein–Barr virus receptor. *J. Gen. Virol.*, **68**, 805–11
7. Greenspan, J. S., Greenspan, D., Lennette, E. T., Abrams, D. I., Conant, M. A., Peterson, V. and Freese, U. K. (1985). Replication of Epstein–Barr virus within the epithelial cells of oral 'hairy' leukoplakia, an AIDS-associated lesion. *N. Engl. J. Med.*, **313**, 1564–71
8. Henle, W. and Henle, G. (1979). Seroepidemiology of the virus. In Epstein, M. A. and Achong, B. G. (eds), *The Epstein–Barr Virus*, pp. 61–78. (Berlin, Heidelberg and New York: Springer Verlag)
9. Rickinson, A. B. (1986). Cellular immunological responses to the virus infection. In Epstein, M. A. and Achong, B. G. (eds), *The Epstein–Barr Virus: Recent Advances*, pp. 75–125. (London: Heinemann)
10. Nilsson, K., Klein, G., Henle, W. and Henle, G. (1971). The establishment of lymphoblastoid lines from adult and fetal human lymphoid tisue and its dependence on EBV. *Int. J. Cancer*, **8**, 443–50
11. Gerber, P., Nonoyama, M., Lucas, S., Perlin, E. and Goldstein, L. I. (1972). Oral excretion of Epstein–Barr virus by healthy subjects and patients with infectious mononucleosis. *Lancet*, **2**, 988–9
12. Chang, R. S., Lewis, J. P. and Abildgaard, C. F. (1973). Prevalence of oropharyngeal excretors of leukocyte-transforming agents among a human population. *N. Engl. J. Med.*, **289**, 1325–9
13. Yao, Q. Y., Rickinson, A. B. and Epstein, M. A. (1985). A re-examination of the Epstein–Barr virus carrier state in healthy seropositive individuals. *Int. J. Cancer*, **35**, 35–42
14. Niederman, J. C., Evans, A. S., Subrahamanyan, L. and McCollum, R. W. (1970). Prevalence, incidence and persistence of EB virus antibody in young adults. N. Engl. J. Med., **282**, 361–5
15. Henle, G. and Henle, W. (1979). The virus as the etiologic agent of infectious mononucleosis. In Epstein, M. A. and Achong, B. G. (eds), *The Epstein–Barr Virus*, pp. 297–320. (Berlin, Heidelberg and New York: Springer Verlag)
16. Weisenburger, D. D. and Purtilo, D. T. (1986). Failure in immunological control of the virus infection: fatal infectious mononucleosis. In Epstein, M. A. and Achong, B. G. (eds), *The Epstein–Barr Virus: Recent Advances*, pp. 127–161. (London: Heinemann)

17. Epstein, M. A. and Morgan, A. J. (1983). Clinical consequences of Epstein–Barr virus infection and possible control by an antiviral vaccine. *Clin. Exp. Immunol.*, **53**, 257–71
18. Whittle, H. C., Brown, J., Marsh, K., Greenwood, B. M., Seidelin, P., Tighe, H. and Wedderburn, L. (1984). T cell control of B cells infected with EB virus is lost during *P. falciparum* malaria. *Nature*, **312**, 449–50
19. Lenoir, G. M. and Bornkamm, G. W. (1987). Burkitt's lymphoma, a human cancer model for the study of the multistep development of cancer; proposal for a new scenario. In Klein, G. (ed.), *Advances in Viral Oncology Series*, Vol. 7, pp. 173–206. (New York: Raven Pres)
20. Klein, G. (1979). The relationship of the virus to nasopharyngeal carcinoma. In Epstein, M. A. and Achong, B. G. (eds), *The Epstein–Barr Virus*, pp. 339–350. (Berlin, Heidelberg and New York: Springer Verlag)
21. Zeng, Y., Zhang, L. G., Li, H. Y., Jan, M. G., Zhang, Q., Wu, Y. C., Wang, Y. S. and Su, G. R. (1982). Serological mass survey for early detection of nasopharyngeal carcinoma in Wuzhou City, China. *Int. J. Cancer*, **29**, 139–41
22. Kinlen, L. J., Sheil, A. G. R., Peto, J. and Doll, R. (1979). Collaborative United Kingdom-Australasian study of cancer in patients treated with immunosuppressive drugs. *Br. Med. J.*, **2**, 1461–6
23. Weintraub, J. and Warnke, R. A. (1982). Lymphoma in cardiac allotransplant recipients: clinical and histological features and immunological phenotype. *Transplantation*, **33**, 347–51
24. Crawford, D. H., Thomas, J. A., Janossy, G., Sweny, P., Fernando, O. N., Moorhead, J. F. and Thompson, J. L. (1980). Epstein–Barr virus nuclear antigen-positive lymphoma after cyclosporin A treatment in a patient with renal allograft. *Lancet*, **1**, 1355–6
25. Hanto, D. W., Frizzera, G., Gajl-Peczalska, K. J., Sakamoto, K., Purtilo, D. T., Balfour, H. H., Simmons, R. L. and Najarian, J. S. (1982). Epstein–Barr virus-induced B-cell lymphoma after renal transplantation: acyclovir therapy and transition from polyclonal to monoclonal B-cell proliferation. *N. Engl. J. Med.*, **306**, 913–18
26. Pope, J. H., Scott, W. and Moss, D. J. (1973). Human lymphoid cell transformation by Epstein–Barr virus. *Nature* (*New Biol.*), **246**, 140–1
27. Miller, G., Shope, T., Coope, D., Waters, L., Pagano, J., Bornkamm, G. W. and Henle, W. (1977). Lymphoma in cotton-top marmosets after inoculation with Epstein–Barr virus; tumor incidence, histologic spectrum, antibody responses, demonstration of viral DNA, and characterization of viruses. *J. Exp. Med.*, **145**, 948–67
28. Cleary, M. L., Epstein, M. A., Finerty, S., Dorfman, R. F., Bornkamm, G. W., Kirkwood, J. K., Morgan, A. J. and Sklar, J. (1985). Individual tumors of multifocal EB virus-induced malignant lymphomas in tamarins arise from different B cell clones. *Science*, **228**, 722–4
29. Epstein, M. A. (1976). Epstein–Barr virus – is it time to develop a vaccine program? *J. Natl. Cancer Inst.*, **56**, 697–700
30. Doll, R. and Peto, R. (1976). Mortality in relation to smoking: 20 years' observation on male British doctors. *Br. Med. J.*, **2**, 1525–36
31. Shanmugaratnam, K. (1971). Studies on the etiology of nasopharyngeal carcinoma. In Richter, G. W. and Epstein, M. A. (eds), *International Review of Experimental Pathology*, Vol. 10, pp. 361–413. (New York and London: Academic Press)
32. Clifford, P. (1970). A review: on the epidemiology of nasopharyngeal carcinoma. *Int. J. Cancer*, **5**, 287–309
33. Cammoun, M., Hoerner, G. W. and Mourali, N. (1974). Tumors of the nasopharynx in Tunisia: an anatomic and clinical study based on 143 cases. *Cancer*, **33**, 184–92
34. Marek, J. (1907). Multiple Nerventzündung (Polyneuritis) bei Hühnern. *Deutsch. Tierärztl. Wschr.*, **15**, 417–21
35. Payne, L. N., Frazier, J. A. and Powell, P. C. (1976). Pathogenesis of Marek's disease. In Richter, G. W. and Epstein, M. A. (eds), *International Review of Experimental Pathology*, Vol. 16, pp. 59–154. (New York, San Francisco, London: Academic Press)
36. Churchill, A. E., Payne, L. N. and Chubb, R. C. (1969). Immunization against Marek's disease using a live attenuated virus. *Nature*, **221**, 744–7
37. Okazaki, W., Purchase, H. G. and Burmester, B. R. (1970). Protection against Marek's disease by vaccination with a herpesvirus of turkeys. *Avian. Dis.*, **14**, 413–29
38. Kaaden, O. R. and Dietzschold, B. (1974). Alterations of the immunological specificity of plasma membranes of cells infected with Marek's disease and turkey herpes viruses. *J. Gen. Virol.*, **25**, 1–10

39. Epstein, M. A. (1984). A prototype vaccine to prevent Epstein–Barr (EB) virus-associated tumours. *Proc. Roy. Soc. B. Lond.*, **221**, 1–20
40. Morgan, A. J., North, J. R. and Epstein, M. A. (1983). Purification and properties of the gp340 component of Epstein–Barr (EB) virus membrane antigen (MA) in an immunogenic form. *J. Gen. Virol.*, **64**, 455–60
41. North, J. R., Morgan, A. J., Thompson, J. L. and Epstein, M. A. (1982). Quantification of an EB virus-associated membrane antigen (MA) component. *J. Virol. Methods*, **5**, 55–65
42. Randle, B. J. and Epstein, M. A. (1984). A highly sensitive enzyme-linked immunosorbent assay to quantitate antibodies to Epstein–Barr virus membrane antigen gp340. *J. Virol. Methods*, **9**, 201–8
43. Moss, D. J. and Pope, J. H. (1972). Assay of the infectivity of Epstein–Barr virus by transformation of human leucocytes *in vitro*. *J. Gen. Virol.*, **17**, 233–6
44. De Schryver, A., Klein, G., Hewetson, J., Rocchi, G., Henle, W., Henle, G., Moss, D. J. and Pope, J. H. (1974). Comparison of EBV neutralization tests based on abortive infection or transformation of lymphoid cells and their relation to membrane reactive antibodies (anti MA),. *Int. J. Cancer*, **13**, 353–62
45. Kirkwood, J. K., Epstein, M. A. and Terlecki, A. J. (1983). Factors influencing population growth of a colony of cotton-top tamarins. *Lab. Animals*, **17**, 35–41
46. Kirkwood, J. K., Epstein, M. A., Terlecki, A. J. and Underwood, S. J. (1985). Rearing of a second generation of cotton-top tamarins (*Saguinus oedipus oedipus*) in captivity. *Lab. Animals*, **19**, 269–72
47. Epstein, M. A., Morgan, A. J., Finerty, S., Randle, B. J. and Kirkwood, J. K. (1985). Protection of cottontop tamarins against Epstein–Barr virus-induced malignant lymphoma by a prototype subunit vaccine. *Nature*, **318**, 287–9
48. Hummel, M., Thorley-Lawson, D. A. and Kieff, E. (1984). An Epstein–Barr virus DNA fragment encodes messages for the two major envelope glycoproteins (gp350/300 and gp220/200). *J. Virol.*, **49**, 413–17
49. Biggin, M., Farrell, P. J. and Barrell, B. G. (1984). Transcription and DNA sequence of the *Bam* HIL fragment of B95-8 Epstein–Barr virus. *EMBO J.*, **3** 1083–90
50. Beisel, C., Tanner, J., Matsuo, T., Thorley-Lawson, D., Kezdy, F. and Kieff, E. (1985). Two major outer envelope glycoproteins of Epstein–Barr virus encoded by the same gene. *J. Virol.*, **54**, 665–74
51. Schultz, L. D., Tanner, J., Hofmann, K., Emini, E., Kieff, E. and Ellis, R. W. (1987). Expression and analysis of EBV gp350 in yeast *Saccharomyces cerevisiae*. In Levine, P. H., Ablashi, D. V., Nonoyama, M., Pearson, G. R. and Glaser, R. (eds), *Epstein–Barr Virus and Human Disease*, pp. 475–478. (Clifton, New Jersey: Humana Press)
52. Whang, Y., Silberklang, M., Morgan, A., Munshi, S., Lenny, A. B., Ellis, R. W. and Kieff, E. (1987). Expression of Epstein–Barr virus gp350/220 gene in rodent and primate cells. *J. Virol.*, **61**, 1796–807
53. Conway, M., Morgan, A. J. and Mackett, M. (1988). Expression of Epstein–Barr virus antigen gp340/220 in mouse fibroblasts using a bovine papilloma virus vector (Submitted)
54. Mackett, M. and Arrand, J. R. (1985). Recombinant vaccinia virus induces neutralising antibodies in rabbits against Epstein–Barr virus membrane antigen gp340. *EMBO J.*, **4** 3229–34
55. Morgan, A. J., Mackett, M., Finerty, S., Arrand, J., Scullion, F. and Epstein, M. A. (1988). Recombinant vaccinia virus expressing Epstein–Barr virus glycoprotein gp340 protects cottontop tamarins against EB virus-induced lymphomas. *J. Med. Virol.*, **25**, 189–95
56. Lowe, R. S., Keller, P. M., Keech, B. J., Davison, A. J., Whang, Y., Morgan, A. J., Kieff, E. and Ellis, R. W. (1987). Varicella-zoster virus as a live vector for the expression of foreign genes. *Proc. Natl. Acad. Sci. USA*, **84**, 3896–900
57. Takahaski, M., Otsuka, T., Okuno, Y., Asano, Y., Yazaki, T. and Isomura, S. (1974). Live varicella vaccine used to prevent the spread of varicella in children in hospital. *Lancet*, **2** 1288–90
58. Weibel, R. W., Neff, B. J., Kuter, B. J., Guess, H. A., Rothenburger, C. A., Fitzgerald, A. J., Connor, K. A., McLean, A. A., Hilleman, M. R. and Buynak, E. B. (1984). Live attenuated varicella virus vaccine: efficiency trial in healthy children. *N. Engl. J. Med.*, **310**, 1409–15
59. Provost, P. J., Keller, P. M., Banker, F. S., Keech, B. J., Klein, H. J., Lowe, R. S., Morton, D. H., Phelps, A. H., McAleer, W. J. and Ellis, R. W. (1987). Successful infection of the

common marmoset (*Callithrix jacchus*) with human varicella-zoster virus. *J. Virol.*, **61**, 2951–5

60. Wedderburn, N., Edwards, J. M. B., Desgranges, C., Fontaine, C., Cohen, B. and de Thé, G. (1984). Infectious mononucleosis-like response in common marmosets infected with Epstein–Barr virus. *J. Infect. Dis.*, **150**, 878–82
61. Morgan, A. J., Smith, A. R., Barker, R. N. and Epstein, M. A. (1984). A structural investigation of the Epstein–Barr (EB) virus membrane antigen glycoprotein, gp340. *J. Gen. Virol.*, **65**, 397–404
62. David, E. M. and Morgan, A. J. (1988). Efficient purification of Epstein–Barr virus membrane antigen gp340 by fast protein liquid chromatography. *J. Immunol. Methods*, **108**, 231–6
63. Hildreth, J. E. K. (1982). *N*-D-Gluco-*N*-methylalkanamide compounds, a new class of non-ionic detergents for membrane biochemistry. *Biochem. J.*, **207**, 363–6
64. Morein, B., Sundquist, B., Höglund, S., Dalsgaard, K. and Osterhaus, A. (1984). Iscom, a novel structure for antigenic presentation of membrane proteins from enveloped viruses. *Nature*, **308**, 457–60
65. Morein, B., Lövgren, K., Höglund, S. and Sundquist, B. (1987). The iscom: an immunostimulating complex. *Immunol. Today*, **8**, 333–8
66. Morgan, A. J., Finerty, S., Lovgren, K., Scullion, F. T. and Morein, B. (1988). Prevention of Epstein–Barr (EB) virus-induced lymphoma in cottontop tamarins by vaccination with the EB virus envelope glycoprotein gp340 incorporated into immune-stimulating complexes. *J. Gen. Virol.*, **69**, 2093–6
67. Speijers, G., Danse, L., Bewary, E., Strik, J. and Vos, J. (1988). Local reactions of the saponin Quil A and a Quil A-containing iscom measles vaccine after intramuscular injection of rats: a comparison with the effects of DPT-polio vaccine. *Fund. Appl. Toxicol.*, **10**, 425–30
68. Allison, A. C. and Byars, N. E. (1986). An adjuvant formulation that selectively elicits the formation of antibodies of protective isotype and cell mediated immunity. *J. Immunol. Methods*, **95**, 157–68
69. Allison, A. C. and Byars, N. E. (1987). Vaccine technology: adjuvants for increased efficiency. *Biotechnology*, **5**, 1041–5
70. Henle, W. and Henle, G. (1969). The relation between the Epstein–Barr virus and infectious mononucleosis, Burkitt's lymphoma and cancer of the postnasal space. *E. African Med. J.*, **46**, 402–6
71. De-Thé, G. (1979). Demographic studies implicating the virus in the causation of Burkitt's lymphoma; prospects for nasopharyngeal carcinoma. In Epstein, M. A. and Achong, B. G. (eds), *The Epstein–Barr Virus*, pp. 417–437. (Berlin, Heidelberg and New York: Springer Verlag)
72. Zuckerman, A. J. (1985). Prevention of hepatocellular carcinoma by immunization against hepatitis B. In Richter, G. W. and Epstein, M. A. (eds), *International Review of Experimental Pathology*, Vol. 25, pp. 59–81. (Orlando, San Diego, New York, London, Toronto, Montreal, Sydney, Tokyo: Academic Press)
73. Deinhardt, F. and Jilg, W. (1986). Vaccines against hepatitis. *Ann. Inst. Pasteur. Virol.*, **137E**, 79–95
74. International Agency for Research on Cancer (1985). An intervention tudy to evaluate the effectiveness of Hepatitis B vaccine for the prevention of hepatocellular carcinoma in a high risk population. *IARC Working Paper*, **3/6**, 1–46
75. Szmuness, W., Stevens, C. E., Zang, E. A., Harley, E. J. and Kellner, A. (1981). A controlled clinical trial of the efficacy of the Hepatitis B vaccine (Hetavax B): a final report. *Hepatology*, **1**, 377–85
76. Bittle, J. L., Houghten, R. A., Alexander, H., Shinnick, T. M., Sutcliffe, J. G., Lerner, R. A., Rowlands, D. J. and Brown, F. (1982). Protection against foot and mouse disease by immunization with a chemically synthesized peptide predicted from the viral nucleotide sequence. *Nature*, **298**, 30–3
77. Epstein, M. A., Achong, B. G. and Barr, Y. M. (1964). Virus particles in cultured lymphoblasts from Burkitt's lymphoma. *Lancet*, **1**, 702–3

13
The development of vaccines against AIDS

P. J. GREENAWAY

INTRODUCTION

AIDS, the acquired immunodeficiency syndrome, is caused by an infection with an exogenous retrovirus now known as the human immunodeficiency virus (HIV)[1-6]. The true incidence of this disease is not known accurately, but the reported cases worldwide continue to accumulate at an ever-increasing rate. Epidemiological surveys indicate that there will be at least 1 million new cases of AIDS within the next 5 years. Clearly, the AIDS pandemic needs to be controlled and prevented. The control of clinical AIDS requires the development of safe, cheap and effective chemotherapeutic drugs. This represents an area of intense research activity, some of which is beginning to bear fruit. However, the drugs developed so far only ameliorate the effects, or delay the onset, of disease; they do not eliminate the virus from infected individuals. Disease prevention is obviously preferable and here there are two avenues for exploration. The first avenue is education. Education, to modify the lifestyles of the populations at risk, has already had a demonstrable beneficial effect but the current indications are that this approach has to be sustained for it to remain effective, and that some members of the community, especially those within the lower socioeconomic groups, are less likely to respond than others[7]. Even so, education programmes can be undertaken immediately, and they will certainly reduce the incidence of infection; they therefore merit considerable investment and continued development. The second avenue to explore involves the development of effective vaccines for use in either selective or mass immunization programmes. Such vaccines are not yet available, although some potential candidates are, perhaps prematurely, now undergoing small-scale human clinical trials. There is no general consensus view on how long it will take for a truly effective AIDS vaccine to be developed, but it is becoming increasingly apparent that a considerable amount of research effort is still needed on the fundamental biology of HIV, particularly on its interactions with the immune system of the host, before one finally emerges. A possible rationale for developing an AIDS vaccine is shown in Table 1. The need and urgency for an AIDS vaccine is reflected by the rapid progress made in many of the areas indicated, and by the vast amount of information already accumulated about AIDS and HIV. A comprehensive review of this entire field is beyond the scope of this chapter, and thus the primary objective is to give a general impression of the current status of AIDS research where it is relevant to vaccine design and to indicate areas where further information is required.

ASPECTS OF AIDS EPIDEMIOLOGY AND HIV TRANSMISSION

Epidemiological monitoring and clinical surveillance of AIDS has been important for identifying the various parameters involved in the epidemic spread of HIV infections, and for assessing morbidity and mortality trends associated with the syndrome. Identifying populations at risk, and determining the incidence of infection, not only enables the course of the pandemic to be predicted but also facilitates the planning of potential vaccination programmes and other public health measures designed to contain the spread of HIV. The available data all clearly indicate that AIDS is mainly a sexually transmitted disease.

In the Western world the populations most at risk to infection with HIV are homosexual or bisexual men, intravenous drug abusers and recipients of contaminated blood or blood products[8,9]. The incidence of HIV infections amongst the more general heterosexual communities is difficult to assess because of the ethical problems associated with mass screening programmes for seroprevalence, but it is known to be low. This contrasts with the situation in Africa where infection amongst the general heterosexual population is more common and not specifically restricted to identifiable risk groups[10–12]. Receptive anal intercourse, as well as vaginal intercourse involving both male to female and female to male routes, are probably all important and equally efficient mechanisms for transmitting HIV. The risk of infection increases with the number of sexual partners and with the number of infected individuals within the population involved[13]. Predisposing factors such as damage to mucous membranes due to trauma or underlying bacterial or

Table 1 A rationale for developing an AIDS vaccine

Studies on the epidemiology, mechanism of transmission and pathogenesis of AIDS
Studies on the immune responses to HIV – the effects of neutralizing antibodies and cell-mediated immune responses
Characterization of HIV isolates
Identification of possible immunogens and studies on their production, biochemical characterization and antigenicity
Studies on the cooperative effects of adjuvants and possible vaccine formulations
Animal testing for safety and efficacy
Human clinical trials and estimation of risk–benefit relationships
Development of large-scale production procedures with in-process quality assurance and control

viral disease may also facilitate both HIV transmission and acquisition[14,15]. HIV has been isolated from a wide range of body fluids and tissues, including whole blood, cell-free plasma, lymphocytes, lymph nodes, cerebrospinal fluid, brain tissue, semen, vaginal secretions, breast milk, saliva and tears. In theory, direct exposure to any contaminated human material may result in an HIV infection, but in practice the risk involved is largely dependent on the route for transmission. Hence the relatively high incidence of AIDS in recipients of unscreened blood or blood products[8,9], the high probability of perinatal or postnatal transmission from an infected mother[16-19] and the concern raised over the potential risks to health-care workers[20,21]. There is no convincing evidence to support the possibility that HIV is spread either by the aerosol route or by casual contact with infected individuals, but hitherto unrecognized or unusual routes of transmission cannot be totally excluded.

These considerations raise two points with respect to vaccine development. First, the route by which an HIV infection is acquired must be taken into account. Prevention of a sexually acquired infection is obviously of greatest importance, and this may indicate a need for inducing mucosal immunity. Second, the population to be vaccinated must be identified. Currently, in the West, it would probably be sufficient to consider a selective programme in which only the relatively small population at highest risk of an HIV infection was vaccinated, whereas in Africa mass vaccination programmes would be essential. Vaccines for use in Africa will have to be cheap, stable and preferably effective after a single dose; those for use in the West will not necessarily have these restrictions placed on them.

PATHOGENESIS OF AIDS

Infection with HIV initially results in a transient viraemia that is closely followed by the induction of antibodies to most, if not all, of the virus proteins[22]; some of these antibodies are capable of neutralizing HIV infectivity *in vitro*[23,24]. There is also some evidence, at least in the initial stages of infection, for the stimulation of some cell-mediated immune responses[25]. Seropositive individuals then enter a long and variable latent or asymptomatic period before progressing to clinical disease. The factors influencing disease development are not clearly understood, but those involving a generally reduced immune competence, the emergence of a more virulent HIV strain by replication *in vivo* as well as activation signals provided by concomitant infections with opportunistic pathogens have all been suggested[26]. A major and characteristic result of an HIV infection is the gradual and eventual catastrophic loss in the total number of circulating T4 helper/inducer lymphocytes with a coincident proliferation of B cells[3,27].

The T4 lymphocyte plays a critical role in the human immune response; it is involved either directly or indirectly in the functioning of cytotoxic T cells, natural killer cells, B cells, monocytes and macrophages, and with the production of various lymphokines. Depletion of T4 lymphocytes therefore produces a multitude of effects on normal immune functions and thereby significantly contributes to the severe immune suppression observed in AIDS patients and their consequent susceptibility to infection with opportunistic pathogens[28,29]. T4 helper/inducer lymphocytes are phenotypically defined by the presence of large amounts of the CD4 surface marker[30]. This antigen, which is a glycoprotein with a molecular weight of 60 000, is also expressed, but to a much smaller and variable extent, on the outer membranes of other cells such as those of the monocyte/macrophage lineage[31], Langerhans cells[32] and glial cells[33,34]. It is now known that the CD4 molecule is a specific and essential component of the receptor for HIV, and that binding to this receptor occurs prior to virus entry into a susceptible cell and its subsequent replication[35,36]. The detailed mechanism for viral entry is not clear, with receptor-mediated endocytosis[37] as well as pH-independent fusion of the cellular and viral surface membranes[38] having both been implicated. However, non-receptor-mediated virus entry cannot be completely excluded, particularly in phagocytic cells or other cell types that are rapidly turning over their outer membranes.

The infection of T4 helper/inducer lymphocytes with HIV results in a characteristic cytopathology and, ultimately, cell death[28,29]. These cytopathic effects are produced *in vitro* by the generation of giant or aggregated multinucleated cells, known as syncytia, through the fusion of both infected and uninfected cells. This undoubtedly contributes to, but does not completely explain, the precipitous loss of T4 lymphocytes in HIV-infected individuals. Similar cytopathic changes are not always observed in the other CD4-bearing cells that are susceptible to infection with HIV. In particular, monocytes appear to be refractile to the cytopathic effects of HIV; because of this they may act as the major reservoir for the virus, and may be responsible for its dissemination to various organs in the body[28,29,39]. This may have important consequences in the development of the other clinical conditions often associated with AIDS. For example, infected monocytes or macrophages may facilitate the secondary spread of HIV to susceptible glial cells in the brain, and thereby promote neurological disorders[40]. Similarly, transport of infected monocytes or macrophages to susceptible cells in the intestinal mucosa[41] may explain the enteropathological consequences of AIDS.

The total number of susceptible cells actually infected with HIV within an infected individual appears to be small, and the amount of free virus present in blood and other excreted body fluids is extremely low[42,43]. It seems quite likely that the number of infected cells increases during the development of AIDS, and this may correlate with the ease with which virus can be isolated from infected individuals as they progress through the disease state and with apparent increases in their infectiousness[22,44]. Not all infected cells actively replicate the virus, and it is now well documented that HIV is able to undergo latency in which a virus genome may be present in an unexpressed form[43,45,46]. The mechanisms involved in latency and subsequent reactivation are not understood, but the available data all indicate that much depends on a complex series of interactions between both cellular and viral derived proteins and the HIV genome[47,48]. There is some evidence to associate virus reactivation with a concomitant infection by other pathogens[49,50]. It is possible that primary infection with HIV is by direct exposure to free virus or, indirectly, by exposure to latently infected cells[51]. The relative efficiency of initiating an infection with these different sources of HIV is unknown.

Studies on the pathogenesis of AIDS raises a number of issues that need to be addressed when developing a candidate vaccine. One important feature is that circulating humoral antibodies with HIV neutralizing capacity can persist, albeit in low levels, throughout the course of clinical AIDS[23,24]. This implies that the stimulation of humoral immunity alone is not sufficient to eliminate HIV from the body following infection. Whether or not these antibodies, if present, are capable of preventing a primary infection remains an open question, but preliminary studies using animal models (see later) indicate that this will not be the case. Similar arguments can be advanced regarding the induction of cell-mediated immune responses as, again, the stimulation of cytotoxic responses against HIV infected cells does not eliminate the virus from infected individuals[25]. In short, it is simply not known what will actually constitute protective immunity to HIV.

This situation is complicated still further by the fact that pathogenic microorganisms are often controlled and eventually eliminated by degradation within phagocytic cells. Yet, as already indicated, these cells, which are members of the monocyte–macrophage lineage, are themselves susceptible to infection with HIV. Hence, antibody-complexed virus could well be delivered to appropriate target cells by normal immune mechanisms. Although it is not known if antibody-complexed virus can initiate an infection in these cells, it does imply that a more unconventional approach to vaccine design may be required[52]. Candidate vaccines will, by necessity, have to prevent both infection and disease, not only by free virus by also by latently infected cells. Thus, despite arguments to the contrary[53], post-infection immunization is unlikely to be effective unless a vaccine capable of eliminating all virus-infected cells is developed.

Another factor that must be taken into account during the development of an AIDS vaccine is that of antibody-dependent enhancement of infection. This has been observed with other viruses[54], and recent evidence indicates that it may occur during an HIV infection[55,56]. Two components in human sera have been shown to enhance an HIV infection and to mask the effect of HIV neutralizing antibodies. Both components are thought to be antibody, with one being heat-stable and uniquely present in sera from HIV-infected individuals, the other being heat-labile and present in normal sera. Cooperative interactions between these components may be responsible for facilitating an HIV infection, but the exact mechanisms involved are not clearly understood. Preliminary evidence indicates that the heat-labile component is complement, whereas the heat-stable enhancing activity is due to antibodies directed against the envelope protein of HIV[55]. The epitopes involved in this latter activity appear to be distinct from those inducing virus neutralization[56]. Thus it may be possible to design a vaccine which retains its capacity to induce virus neutralization but which does not induce antibody-dependent enhancement of infectivity.

One further point to consider during vaccine development is that of autoimmunity[26,29]. Evidence for an involvement of autoimmune responses in the pathogenesis of AIDS is far from clear and, at best, only suggestive[57,58]. Nevertheless, polyclonal B-cell activation leading to hyperglobulinaemia and the increased presence of antilymphocyte antibodies is often observed in AIDS patients; this could well lead to the formation of the immune complexes that are often associated with the clinical consequences of other autoimmune disorders[59,60]. In addition, infection with HIV augments the number of HIV-specific HLA class I restricted cytotoxic T cells and lymphokine-activated killer cells which may also be capable of producing autoimmune reactions[61]. Finally, because CD4 recognizes part of the class II major histocompatibility complex, and because the outer membrane of HIV binds to CD4, it has been proposed that the HIV envelope mimics the configuration of antigenic sites within the class II major histocompatibility complex molecule. Thus antibodies and cytotoxic responses induced by immunization with the envelope protein of HIV may induce autoimmune responses by cross-reacting with the class II major histocompatibility complex[29,62]. Clearly, candidate AIDS vaccines should not contain components that may be capable of inducing autoimmune responses.

STUDIES ON HIV REPLICATION AND CHARACTERIZATION

HIV is a member of the lentivirus subfamily of the retroviridae[63]. Other lentiviruses include visna virus of sheep[64] and caprine arthritis encephalitis virus of goats[65], both of which produce a progressive neurodegenerative disease, equine infectious anaemia virus[66] which causes haemolytic anaemia in horses and the feline[67], bovine[68] and simian[69] immunodeficiency viruses, which all produce similar pathogenic responses to HIV but in the corresponding animals. These viruses are all exogenous, non-transforming and cytopathic; they each have a restricted replication which leads to a latent infection of susceptible cells *in vivo*, and which probably contributes to their persistence in the host and to the slow, progressive nature of the diseases they cause.

Electronmicroscopy of HIV shows that the virus particle is approximately 100 nm in diameter[70–74]. A schematic representation of a mature HIV particle is shown in Figure 1. Each particle has an electron-dense cone-shaped core which contains two copies of a positive-sense RNA genome[75] in close association with the virus-encoded reverse transcriptase. Surrounding this there is a capsid, probably with icosahedral symmetry, composed of a protein with an aproximate molecular weight of 24 000 (p24). A coat composed of a protein with an approximate molecular weight of 17 000 (p17) surrounds the capsid, and finally there is an outer membrane composed of a lipid bilayer acquired during assembly of the virus particle on membrane surfaces of an infected cell. The outer virus membrane or envelope contains two virus-encoded glycoproteins with molecular weights of approximately 120 000 (gp120) and 41 000 (gp41); gp41 is a totally integrated transmembrane protein which is non-covalently bound to gp120, the outer envelope protein responsible for the external surface topography observed during electron microscopy of mature HIV particles. The outer envelope protein is either spontaneously shed during virus ageing or easily lost during the manipulation

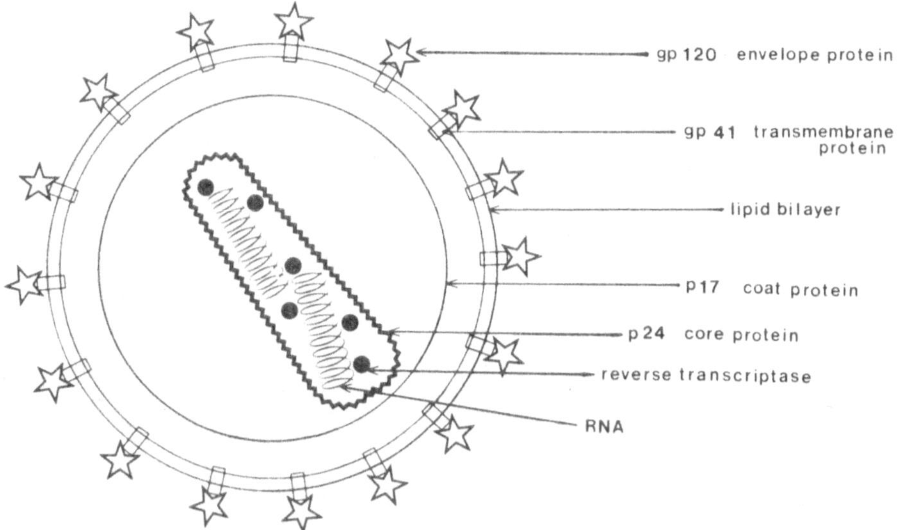

Figure 1 Schematic representation of the mature HIV particle

of virus preparations *in vitro*. The ease with which this occurs appears to depend on the virus strain under investigation; as gp120 is responsible for binding HIV to the CD4 receptor this observation may account for the high ratio of physical to infectious particles detected in virus preparations[76,77]. The outer membrane of HIV also contains variable amounts of cellular-derived proteins, but these have not been extensively characterized and their exact composition could well depend on the cell in which the virus was grown[73].

As indicated previously, the virus replicative cycle (Figure 2) which has both nuclear and cytoplasmic involvements is initiated by the binding of the envelope protein of HIV (gp120) to the CD4 receptor on susceptible cells[35,36]. After penetration into the cytoplasm the virus is uncoated and its RNA genome copied by reverse transcription first into single-stranded complementary DNA and then into a double-stranded molecule which is eventually circularized. The newly replicated virus nucleic acid is transported to the nucleus and is integrated into the host chromosome, possibly during cell division. Integration is a random event and each infected cell may contain several copies of the integrated provirus DNA; large amounts of unintegrated HIV DNA can also accumulate within infected T cells. Virus replication often stops at this stage to produce a latently infected cell in which there is little or no expression of the virus genetic information. The replicative cycle continues when mRNA and full-length copies of the virus genome are transcribed from the integrated provirus DNA, and when the virus-encoded gene products necessary for virus assembly and maturation are produced.

The assembly of mature HIV particles has been observed at two sites within infected cells. The first site, and the one most commonly reported in the literature, is the outer surface membrane of infected cells (Figure 3)[28,42,63,70,78,79]. Viruses with dense cores are rarely, if ever, seen connected

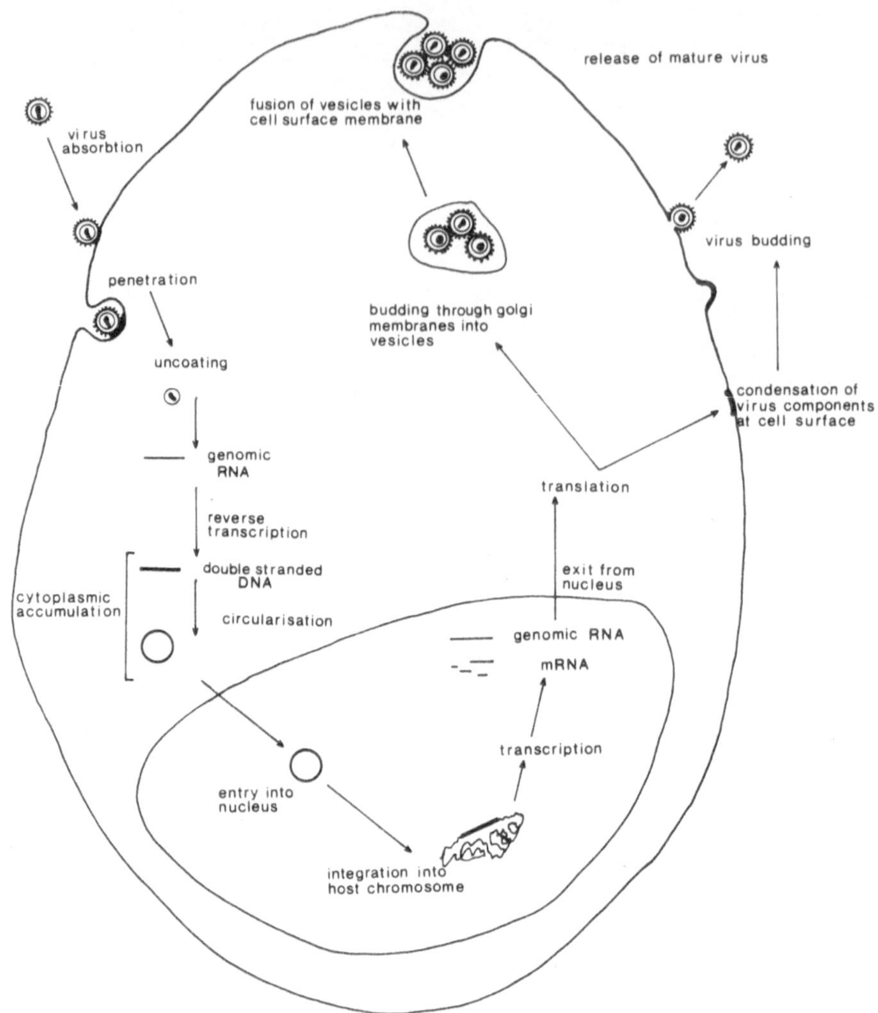

Figure 2 Replicative cycle of HIV

to the cell surface and it has been proposed that the last step in the maturation of HIV particles occurs outside the cell and involves the rearrangement of the inner structural components[79]. It has also been suggested that the localized assembly of virus particles at different regions of the cell surface contributes to the cytopathic effect of HIV by increasing the permeability of the surface membrane. The second site for the assembly of HIV particles is at the inner membranes of intracytoplasmic vesicles (Figure 4a). This has been observed in syncytia formed by the fusion of infected T lymphocytes *in vitro*[80], in macrophages[81], in macrophage-derived multinucleated giant cells from brain tissue[82] and in human rhabdomyosarcoma cells transfected with a full-length molecular clone of HIV[83]. Intracytoplasmic vesicles

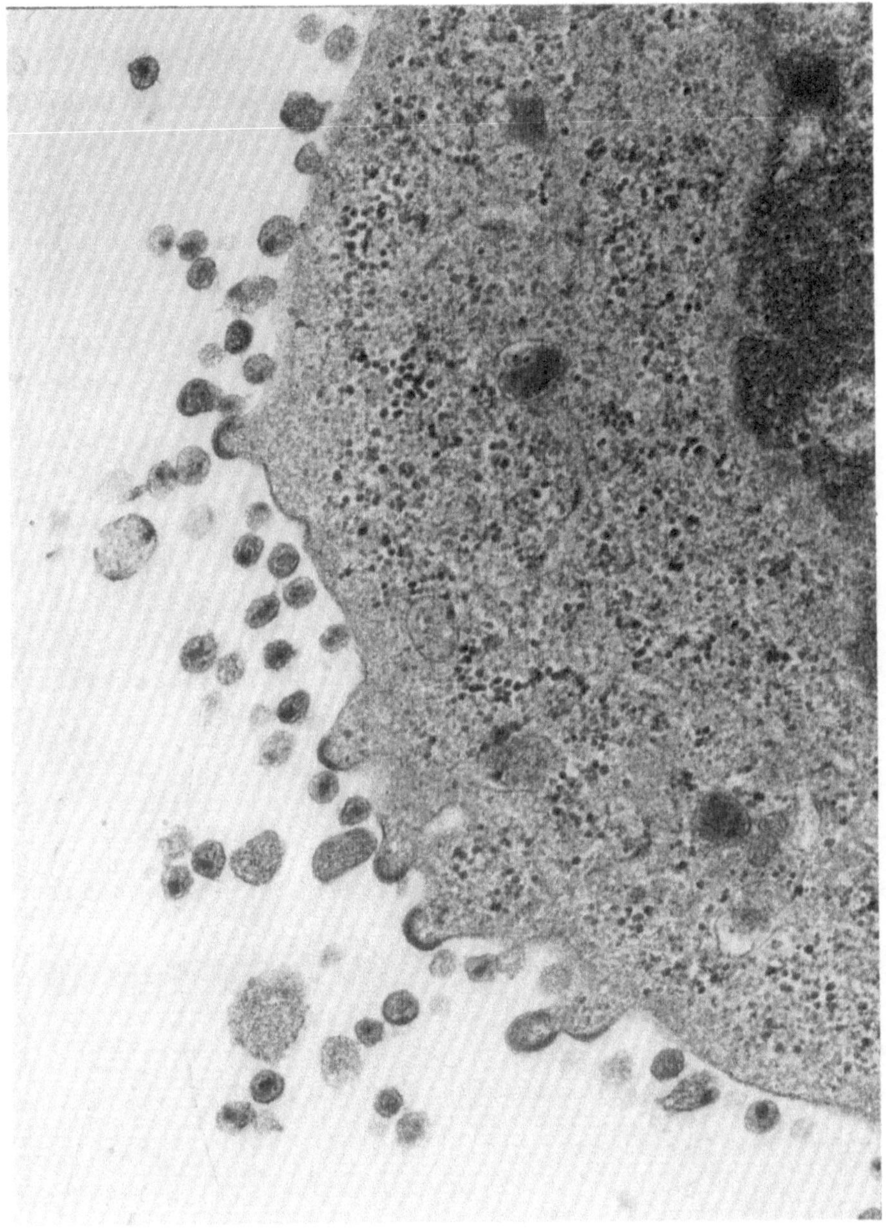

Figure 3 Assembly of mature HIV particles on the surface membrane of infected cells

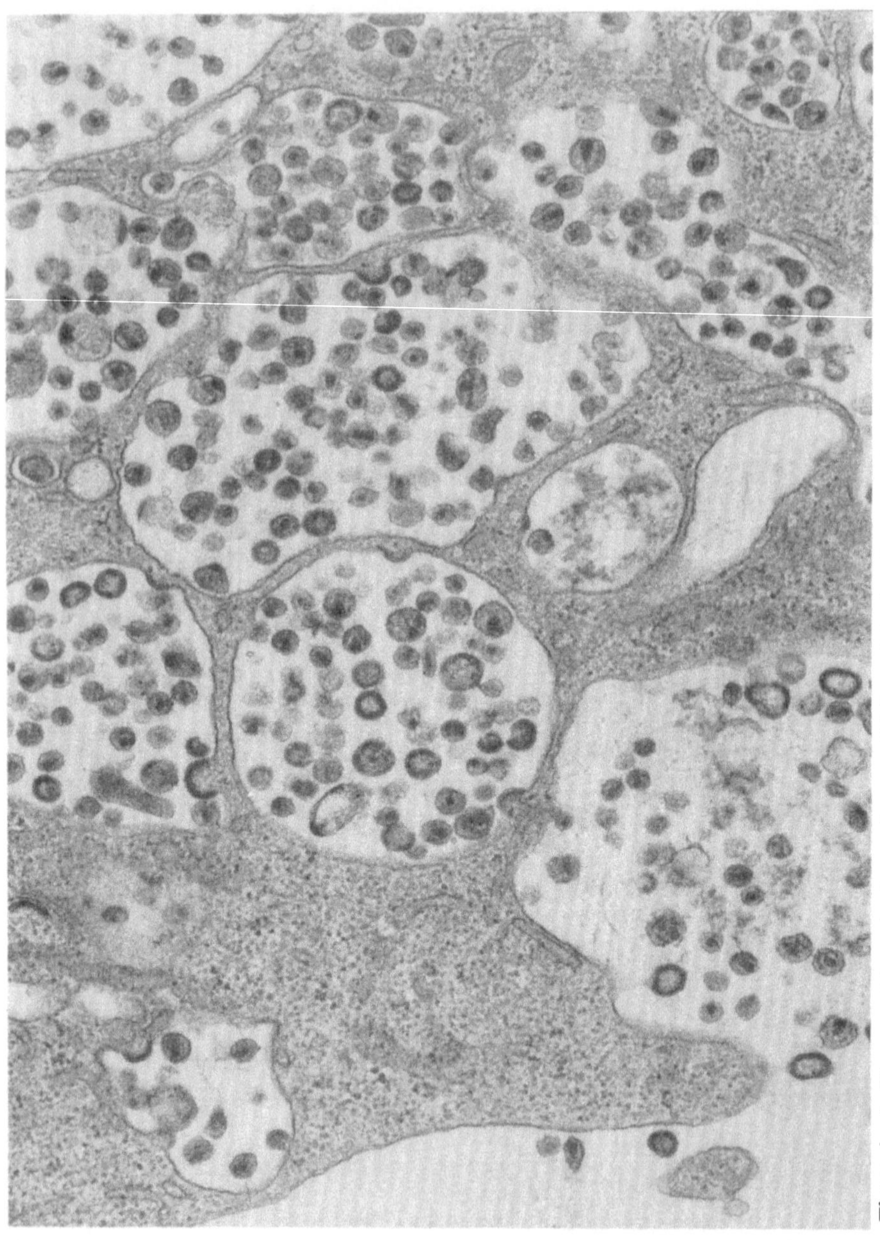

Figure 4 A: The assembly and release of mature HIV particles into intracytoplasmic vesicles

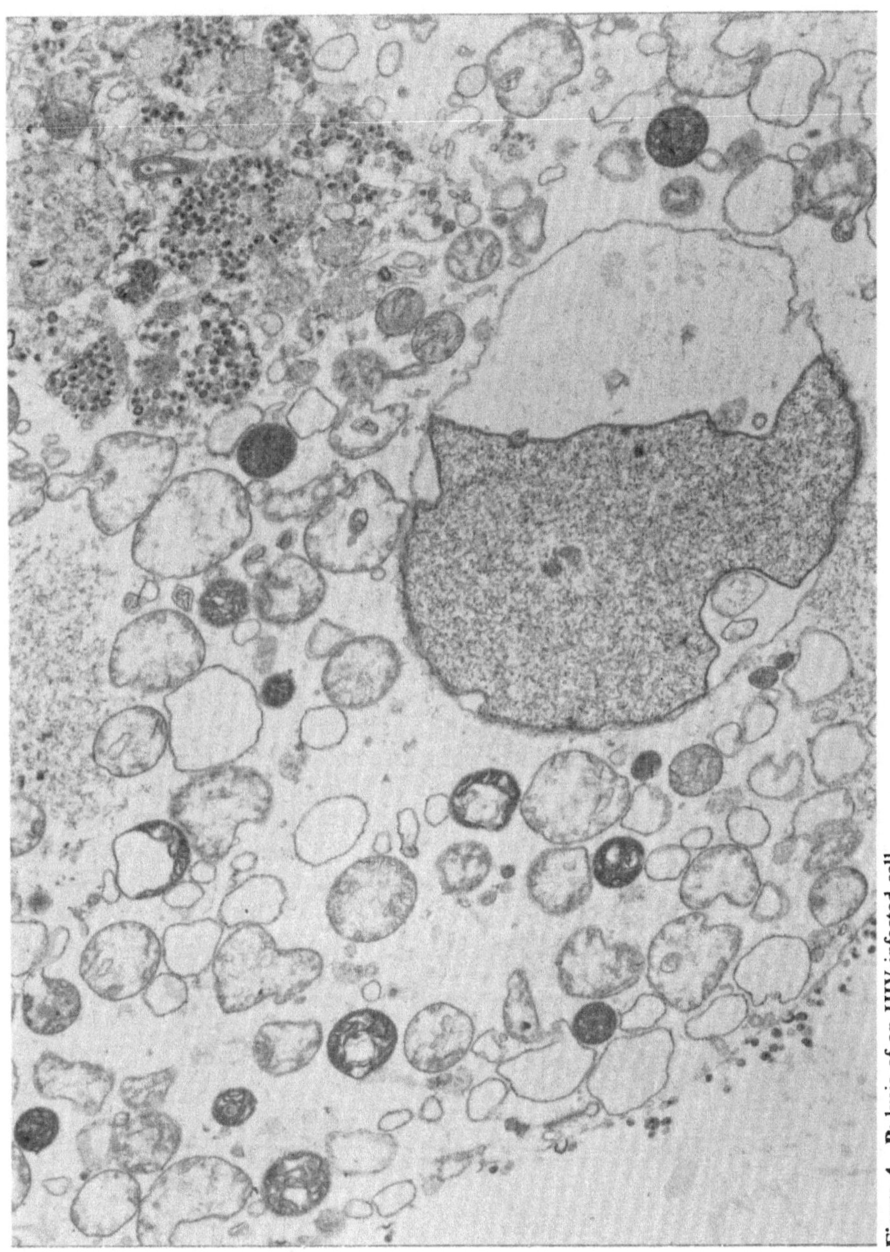

Figure 4 **B**: lysis of an HIV-infected cell

containing mature HIV particles are able to fuse with the outer membrane of infected cells and thereby release virus into the tissue spaces; the accumulation of large numbers of vesicles eventually results in the breakdown of membrane surfaces and the lysis of infected cells (Figure 4b). This morphogenetic pathway is often associated with the overproduction of HIV.

The formation of Golgi-derived multivesicular bodies has been observed in uninfected monocytes during differentiation[84]; thus those observed in HIV-infected cells may well have the same origin. Indeed, the condensation of HIV structural components has been observed directly on Golgi cisternae (Farrar, Dowsett and Greenaway, unpublished observations). In addition, enhanced production of tuboreticular structures, tubular confronting cisternae and intracytoplasmic vacuoles has been observed in the lymphocytes of AIDS patients but not asymptomatic carriers, and this may be related to disease progression[85].

Two major and readily distinguishable strains of human immunodeficiency virus, designated HIV-1 and HIV-2 have been isolated[4,5,6,86]. The genomes of these viruses differ slightly in size, but with one exception, contain the same genes in the same relative order (Figure 5 and Table 2). Each genome is flanked by long terminal repeat sequences which contain a variety of genetic control elements[87,88]. The virus encodes three major structural genes known as gag, pol and env. The gag gene is expressed via precursor polyproteins with approximate molecular weights of 200 000 (p200) and 55 000 (p55) which are subsequently processed into three proteins with molecular weights of 17 000 (p17), 24 000 (p24) and 15 000 (p15)[89,90]. p17 is associated with the virus capsid; it is myristylated and may therefore be required for the intracytoplasmic transport of the capsid to the site of virus assembly[90]. p24 is phosphorylated and carries the major group specific antigenic determinants. p15 is further processed to give two smaller peptides with molecular weights of 9000 (p9) and 7000 (p7)[89]; p9 is a proline-rich protein, whereas p7 has nucleic acid binding properties. The 5′-terminus of the pol gene overlaps the 3′-terminus of the gag gene out of frame by about 250 nucleotides[90–93]. These genes share a common mRNA and a ribosomal frameshifting mechanism operates to generate the pol gene precursor

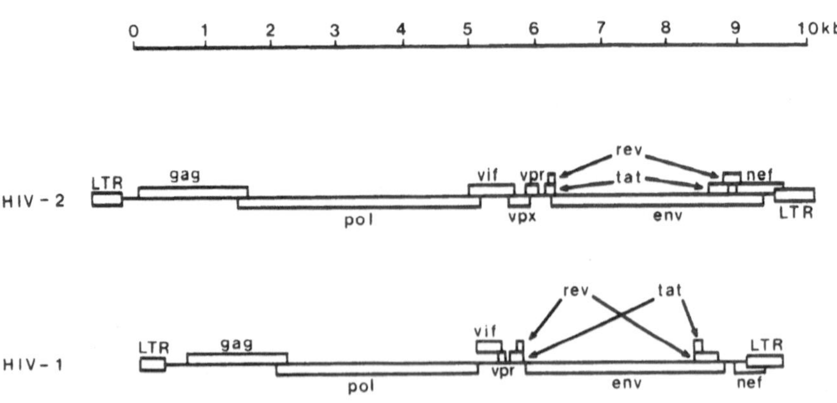

Figure 5 Organization of the HIV-1 and HIV-2 genomes

Table 2 The protein products of HIV genes and their proposed functions

HIV genes	*Molecular weights of protein product*	*Function*
gag	200 000	Precursor
	55 000	Precursor
	17 000	Capsid coat; possible transport function
	24 000	Major core protein; group-specific antigenic determinants
	15 000	Precursor
	9000	Proline- rich
	7000	Nucleic acid binding
pol	160 000	Precursor
	92 000	Precursor
	9000	Protease
	66 000	Reverse transcriptase/RNaseH
	51 000	Processing product
	15 000	RNaseH
	34 000	Endonuclease/Integrase
env	160 000	Precursor
	120 000	Outer envelope protein
	41 000	Transmembrane protein
tat	14 000	Transactivator
rev	20 000	Upregulator
vif	23 000	Facilitates virus transmission and production of infectious particles
nef	27 000	Negative regulator, involved with packaging of virus particles
vpr	15 000	Unknown
vpx (HIV-2 only)	16 000	Unknown

polyprotein which has a predicted molecular weight of approximately 160 000[94]. The cleavage sequence to generate the functional proteins encoded by pol has not been determined unequivocally, but probably involves at least one additional precursor with a molecular weight of 92 000[95]. The pol gene encodes four distinct enzymic activities – a protease, a reverse transcriptase with an associated RNaseH activity and an endonuclease or integrase. The mature protease has a molecular weight of approximately 9000 (p9) and is activated autocatalytically[95,96]; it is a member of the aspartic family of proteases and may function as a dimer[97]. p9 is responsible for the processing of the gag gene and, probably, the pol gene precursor polyproteins. Proteins with molecular weights of 66 000 (p66) and 51 000 (p51) were initially identified as being associated with the HIV reverse transcriptase[98]. Recent data[99,100] indicate that the reverse transcriptase activity is associated mainly with p66 but that processing of this molecule at its C-terminus occurs to release p51 and a further 15 000 molecular weight protein (p15)[100]. In addition to a reverse transcriptase activity p66 also has an RNaseH activity which is the processive exonuclease responsible for degrading HIV genomic RNA when duplexed to its complementary DNA after synthesis by reverse transcription. p15 also has RNaseH activity, but when free of p66 it has a lower template-binding ability and is non-processive or random in its mode of action. The relative abundance of p15, exceeding or equivalent to that of p66, suggests that it may be biologically relevant during HIV replication. Finally, the endonuclease encoded by the pol gene, which is responsible for integrating the HIV provirus into the host chromosome, has a molecular weight[101] of 34 000.

The primary product of the third major structural gene, env, is a glycosylated precursor protein with an approximate molecular weight of 160 000 (gp160) which is subsequently processed by proteolysis into a heterodimer containing the major envelope (gp120) and transmembrane (gp41) protein species referred to previously[102–105]. gp120 contains the CD4 binding site[35,36,106] and type-specific neutralizing determinants[23,24]; it may also be toxic to some cell types with an inherent ability to alter normal cell functions *in vitro*[107]. The carbohydrate moeities present on gp120 may be important for interactions with the CD4 receptor and, by analogy with other lentiviruses, for protecting the protein from proteolytic degradation and from rapid access by neutralizing antibodies[108,109]. In contrast, gp41 contains group specific antigenic determinants[110,111] and is responsible for the fusion of HIV and cellular membranes during entry of the virus into susceptible cells[112,113]. Non-covalent interactions between the amino terminus of gp120 and an exterior portion of gp41 are probably responsible for the association of these molecules after proteolytic cleavage of the gp160 precursor[112].

HIV also has at least five other non-structural genes; three of these have regulatory functions which control HIV gene expression and, ultimately, the mechanisms by which the virus exerts its pathogenic effects[87]. The first, and perhaps the most important, of these genes is tat. Tat is a spliced gene which overlaps part of the 3′-terminus of env in a different reading frame and which encodes a protein with an approximate molecular weight of 14 000[114,115]. This gene product is required for high-level expression of HIV genes in infected cells[116], and acts by binding to the TAR sequences present in the HIV LTR[117]. Effects on the rate of transcription, the stability of mRNA and on the derepression of translation have all been proposed as possible mechanisms for the mode of action of this protein[87]. The rev gene, which was previously known as art or trs, and which contains two exons that partially overlap the 3′-terminus of env and parts of tat in the third reading frame, encodes a protein with an approximate molecular weight of 20 000[118,119]. This protein is necessary for the synthesis of the gag, pol and env proteins, upregulating their expression by a trans-activating anti-repression mechanism[120] that may control the extent of mRNA processing. The sequence elements responsive to the rev gene product have not yet been identified.

The vif gene, also known as either sor, A, P′ or Q, overlaps the 3′-terminus of the pol gene in a different reading frame and encodes a protein with an approximate molecular weight of 23 000[91–93,121–123]. The function of the vif gene product is not clearly understood, for although it is necessary for the efficient generation of infectious particles it is not directly required for their formation. The vif gene product also apparently enhances HIV transmission *in vitro*, but this effect appears to depend on the cell type infected[124,125]. The nef gene, previously known as either 3′-orf, B, E′ or F, overlaps the HIV LTR and, in the case of HIV-2, also overlaps the 3′-terminus of env[91–93,126]. The gene encodes a myristylated protein with a molecular weight of approximately 27 000 which, although not essential for either the replication or cytopathogenicity of HIV, probably functions by being a negative regulator of virus gene expression[127–129], and by being involved with the packaging of virus particles at the inner surface of the outer membrane of infected cells[130]. The protein is antigenic *in vivo*[129,131]. A further gene, vpr, previously known as R, has also been identified[91–93,132] and is located between the pol and env genes. It probably encodes a protein with an anticipated molecular weight of 15 000. Although the function of this protein is unknown it is immunogenic, and is recognized by sera from some HIV-seropositive individuals; it is unlikely to be required for HIV replication. Finally, two other genes need to be considered. The first, which is known as vpx and which is unique to HIV-2, encodes a protein with a predicted molecular weight of 16 000[126]; the function of this protein remains to be determined. The second, identified by inspection of HIV genomic nucleotide sequences, is located on the opposite (plus) strand to that of the env gene, and has a coding capacity sufficient to produce a protein with a molecular weight of 20 000[133]. It is not known whether this potential open reading frame is utilized during an HIV infection and, if so, whether the protein has a functional role. Bidirectional transcription of the same fragment of genetic information is not without precedent in eukaryotic viruses[134,135] and this may restrict the evolutionary capacity of the genes concerned. It is possible that the production of an RNA species complementary in sequence to env mRNA may, by base-pairing, reduce the efficiency of its translation and hence control the level of gp160 produced.

As indicated above, most, if not all, of the HIV gene products are immunogenic, and some induce antibodies that are able to neutralize the virus *in vitro*. There may be some correlation between the presence of antibodies against different HIV-encoded proteins and the clinical status of infected individuals[22,136]. Some of the HIV gene products are also capable of directly inducing cell-mediated immune responses to HIV antigen-presenting cells[137,139]. Hence most of the HIV gene products, either individually or in combination, are legitimate candidates for inclusion in potential AIDS vaccine formulations. However, the inherent toxicity of some of these proteins, and the possibility of immune responses to down-regulating proteins such as nef facilitating HIV replication, provide counter-arguments, or at least cautionary arguments, against this.

Nucleotide sequence analyses on different isolates of HIV show that the virus is rapidly evolving[140] such that significant genetic variation can be detected between isolates obtained not only from different geographical locations[91–93] but also from the same individual at different times[141]. These sequence changes often result in changes to the translation products of the different HIV genes[142]. The pattern of sequence variation is not constant over the entire HIV genome, with the gag, pol and the non-structural genes all being more conserved than env. Even within env the observed variations are not uniformly distributed, as both highly conserved and hypervariable regions can be identified[141,143–145]. Recombination between unintegrated provirus variants and reverse transcription, which is known to be associated with high rates of mutation, have both been proposed as possible mechanisms for generating this observed genetic variation[146].

One of the consequences of genetic variation is the generation of HIV variants which have a differential sensitivity to serum neutralization[147] and an altered ablity to induce the synthesis of cross-neutralizing antibodies[148]. Epitopes encoded by different regions of the env gene[148–152] are likely to be responsible for the selection of HIV variants with a capacity to evade immune surveillance within the host. Other biological features that show a similar variation have also been detected amongst different HIV isolates. These include the isolation of HIV subtypes from the central nervous system which replicate more efficiently in macrophages than in T lymphocytes[39], the isolation of variants with a differential capacity to induce the formation of syncytia[153]or to produce other cytopathogenic responses[154,155], and the isolation of subtypes with altered virulence[156].

It is clear that a wide spectrum of genetic variation exists between the two prototype strains designated HIV-1 and HIV-2, and that this variation is reflected by changes in the biological properties of different isolates. The true effect of this on the pathogenesis of AIDS remains to be established, and it obviously has to be taken into account during the development of an AIDS vaccine so that protection can be obtained not only against variants which do not show close antigenic relationships and which do not cross-neutralize, but also against those showing different tropisms or capable of inducing different cytopathic effects. This may mean that the 'ideal' vaccine will have to contain immunogens derived from representative examples of all the identifiable HIV subtypes or, more speculatively, that vaccine formulations will have to be 'custom-made' to suit the population for which protection is required. Clearly, vigilant monitoring and detailed biological characterization of the HIV subtypes circulating within either defined or more general communities is necessary, until the consequences of the high evolutionary rate of this virus has been fully evaluated.

CANDIDATE AIDS VACCINES

Current attempts to formulate an effective AIDS vaccine are based largely on a historical perspective of approaches that have been successfully used with other pathogenic microorganisms. Some of these approaches are unlikely to succeed, due to inherent problems associated with the pathogenesis of HIV, and more innovative developments are likely to be required. These will undoubtedly depend on advances in molecular biology and immunology, but until the mechanisms for inducing protective immunity to HIV have been defined unequivocally the development of an AIDS vaccine has to remain only a theoretical possibility. However, this has not prevented a variety of potential vaccine formulations from being produced, some of which are now undergoing evaluation in both *in vitro* and *in vivo* systems.

Some of the more common vaccines generally available are based on an inactivated preparation of the corresponding bacterial or viral pathogen. Inactivation procedures using such chemical inactivants as formalin, psoralen or 4β-propiolactone, which destroy infectivity yet retain at least some immunogenicity, are well documented. Although simple to adopt, this approach has a number of drawbacks which make it unsuitable for HIV[157]. These include having to grow large amounts of virus using secure physical containment, and having a totally reliable indicator of complete inactivation; the virus may also need to be highly purified to prevent unwanted side-reactions due to cellular contaminants. In addition, there would have to be safeguards to ensure that there was no possibility of unmodified virus nucleic acid becoming inserted into the host chromosome or recombining with endogenous virus sequences to reactivate or to otherwise generate mutant infectious virus with an unknown pathogenesis. Some of these difficulties might be circumvented by the use of genetically inactivated, replication-deficient strains, but the general approach is receiving little current attention due to the logistical problems involved. However, killed or inactivated vaccines may yet prove useful in animal challenge systems, so that a better understanding of protective immunity can be obtained.

Similar arguments have been advanced against the use of live, attenuated virus vaccines which have additional major problems because of their potential to revert back to a virulent phenotype during replication in the recipient and because of the possbility of establishing a persistent or latent infection. Hence live attenuated vaccines based on HIV itself are, at present, considered totally impracticable. However, antigens presented to the immune system during attenuated virus replication have been shown to be one of the most efficient ways to produce long-lasting protective immunity against a number of other pathogens. Hence the use of live but recombinant or hybrid viruses capable of expressing specific HIV antigens and presenting them to the immune system during replication, in the same way as they would be during a natural infection, is being actively investigated. The construction of recombinant viruses based on adenovirus, herpesvirus and vaccinia virus have all been proposed, but at present work is concentrating on the use of the latter agent. Some of the advantages for developing a live recombinant AIDS vaccine based on vaccinia virus include a well-defined history of use in mass immunization programmes, ease of production and administration, and good stability. The disadvantages to its use centre largely on the toxic side-effects that can occur, especially after primary immunization of adults. Several groups have now constructed recombinant vaccinia viruses that contain and express different HIV gene products[139,158,159]; those containing the HIV env gene have been shown to glycosylate, process and transport the corresponding gene product to the plasma membrane of infected cells[158]. These recombinants also induce both humoral and cell-mediated immune responses in macaques[160], chimpanzees[161,162] and humans[163,164]; however, preliminiary results indicate that immunized monkeys are not protected from a subsequent HIV challenge[160–162]. Further work is clearly needed to evaluate fully this approach as a means of developing an AIDS vaccine.

The adverse safety implications associated with the use of either attenuated or killed AIDS vaccines has resulted in a considerable amount of effort being placed in the development of a subunit vaccine. As indicated above, most of the HIV-encoded gene products are antigenic *in vivo*, and each is therefore a candidate for use as an immunizing reagent. However, gp120, which has an external location on the virus particle and a unique involvement with both virus adsorption and the immune system, is considered to be the prime candidate for a subunit vaccine. The most obvious source of material for use in subunit vaccine preparations is either HIV-infected cells or purified virus[90,165–167]. This immediately presents the problem of the need to grow large amounts of virus under secure physical containment and, subsequently, of developing purification procedures that will ensure that the product is free of virus nucleic acid and other unwanted cellular contaminants. The techniques of genetic manipulation, to transfer and express relevant parts of the HIV genome in more suitable host cell systems, can be utilized to overcome these particular problems. There is now a wealth of literature describing the cloning and expression of different HIV genes in a variety of sytems that range from prokaryotes, such as *Escherichia coli*[89,90,95,96,99,111,123,131,168–177] or *Bacillus subtilis*[178], through simple eukaryotes, such as yeasts[179,180] to insect[181,182] and mammalian cells[158,159,183–185]. Thus, relatively simple fermentation procedures can now be used to produce large amounts of individual HIV proteins. Each host system used for genetic manipulation is associated with its own advantages and disadvantages, but one of the factors that may determine which is used is whether or not the protein produced is subjected to post-translational modification. Proteins produced in prokaryotic environments are not glycosylated and hence, if carbohydrate groups prove to be necessary for inducing the correct immune response, other sources of these proteins will be required. Although yeast and insect cells can produce glycosylated proteins this, in turn, may not be sufficient, as the pattern of glycosylation differs quite significantly from that which occurs in mammalian cells.

The HIV proteins obtained via genetic manipulation techniques have been shown to produce similar immune responses to their native counterparts when inoculated into experimental animals[96,111,139,151,160–162,169,171,176]. Hence, this approach to the production of an AIDS subunit vaccine seems a reasonable proposition. However, some problems are anticipated because of the observed genetic variability between different HIV isolates. Proteins produced using the genetic information of one strain may not induce a cross-protective immune response during a challenge with a different variant. Possible ways around this problem include placing greater emphasis on proteins with conserved sequences between different HIV isolates, and on making subunit vaccine preparations that contain mixtures of proteins derived from the genetic sequences of a number of strains.

A further refinement to this approach has been made possible by the identification of immunodominant domains (or epitopes) on various HIV proteins[110–112,143,144,148–151]. If specific linear (or continuous) epitopes present on individual HIV proteins are shown to be able to induce protective immunity then chemical synthesis can be used to produce a peptide for use in a purely synthetic vaccine preparation[186–188]. This offers many advantages, as the required components would be stable, cheap to produce in high purity, and any amino acid sequences associated with toxic side-effects could be eliminated. Such synthetic vaccines would have to take into account the genetic variability of HIV, but this may not turn out to be important if the epitopes concerned were conserved between different isolates. A potential disadvantage to the use of a single peptide within a vaccine preparation may result from the fact that cell-mediated immune responses to HIV are HLA restricted. Hence, cytotoxic T-lymphocyte responses in different individuals may not always be induced by the same epitope within a given protein species. Even so, synthetic peptides containing linear epitopes from, in particular gp120, have been shown to induce virus-neutralizing antibodies when inoculated into experimental animals, thus demonstrating the feasibility of this approach[186,187].

Whilst synthetic peptides, like whole proteins, may possess the specificity demanded from a vaccine preparation, they are often associated with a low antigenicity and may therefore require adjuvants to enhance their potency[189,190]. Although many adjuvants are now known, relatively few have been clinically evaluated for toxic side-reactions and even fewer have been accepted for human use. Some adjuvants, such as aluminium hydroxide, aluminium phosphate and muramyl dipeptide, are relatively simple and defined chemical compounds, whereas others are quite complex and are basically ill-defined extracts from plant or bacterial sources. Natural immuno-potentiators such as human interleukin-1, which is able to enhance the presentation of soluble antigens to T cells and thereby stimulate antibody production, are also under active consideraton as potential adjuvants.

The ways in which adjuvants function are not fully understood, but novel ways of presenting the antigen to the immune system are likely to be involved. In this respect the presentation of an antigen as a defined multimeric complex may be one of the most efficient ways of stimulating an immune response. Thus the generation of protein micelles which represent an aggregation of antigenic components, the formation of liposomes in which proteins or peptides are embedded within phospholipid vesicles or the production of immunostimulating complexes based on the glycoside Quil A, in which antigens are incorporated into a defined clathrin or cage-like multimeric structure, have all been considered as possible ways of enhancing the immunogenicity of either isolated HIV proteins or synthetic peptides[191,192]. Yet more sophisticated approaches, again utilizing the techniques of genetic manipulation, have also been used to produce novel multimolecular structures with immune enhancing properties. The incorporation of HIV genetic information into the yeast Ty transposon[180] or into hepatitis B virus genetic sequences[193], to generate non-replicative, assembled particles, offer two such possibilities for increasing the immunogenicity of defined epitopes derived from HIV proteins. With such great emphasis being placed on the development of subunit vaccines further work is clearly needed on the use of adjuvants, and on the development of more efficient antigen presentation systems, as these will be critical for the induction of an effective protective immune response.

One further and more theoretical approach to the development of an

AIDS vaccine is based on the idiotypic–anti-idiotypic network theory[194], and on the molecular mimicry that is thought to be involved. In this approach antibodies to the gp120 binding site on the CD4 receptor (idiotypic antibodies) are themselves used in vaccine formulations to induce the synthesis of further antibodies (anti-idiotypic antibodies). The induced anti-idiotypic antibodies should, in theory, mimic the conformation of the CD4 receptor and thereby bind to the CD4 binding site on gp120 to facilitate virus neutralization and to prevent infection. Although this represents a somewhat complex approach it is technically feasible, and its adoption circumvents the safety problems associated with immunization schedules involving live HIV or purified virus components[195]. Some advances in this area have already been made using murine monoclonal antibodies directed against the leu 3A epitope on the CD4 receptor[196]. The anti-idiotypic antibodies induced by inoculation of these monoclonal antibodies into experimental animals not only neutralize different isolates of HIV-1 but also neutralize one isolate of HIV-2[197]. Hence, anti-idiotype vaccines may provide a mechanism for overcoming the difficulties associated with the genetic variability of HIV.

ANIMAL MODELS

As indicated above, there is no shortage of either ideas or potential immunogens for candidate AIDS vaccine preparations. However, the real key to the development of an effective AIDS vaccine rests on the identification of a suitable animal model that can be utilized in challenge experiments to investigate the most effective way of stimulating protective immunity. An ideal model would be one in which HIV infects a readily available laboratory animal to reproducibly produce a disease with an AIDS-like pathogenesis within a reasonable time. Unfortunately, as yet, no such model exists as the only animal, apart from man, that can be infected with HIV is the chimpanzee[198–200]. Infected chimpanzees consistently produce both humoral[200–202] and cell-mediated[203] immune responses against various HIV-encoded proteins, but despite the fact that virus can be repeatedly re-isolated from them[202], they do not apparently progress to produce the clinical symptoms associated with human AIDS. Although inappropriate as a disease model, it is the only system in which HIV can be used in challenge experiments to investigate the ability of vaccine preparations to stimulate protective immunity and to prevent infection. As a consequence, a number of potential AIDS vaccines have been used in the chimpanzee model but, as yet, none has proved effective at protecting immunized animals from infection[203–206]. Although disappointing, it is probably fair to say that this failure may be due as much to the small numbers of animals used with inappropriate doses of challenge virus as to the inadequacies of the vaccine preparations themselves.

The general lack of large numbers of chimpanzees, along with the constraints of expense and general husbandry, also make this an unsuitable animal model for routine use during the initial stages of vaccine development. Hence serious consideration is being given to the use of the other immunodeficiency viruses, particularly the simian immunodeficiency viruses, and their corresponding susceptible animals as alternative model systems[67–69]. Simian immunodeficiency viruses have been isolated from a number of Old World primate species[69,207–210]; they are similar to HIV in terms of genetic structure, morphology, growth characteristics and cell tropisms[211,212]. Some of these viruses will, on inoculation into rhesus macaques, produce a disease with a relatively short incubation period and with a pathogenesis that closely resembles human AIDS[213–216]. Clinically, infected animals develop lymphadenopathy, diarrhoea and weight loss soon after seroconversion, and some also develp neuropathological symptoms. Concomitant changes in immune function increase the susceptibility of infected animals to infection with a variety of opportunistic pathogens. The induced disease is therefore associated with a high rate of morbidity and mortality, and it has been shown that the strength of the immune response to SIV antigenic determinants directly correlates with the ability of infected animals to survive. Hence, although it has to remain a less-than-perfect model for developing a human AIDS vaccine, it does provide an excellent system for pathogenicity studies, and for investigating the potential of different immunogenic preparations, based on material derived from SIV, to protect against both infection and disease. The major limitation of the SIV model is that it has to be assumed that any data obtained will directly correlate with HIV in the corresponding human situation. However, a compromise may be possible if it can be demonstrated that candidate vaccines based on HIV immunogens are capable of preventing a SIV-induced disease in the rhesus macaque. Considerable groundwork is still needed to establish the SIV rhesus macaque model but, as with the chimpanzee model, initial experiments using a range of potential vaccine formulations have been unable to demonstrate that protective immunity can be induced.

Other animal models based on the infection of cats with the feline immunodeficiency virus (FIV)[67] or cattle with the bovine immunodeficiency virus (BIV)[68] are much less advanced than the primate models. That based on FIV has the obvious advantages associated with the availability and the relatively low costs of maintaining infected animals. Its disadvantages are that it produces fewer disease symptoms characteristic of an AIDS-like illness, and that it does not apparently have a tropism for $CD4^+$ bearing cells[68,217,218]. Obviously, further work on this and other potential animal model systems is urgently needed.

VACCINE EVALUATION

It goes without saying that before a vaccine can be properly evaluated methods for its large-scale production should be fully established so that sufficient amounts can be reproducibly obtained under conditions appropriate for the manufacture of human therapeutic substances. Suitable quality control and quality assurance procedures should also be in place to ensure that there is standardization of purity and composition from batch to batch, and that the product remains sterile and stable for a specified period of time.

The actual procedures adopted for this will depend not only on the manufacturing process but also on the materials used to generate the viral antigen incorporated into the vaccine formulation. Of particular concern are in-process control procedures to ensure that products generated by recombinant DNA methods have the required amino acid sequence and do not contain unwanted contaminants due to, for example, premature termination of transcription or translation of the manipulated virus genetic information. Obviously adequately sized and suitably characterized seed lots of any cells, virus strains or recombinant microorganisms used in the manufacture of the vaccine preparation under consideration need to be established.

Procedures necessary for vaccine manufacture, standardization and control are usually developed during the preclinical testing period that precedes the clinical trials for effectivensess and potency[219]. Generally, preclinical testing of vaccine preparations in animals is a prerequisite for their subsequent evaluation in humans. This testing provides data not only on the types of immune response that can be induced, but also on the dose and immunization regime necessary to achieve this response. The data obtained can then be used to estimate an effective immunizing dose for humans, and to provide some form of assurance that the product under consideration is unlikely to produce extreme toxic side-reactions. However, because of the lack of a well-characterized animal model for preclinical evaluation at least six separate human trials have begun. These trials involve vaccine preparations based on killed, whole virus[220], vaccinia recombinants containing the gp120 gene[164], baculovirus derived gp160[221], gp120[222], a synthetic peptide from p18 using keyhole limpet haemocyanin as adjuvant[223] and an anti-idiotype antibody[224]. These trials currently involve only small numbers of volunteers, and may not therefore be sufficiently controlled to provide anything other than anecdotal evidence on the safety and efficacy of each preparation.

Under more usual circumstances clinical trials of potential vaccine preparations proceed in three defined phases. The first phase usually involves small numbers of healthy volunteers derived from a low-risk population, and is specifically designed to assess the safety of the vaccine preparation. A limited amount of information on immunogenicity is generally obtained, but this is studied more intensively during the second phase, which involves a larger group of individuals drawn from the target population but who are at low risk for disease acquisition. Broader issues such as dose–response, immunization regimes, the extent and quality of the immune response and a more in-depth assessment of both local and systemic side-reactions are all addressed during this phase. The efficacy of a vaccine preparation is really only considered during the third and final phase of a clinical trial. This is normally done with a relatively large group of volunteers derived from a target group with a high incidence of AIDS. The actual size of the trial group will be determined by the anticipated incidence of HIV infection amongst the unvaccinated control group during the trial, on whether the vaccine is to prevent infection or disease, and on the confidence limits set for estimating vaccine efficacy. The actual design of a phase three clinical trial for a candidate AIDS vaccine will be complex, because the ethical issues involved may ultimately bias the conclusions made. This is almost inevitable, as the very population in which the vaccine is to be evaluated must, ethically, receive continuous in-depth counselling on ways to modify high-risk behaviour and thereby reduce exposure to HIV. It may therefore be difficult to differentiate between the effectiveness of the vaccine and the effectiveness of the associated education programme.

Any phase three vaccine trial requires meticulous planning, independent monitoring and long-term follow-up, but an AIDS vaccine trial, if it is to be effective, must also take into account the genetic variability of HIV, the different mechanisms for transmission and the various clinical manifestations of the disease. It may also be necessary to conduct independent trials in different parts of the world, so that a range of socioeconomic factors involved in disease development, such as nutritional status, level of hygiene and exposure to different populations of opportunistic pathogens can all be taken into account. These are not insurmountable problems but, coupled with the fact that more information is still required regarding the induction of protective immunity to HIV, they clearly demonstrate that the general availability of a truly effective AIDS vaccine is still some considerable time away. Unfortunately time is not on our side, and it is a cruel fact of life that short cuts will be taken, bad science will be supported, and many false hopes will be raised as many members of the scientific community race to develop a vaccine that will protect the human population from the devastating consequences of AIDS.

ACKNOWLEDGEMENTS

I wish to thank Dr G. Farrar for a critical appraisal of this article, Barry Dowsett for the electron micrographs and Miss T. M. Gallagher for patience and care in preparing the manuscript. I also wish to acknowledge the continuing financial support from the AIDS Directed Programme of the Medical Research Council which has enabled this article to be written.

REFERENCES

1. Gottlieb, M. S., Schroff, R., Schanker, H. M., Weisman, J. D., Fan, P. T., Wolf, R. A. and Saxon, A. (1981). *Pneumocystis carinii* pneumonia and mucosal candidiasis in previously healthy homosexual men: evidence of a new acquired cellular immunodeficiency. *N. Engl. J. Med.*, **305**, 1425–31
2. Masur, H., Michelis, M. A., Greene, J. B., Onorato, I., Van de Stouwe, R. A., Holzman, R. S., Wormser, G., Brettman, L., Lange, M., Murray, H. W. and Cunningham-Rundles, S. (1981). An outbreak of community-acquired *Pneumocystis carinii* pneumonia: initial manifestation of cellular immune dysfunction. *N. Engl. J. Med.*, **305**, 1431–8
3. Siegal, F. P., Lopez, C., Hammer, G. S., Brown, A. E., Kornfeld, S. J., Gold, J., Hassett, J., Hirschman, S. Z., Cunningham-Rundles, C., Adelsberg, B. R., Parham, D. M., Siegal, M., Cunningham-Rundles, S. and Armstrong, D. (1981). Severe acquired immunodeficiency in male homosexuals manifested by chronic perianal ulcerative herpes simplex lesions. *N. Engl. J. Med.*, **305**, 1439–44
4. Barre-Sinoussi, F., Chermann, J. C., Rey, F., Nugeyre, M. T., Chamaret, S., Gruest, J., Dauguet, C., Axler-Blin, C., Vezinet-Brun, F., Rouzioux, C., Rozenbaum, W. and Montagn-

ier, L. (1983). Isolation of a T-lymphotropic retrovirus from a patient at risk for acquired immune deficiency syndrome (AIDS). *Science*, **220**, 868–71
5. Gallo, R. C., Salahuddin, S. Z., Popovic, M., Shearer, G. M., Kaplan, M., Haynes, B. F., Palker, T. J., Redfield, R., Oleske, J., Safai, B., White, G., Foster, P. and Markham, P. D. (1984). Frequent detection and isolation of cytopathic retroviruses (HTLV-III) from patients with AIDS and at risk for AIDS. *Science*, **224**, 500–3
6. Levy, J. A., Hoffman, A. D., Kramer, S. M., Landis, J. A., Shimabukuro, J. M. and Oshiro, L. S. (1984). Isolation of lymphocytopathic retroviruses from San Francisco patients with AIDS. *Science*, **225**, 840–2
7. Fineberg, H. V. (1988). Education to prevent AIDS: prospects and obstacles. *Science*, **239**, 592–6
8. Curran, J. W., Jaffe, H. W., Hardy, A. M., Morgan, W. M., Selik, R. M. and Dondero, T. J. (1988). Epidemiology of HIV infection and AIDS in the United States. *Science*, **239**, 610–16
9. McCormick, A., Tillet, H., Bannister, B. and Emslie, J. (1987). Surveillance of AIDS in the United Kingdom. *Br. Med. J.*, **234**, 1466–9
10. Quinn, T. C., Mann, J. C., Curran, J. W. and Piot, P. (1986). AIDS in Africa: an epidemiologic paradigm. *Science*, **234**, 955–63
11. Mann, J. (1987). AIDS in Africa. *New. Sci.*, **113**(1553), 40–43
12. Piot, P., Plummer, F. A., Mhalu, F. S., Lamboray, J.L., Chin, J. and Mann, J. M. (1988). AIDS: an international perspective. *Science*, **239**, 573–9
13. Anderson, R. M. and May, R. M. (1988). Epidemiological parameters of HIV transmission. *Nature*, **333**, 514–19
14. Archer, D. L. and Glinsmann, W. H. (1985). Enteric infections and other cofactors in AIDS. *Immunol. Today*, **6**, 292–5
15. Weber, J. N., McCreaner, A., Berrie, E., Wadsworth, J., Jeffries, D. J., Pinching, A. J. and Harris, J. R. W. (1986). Factors affecting seropositivity of human T-cell lymphotropic virus type III (HTLV-III) or lymphadenopathy associated virus (LAV) and progression of disease in sexual partners with AIDS. *Genitoruin. Med.*, **62**, 177–80
16. Pahwa, S., Kaplan, M., Fikrig, S., Pahwa, R., Sarngadharan, M. G., Popovic, M. and Gallo, R. C. (1986). Spectrum of human T cell lymphotrophic virus type III infection in children. *J. Am. Med. Assoc.*, **255**, 2299–305
17. Mok, J. Q., Giaquinto, C., De Rossi, A., Grosch-Worner, I., Ades, A. E. and Peckham, C. S. (1987). Infants born to mothers seropositive for human immunodeficiency virus. *Lancet*, **1**, 1164–8
18. Borkowsky, W., Krasinski, W. K., Paul, D., Moore, T., Benenroth, D. and Chandwani, S. (1987). Human immunodeficiency virus infections in infants negative for anti-HIV by enzyme linked immunoassay. *Lancet*, **1**, 1168–71
19. Hoff, R., Berardi, V. P., Weiblen, B. J., Mahoney-Trout, L., Mitchell, M. L. and Grady, G. F. (1988). Seroprevalence of human immunodeficiency virus among childbearing women: estimation by testing samples of blood from newborns. *N. Engl. J. Med.*, **318**, 525–30
20. McEnvoy, M., Porter, K., Mortimer, P., Simmons, N. and Shanson, D. (1987). Prospective study of clinical, laboratory and ancilliary staff with accidental exposure to blood or body fluids from patients infected with HIV. *Br. Med. J.*, **294**, 1595–7
21. Weiss, S. H., Goedert, J. J., Gartner, S., Popovic, M., Waters, D., Markham, P., Veronese, F. D. M., Gail, M. H., Barkley, W. E., Gibbons, J., Gill, F. A., Leuther, M., Shaw, G. M., Gallo, R. C. and Blattner, W. A. (1988). Risk of human immunodeficiency virus (HIV-1) infection among laboratory workers. *Science*, **239**, 68–71
22. Pederson, C., Nielsen, C. M., Vestergaard, B. F., Gerstoft, J., Krogsgaard, K. and Nielsen, J. O. (1987). Temporal relation of antigenaemia and loss of antibodies to core antigens to development of clinical disease in HIV infection. *Br. Med. J.*, **295**, 567–9
23. Weiss, R. A., Clapham, P. R., Cheingsong-Popov, R., Dalgleish, A. G., Carne, C. A., Weller, I. V. D. and Tedder, R. S. (1985). Neutralization of human T-lymphotropic virus type III by sera of AIDS and AIDS-risk patients. *Nature*, **316**, 69–72
24. Robert-Guroff, M., Brown, M. and Gallo, R. C. (1985). HTLV-III neutralizing antibodies in patients with AIDS and AIDS-related complex. *Nature*, **316**, 72–4
25. Spickett, G. P. and Dalgleish, A. G. (1988). Cellular immunology of HIV-infection. *Clin. Exp. Immunol.*, **71**, 1–7

26. Levy, J. A. (1988). Mysteries of HIV: challenges for therapy and prevention. *Nature*, **333**, 519–22
27. Lane, H. C. and Fauci, A. S. (1985). Immunologic abnormalities in the acquired immunodeficiency syndrome. *Ann. Rev. Immunol.*, **3**, 477–500
28. Ho, D. D., Pomerantz, R. J. and Kaplan, J. C. (1987). Pathogenesis of infection with human immunodeficiency virus. *N. Engl. J. Med.*, **317**, 278–86
29. Fauci, A. S. (1988). The human immunodeficiency virus: infectivity and mechanisms of pathogenesis. *Science*, **239**, 617–22
30. Terhost, C., van Agthoven, A., Reinherz, E. and Schlossman, S. (1980). Biochemical analysis of human T-lymphocyte differentiation antigens T4 and T5. *Science*, **209**, 520–1
31. Talle, M. A., Rao, P. E., Westberg, E., Allegar, N., Makowski, M., Mittler, R. S. and Goldstein, G. (1983). Patterns of antigenic expression on human monocytes as defined by monoclonal antibodies. *Cell. Immunol.*, **78**, 83–99
32. Niedecken, H., Lutz, G., Bauer, R. and Kreysel, H. W. (1987). Langerhans cell as primary target and vehicle for transmission of HIV. *Lancet*, **2**, 519–20
33. Cheng-Mayer, C., Rutka, J. T., Rosenblum, M. L., McHugh, T., Stites, D. P. and Levy, J. A. (1987). Human immunodeficiency virus can productively infect cultured human glial cells. *Proc. Natl. Acad. Sci. USA*, **84**, 3526–30
34. Dewhurst, S., Bresser, J., Stevenson, M., Sakai, K., Evinger-Hodges, M. J. and Volsky, D. J. (1987). Susceptibility of human glial cells to infection with human immunodeficiency virus (HIV). *FEBS Lett.*, **213**, 138–43
35. Dalgleish, A. G., Beverley, P. C. L., Clapham, P. R., Crawford, D. H., Greaves, M. F. and Weiss, R. A. (1984). The CD4 (T4) antigen is an essential component of the receptor for the AIDS retrovirus. *Nature*, **312**, 763–7
36. Klatzmann, D., Champagne, E., Chamaret, S., Gruest, J., Guetard, D., Hercend, T., Gluckman, J.-C. and Montagnier, L. (1984). T-lymphocyte T4 molecule behaves as the receptor for human retrovirus LAV. *Nature*, **312**, 767–8
37. Maddon, P. J., Dalgleish, A. G., McDougal, J. S., Clapham, P. R., Weiss, R. A. and Axel, R. (1986). The T4 gene encodes the AIDS virus receptor and is expressed in the immune system and the brain. *Cell*, **47**, 333–48
38. Stein, B. S., Gowda, S. D., Lifson, J. D., Penhallow, R. C., Bensch, K. G. and Engleman, E. G. (1987). pH-dependent HIV entry into CD4-positive T-cells via virus envelope fusion to the plasma membrane. *Cell*, **49** 659–68
39. Gartner, S., Markovits, P., Markovitz, D. M., Kaplan, M. H., Gallo, R. C. and Popovic, M. (1986). The role of mononuclear phagocytes in HTLV-III/LAV infection. *Science*, **233**, 215–19
40. Price, R. W., Brew, B., Sidtis, J., Rosenbaum, M., Scheck, A. C. and Cleary, P. (1988). The brain in AIDS: central nervous system HIV-I infection and AIDS dementia complex. *Science*, **239**, 586–92
41. Nelson, J. A., Wiley, C. A., Reynolds-Kohler, C., Reese, C. E., Margaretten, W. and Levy, J. A. (1988). Human immunodeficiency virus detected in bowel epithelium from patients with gastrointestinal symptoms. *Lancet*, **1**, 259–62
42. Klatzmann, D., Barre-Sinoussi, F., Nugeyre, M. T., Dauguet, C., Vilmer, E., Griscelli, C., Brun-Vezinet, F., Rouzioux, C., Gluckman, J. C., Chermann, J. C. and Montagnier, L. (1984). Selective tropism of lymphadenopathy associated virus (LAV) for helper-inducer T-lymphocytes. *Science*, **225**, 59–63
43. Harper, M. E., Marselle, L. M., Gallo, R. C. and Wong-Staal, F. (1986). Detection of lymphocytes expressing human T-lymphotropic virus type III in lymph nodes and peripheral blood from infected individuals by *in situ* hybridization. *Proc. Natl. Acad. Sci. USA*, **83**, 772–6
44. Falk, L. A., Paul, D., Landay, A. and Kessler, H. (1987). HIV isolation from plasma of HIV-infected persons. *N. Engl. J. Med.*, **316**, 1547–8
45. Hoxie, J. A., Haggarty, B. S., Rackowski, J. L., Pillsbury, N. and Levy, J. A. (1985). Persistent noncytopathic infection of normal human T lymphocytes with AIDS associated retrovirus. *Science*, **229**, 1400–2
46. Folks, T., Powell, D. M., Lightfoote, M. M., Benn, S., Martin, M. A. and Fauci, A. S. (1986). Induction of HTLV III/LAV from a non virus-producing T cell line: implications for latency. *Science*, **231**, 600–2

47. McDougal, J. S., Mawle, A., Cort, S. P., Nicholson, J. K. A., Cross, G. D., Scheppler-Campbell, J. A., Hicks, D. and Sligh, J. (1985). Cellular tropism of the human retrovirus HTLV-III/LAV (1) role of T-cell activation and expression of the T4 antigen. *J. Immunol.*, **135**, 3151–62
48. Folks, T. M., Kelly, J., Benn, S., Kinter, A., Justement, J., Gold, J., Redfield, R., Sell, K. W. and Fauci, A. S. (1986). Susceptibility of normal human lymphocytes to infection with HTLV-III/LAV. *J. Immunol.*, **136**, 4049–53
49. Mosca, J. D., Bednarik, D. P., Raj, N. B. K., Rosen, C. A., Sodroski, J. G., Haseltine, W. A. and Pitha, P. M. (1987). Herpes simplex virus type-1 can reactivate transcription of latent human immunodeficiency virus. *Nature*, **355**, 67–70
50. Skolnik, P. R., Kosloff, B. R. and Hirsch, M. S. (1988). Bidirectional interactions between human immunodeficiency virus type 1 and cytomegalovirus. *J. Infect. Dis.*, **157**, 508–14
51. Bloom, B. R. (1987). AIDS vaccine strategies. *Nature*, **327**, 193
52. Langley, D. and Spier, R. E. (1988). Is a vaccine against AIDS possible? *Vaccine*, **6**, 3–5
53. Salk, J. (1987). Prospects for the control of AIDS by immunizing seropositive individuals. *Nature*, **327** 473–6
54. Porterfield, J. S. (1986). Antibody-dependent enhancement of viral infectivity. *Adv. Virus Res.*, **31**, 335–55
55. Robinson, W. E., Montefiori, D. C. and Mitchell, W. M. (1988). Antibody-dependent enhancement of human immunodeficiency virus type 1 infection. *Lancet*, **1**, 790–5
56. Robinson, W. E., Montefiori, D. C. and Mitchell, W. M. (1988). Will antibody-dependent enhancement of HIV-1 infection be a problem with AIDS vaccines? *Lancet*, **1**, 830–1
57. Lepe-Zuniga, J. L. and Mansell, P. W. A. (1986). AIDS: From immunity to infection to autoimmunity. A comprehensive hypothesis of the pathogenesis of the disease. *AIDS Res.*, **2**, 363–8
58. Solinger, A. M., Adams, L. E., Friedman-Kien, A. E. and Hess, E. V. (1988). Acquired immune defiency syndrome (AIDS) and autoimmunity – mutually exclusive entities? *J. Clin. Immunol.*, **8**, 32–41
59. Fauci, A. S. (1984). Immunologic abnormalities in the acquired immunodeficiency syndrome (AIDS). *Clin. Res.*, **32**, 491–9
60. Fahey, J. L. (1986). Immunologic aspects of human immunodeficiency virus infection and AIDS. *Clin. Aspects Autoimmun.*, **1**, 12–23
61. Klatzmann, D. and Gluckman, J. C. (1986). HIV infection: facts and hypotheses. *Immunol. Today*, **7**, 291–6
62. Ziegler, J. L. and Stites, D. P. (1986). Hypothesis: AIDS is an autoimmune disease directed at the immune system and triggered by a lymphotropic retrovirus. *Clin. Immunol. Immunopathol.*, **41**, 305–13
63. Gonda, M. A., Wong-Staal, F., Gallo, R. C., Clements, J. E., Narayan, O. and Gilden, R. V. (1985). Sequence homology and morphologic similarity of HTLV-III and Visna virus, a pathogenic lentivirus. *Science*, **227**, 173–7
64. Nathanson, N., Georgsson, G., Palsson, P. A., Najjar, J. A., Lutley, R. and Petursson, G. (1985). Experimental visna in Icelandic sheep: the prototype lentiviral infection. *Rev. Infect. Dis.*, **7**, 75–82
65. Narayan, O. and Cork, L. C. (1985). Lentiviral diseases of sheep and goats: chronic pneumonia leukoencephalomyelitis and arthritis. *Rev. Infect. Dis.*, **7**, 89–98
66. Cheevers, W. P. and McGuire, T. C. (1985). Equine infectious anemia virus: immunopathogenesis and persistence. *Rev. Infect. Dis.*, **7**, 83–8
67. Pedersen, N. C., How, E. W., Brown, M. L. and Yamamoto, J. K. (1987). Isolation of a T-lymphotropic virus from domestic cats with an immunodeficiency-like syndrome. *Science*, **235**, 790–3
68. Gonda, M. A., Braun, M. J., Carter, S. G., Kost, T. A., Bess, J. W., Arthur, L. O., Van Der Maaten, M. J. (1987). Characterization and molecular cloning of a bovine lentivirus related to human immunodeficiency virus. *Nature*, **330**, 388–91
69. Daniel, M. D., Letvin, N. L., King, N. W., Kannagi, M., Sehgal, P. K., Hunt, R. D., Kanki, P. J., Essex, M. and Desrosiers, R. C. (1985). Isolation of a T-cell tropic HTLV-III-like retrovirus from macaques. *Science*, **228**, 1201–4
70. Palmer, E., Sporborg, C., Harrison, A., Martin, M. L. and Feorino, P. (1985). Morphology and immunoelectron microscopy of AIDS virus. *Arch. Virol.*, **85**, 189–96

71. Munn, R. J., Marx, P. J., Yamamoto, K. J. and Gardner, M. B. (1985). Ultrastructural comparison of the retroviruses associated with human and simian acquired immunodeficiency syndrome. *Lab. Invest.*, **53**, 194–9
72. Gelderblom, H. R., Hausmann, E. H. S., Ozel, M., Pauli, G. and Koch, M. A. (1987). Fine structure of human immunodeficiency virus (HIV) and immunolocalization of structural proteins. *Virology*, **156**, 171–6
73. Koch, M. (1987). The anatomy of the virus. *New Sci.*, **113**(1553), 46–51
74. Stannard, L. M., Van Der Riet, F. De S. T. J. and Moodie, R. W. (1987). The morphology of human immunodeficiency virus particles by negative staining electron microscopy. *J. Gen. Virol.*, **68**, 919–23
75. Rabson, A. B. and Martin, M. A. (1985). Molecular organization of the AIDS retrovirus. *Cell*, **40**, 477–80
76. Gelderblom, H. R., Reupke, H. and Pauli, G. (1985). Loss of envelope antigens of HTLV III/LAV, a factor in AIDS pathogenesis? *Lancet*, **2**, 1016–17
77. Hausmann, E. H. S., Gelderblom, H. R., Clapham, P. R., Pauli, G. and Weiss, R. A. (1987). Detection of HIV envelope specific antibodies by immunoelectron microscopy and correlation with antibody titer and virus neutralizing activity. *J. Virol. Methods*, **16**, 125–37
78. Tsuchie, H., Katsumoto, T., Hattori, N., Kawatani, T., Kurimura, T. and Hinuma, Y. (1986). Budding process and fine structure of lymphadenopathy-associated virus (LAV). *Microbiol. Immunol.*, **30**, 545–52
79. Katsumoto, T., Hattori, N. and Kurimura, T. (1987). Maturation of human immunodeficiency virus, strain LAV, *in vitro. Intervirology*, **27**, 148–53
80. Dowsett, A. B., Roff, M. A., Greenaway, P. J., Elphick, E. R. and Farrar, G. H. (1987). Syncytia – a major site for the production of human immunodeficiency virus? *AIDS*, **1**, 147–50
81. Gendelman, H. E., Orenstein, J. M., Martin, M. A., Ferrua, C., Mitra, R., Phipps, T., Wahl, L. A., Lane, H. C., Fauci, A. S., Burke, D. S., Skillman, D. and Meltzer, M. S. (1988). Efficient isolation and propagation of human immunodeficiency virus on recombinant colony-stimulating factor 1-treated monocytes. *J. Exp. Med.*, **167**, 1428–41
82. Meyenhofer, M. F., Epstein, L. G., Cho, E.-C. and Sharer, L. R. (1987). Ultrastructural morphology and intracellular production of human immunodeficiency virus (HIV) in brain. *J. Neuropathol. Exp. Neurol.*, **46**, 474–84
83. Srinivasan, A., Goldsmith, C. S., York, D., Anand, R., Luciw, P., Schochetman, G., Palmer, E. and Bohan, C. (1988). Studies on human immunodeficiency virus-induced cytopathic effects: use of human rhabdomyosarcoma (RD) cells. *Arch. Virol.*, **99**, 21–30
84. Forsbeck, K., Nygren, P., Larsson, R., Nilsson, M., Nilsson, K. and Gylfe, E. (1988). Cytoplasmic pH is differently regulated in the monoblastic U-937 and erythroleukemic K-562 cell lines. *Exp. Cell Res.*, **176**, 96–106
85. Feremans, W. W., Huygen, K., Menu, R., Farber, C. M., De Caluwe, J. P., Van Vooren, J. P., Marcelis, L., Andre, L., Brasseur, M., Bondue, H., Lebon, B. and Clumeck, N. (1988). Fifty cases of human immunodeficiency virus (HIV) infection: immunoultrastructural study of circulating lymphocytes. *J. Clin. Pathol.*, **41**, 62–71
86. Clavel, F., Guetard, D., Brun-Vezinet, F., Chamaret, S., Rey, M.-A., Santos-Ferreira, M. O., Laurent, A. G., Dauguet, C., Katlama, C., Rouzioux, C., Klatzmann, D., Champalimaud, J. L. and Montagnier, L. (1986). Isolation of a new human retrovirus from West African patients with AIDS. *Science*, **233**, 343–6
87. Chen, I. S. Y. (1986). Regulation of AIDS virus expression. *Cell*, **47**, 1–2
88. Tong-Starksen, S. E., Luciw, P. A. and Peterlin, B. M. (1987). Human immunodeficiency virus long terminal repeat responds to T-cell activation signals. *Proc. Natl. Acad. Sci. USA*, **84**, 6845–9
89. Ghrayeb, J., Kato, I., McKinney, S., Huang, J. J., Chanda, P. K., Ho, D. D., Sarngadharan, M. G., Chang, T. W. and Chang, N. T. (1986). Human T-cell lymphotropic virus type III (HTLV-III) core antigens: synthesis in *Escherichia coli* and immunoreactivity with human sera. *DNA*, **5**, 93–9
90. Di Marzo Veronese, F., Copeland, T. D., Oroszlan, S., Gallo, R. C. and Sarngadharan, M. G. (1988). Biochemical and immunological analysis of human immunodeficiency virus gag gene products p17 and p24. *J. Virol.*, **62**, 795–801
91. Ratner, L., Haseltine, W., Patarca, R., Livak, K. J., Starcich, B., Josephs, S. F., Doran, E.

R., Rafalski, J. A., Whitehorn, E. A., Baumeister, K., Ivanoff, L., Petteway, S. R., Pearson, M. L., Lautenberger, J. A., Papas, T. S., Ghrayeb, J., Chang, N. T., Gallo, R. C. and Wong-Staal, F. (1985). Complete nucleotide sequence of the AIDS virus, HTLV-III. *Nature*, **313**, 277–83

92. Wain-Hobson, S., Sonigo, P., Danos, O., Cole, S. and Alizon, M. (1985). Nucleotide sequence of the AIDS virus, LAV. *Cell*, **40**, 9–17
93. Sanchez-Pescador, R., Power, M. D., Barr, P. J., Steimer, K. S., Stempien, M. M., Brown-Shimer, S. L., Gee, W. W., Renard, A., Randolph, A., Levy, J. A., Dina, D. and Luciw, P. A. (1985). Nucleotide sequence and expression of an AIDS-associated retrovirus (ARV-2). *Science*, **227**, 484–92
94. Jacks, T., Power, M. D., Masiarz, F. R., Luciw, P. A., Barr, P. J. and Varmus, H. E. (1988). Characterization of ribosomal frameshifting in HIV-I gag-pol expression. *Nature*, **331**, 280–3
95. Mous, J., Heimer, E. P. and LeGrice, S. F. J. (1988). Processing protease and reverse transcriptase from human immunodeficiency virus type 1 polyprotein in *Escherichia coli. J. Virol.*, **62**, 1433–6
96. Hansen, J., Billich, S., Schulze, T., Sukrow, S. and Moelling, K. (1988). Partial purification and substrate analysis of bacterially expressed HIV protease by means of monoclonal antibody. *EMBO J.*, **7**, 1785–91
97. Pearl, L. H. and Taylor, W. R. (1987). A structural model for the retroviral proteases. *Nature*, **329**, 351–4
98. Di Marzo Veronese, F., Copeland, T. D., DeVico, A. L., Rahman, R., Oroszlan, S., Gallo, R. C. and Sarngadharan, M. G. (1986). Characterization of highly immunogenic p66/p51 as the reverse transcripase of HTLV-III/LAV. *Science*, **231**, 1289–91
99. Larder, B., Purifoy, D., Powell, K. and Darby, G. (1987). AIDS virus reverse transcriptase defined by high level expression in *Escherichia coli. EMBO J.* **6**, 3133–7
100. Hansen, J., Schulze, R. T., Mellert, W. and Moelling, K. (1988). Identification of HIV-specific RNase H by monoclonal antibody. *EMBO J.*, **7** 239–43
101. Lightfoote, M. M., Coligan, J. E., Folks, T. M., Fauci, A. S., Martin, M. A. and Venkatesan, S. (1986). Structural characterization of reverse transcriptase and endonuclease polypeptides of the acquired immunodeficiency syndrome retrovirus. *J. Virol.*, **6**, 771–5
102. Robey, W. G., Safai, B., Oroszlan, S., Arthur, L. O., Gonda, M. A., Gallo, R. C. and Fischinger, P. (1985). Characterization of envelope and core structural gene products of HTLV-III with sera from AIDS patients. *Science*, **228**, 593–5
103. Allan, J. S., Coligan, J. E., Barin, F., McLane, M. F., Sodroski, J. G., Rosen, C. A., Haseltine, W. A., Lee, T. H. and Essex, M. (1985). Major glycoprotein antigens that induce antibodies in AIDS patients are encoded by HTLV-III. *Science*, **228**, 1091–4
104. Barin, F., McLane, M. F., Allan, J. S., Lee, T. H., Groopman, J. E. and Essex, M. (1985). Virus envelope proteins of HTLV-III represents major target antigen for antibodies in AIDS patients. *Science*, **228**, 1094–6
105. Di Marzo Veronese, F., DeVico, A. L., Copeland, T. D., Oroszlan, S., Gallo, R. C. and Sarngadharan, M. G. (1985). Characterization of gp41 as the transmembrane protein coded by the HTLV-III/LAV envelope gene. *Science*, **229**, 1402–5
106. Lifson, J. D., Feinberg, M. B., Reyes, G. R., Rabin, L., Banapour, B., Chakrabarti, S., Moss, B., Wong-Staal, F., Steimer, K. S. and Engleman, E. G. (1986). Induction of CD4-dependent cell fusion by the HTLV-III/LAV envelope glycoprotein. *Nature*, **323**, 725–8
107. Barnes, D. M. (1987). Solo actions of AIDS virus coat. *Science*, **237**, 971–3
108. Lifson, J., Coutre, S., Huang, E. and Engelman, E. (1986). Role of envelope glycoprotein carbohydrate in human immunodeficiency virus (HIV) infectivity and virus-induced cell fusion. *J. Exp. Med.*, **164**, 2101–6
109. Huso, D. L., Narayan, O. and Hart, G. W. (1988). Sialic acids on the surface of caprine arthritis-encephalitis virus determine the biological properties of the virus. *J. Virol.*, **62**, 1974–80
110. Folks, T. M. (1987). Epitope mapping of human immunodeficiency virus: a monoclonal approach. *J. Immunol.*, **139**, 3913–14
111. Windheuser, M. G. and Wood, C. (1988). Characterization of immunoreactive epitopes of the HIV-I gp41 envelope protein using fusion proteins synthesized in *Escherichia coli. Gene*, **64**, 107–19

112. Kowalski, M., Potz, J., Basiripour, L., Dorfman, T., Goh, W. C., Terwilliger, E., Dayton, A., Rosen, C., Haseltine, W. and Sodroski, J. (1987). Functional regions of the envelope glycoprotein of human immunodeficiency virus type 1. *Science*, **237**, 1351–5
113. McCune, J. M., Rabin, L. B., Feinberg, M. B., Lieberman, M., Kosek, J. C., Reyes, G. R. and Weissman, I. L. (1988). Endoproteolytic cleavage of gp160 is required for the activation of human immunodeficiency virus. *Cell*, **53**, 55–67
114. Arya, S. K., Guo, C., Josephs, S. F. and Wong-Staal, F. (1985). Transactivator gene of human T-lymphotropic virus type III (HTLV-III). *Science*, **229**, 69–73
115. Sodroski, J., Patarca, R., Rosen, C., Wong-Staal, F. and Haseltine, W. (1985). Location of the trans-activating region on the genome of human T-cell lymphotropic virus type III. *Science*, **229**, 74–7
116. Fisher, A. G., Feinberg, M. B., Josephs, S. F., Harper, M. E., Marselle, L. M., Reyes, G., Gonda, M. A., Aldovini, A., Debouk, C., Gallo, R. C. and Wong-Staal, F. (1986). The trans-activator gene of HTLV-III is essential for virus replication. *Nature*, **320**, 367–71
117. Rosen, C. A., Sodroski, J. G. and Haseltine, W. A. (1985). The location of cis-acting regulatory sequences in the human T-cell lymphotropic virus type III (HTLV-III/LAV) long terminal repeat. *Cell*, **41**, 813–23
118. Sodroski, J., Goh, W. C., Rosen, C., Dayton, A., Terwilliger, E. and Haseltine, W. (1986). A second post-transcriptional trans-activator gene required for HTLV-III replication. *Nature*, **321**, 412–17
119. Feinberg, M. B., Jarrett, R. F., Aldovini, A., Gallo, R. C. and Wong-Staal, F. (1986). HTLV-III expression and production involve complex regulation at the levels of splicing and translation of viral RNA. *Cell*, **46**, 807–17
120. Terwilliger, E., Burghoff, R., Sia, R., Sodroski, J., Haseltine, W. and Rosen, C. (1988). The art gene product of human immunodeficiency virus is required for replication. *J. Virol.*, **62**, 655–8
121. Lee, T.-H., Coligan, J. E., Allan, J. S., McLane, M. F., Groopman, J. E. and Essex, M. (1986). A new HTLV-III/LAV protein encoded by a gene found in cytopathic retroviruses. *Science*, **231**, 1546–9
122. Sodroski, J., Goh, W. C., Rosen, C., Tartar, A., Portetelle, D., Burny, A. and Haseltine, W. (1986). Replicative and cytopathic potential of HTLV-III/LAV with sor gene deletions. *Science*, **231**, 1549–53
123. Kan, N. C., Franchini, G., Wong-Staal, F., DuBois, G. C., Robey, W. G., Lautenberger, J. A. and Papas, T. S. (1986). Identification of HTLV-III/LAV sor gene product and detection of antibodies in human sera. *Science*, **231**, 1553–5
124. Fisher, A. G., Ensoli, B., Ivanoff, L., Chamberlain, M., Petteway, S., Ratner, L., Gallo, R. C. and Wong-Staal, F. (1987). The sor gene of HIV-I is required for efficient virus transmission *in vitro*. *Science*, **237**, 888–93
125. Strebel, K., Daugherty, D., Clouse, K., Cohen, D., Folks, T. and Martin, M. A. (1987). The HIV 'A' (sor) gene product is essential for virus infectivity. *Nature*, **328**, 728–30
126. Guyader, M., Emerman, M., Sonigo, P., Clavel, F., Montagnier, L. and Alizon, M. (1987). Genome organization and transactivation of the human immunodeficiency virus type 2. *Nature*, **326**, 622–69
127. Terwilliger, E., Sodroski, J. G., Rosen, C. A. and Haseltine, W. A. (1986). Effects of mutations within the 3′-orf open reading frame region of human T-cell lymphotropic virus type III (HTLV-III/LAV) on replication and cytopathogenicity. *J. Virol.*, **60**, 754–60
128. Fisher, A. G., Ratner, L., Mitsuya, H., Marselle, L. M., Harper, M. E., Broder, S., Gallo, R. C. and Wong-Staal, F. (1986). Infectious mutants of HTLV-III with changes in the 3′-region and markedly reduced cytopathic effects. *Science*, **233**, 655–9
129. Allan, J. S., Coligan, J. E., Lee, T. H., McLane, M. F., Kanki, P. J., Groopman, J. E. and Essex, M. (1985). A new HTLV-III/LAV encoded antigen detected by antibodies from AIDS patients. *Science*, **230**, 810–13
130. Franchini, G., Robert-Guroff, M., Ghrayeb, J., Chang, N. T. and Wong-Staal, F. (1986). Cytoplasmic localization of the HTLV-III 3′-orf protein in cultured T cells. *Virology*, **155**, 593–9
131. Franchini, G., Robert-Guroff, M., Wong-Staal, F., Ghrayeb, J., Kato, I., Chang, T. W. and Chang, N. T. (1986). Expression of the protein encoded by the 3′-open reading frame of human T-cell lymphotropic virus type III in bacteria: demonstration of its immunoreactivity with human sera. *Proc. Natl. Acad. Sci. USA*, **83**, 5282–5

132. Wong-Staal, F., Chanda, P. K. and Ghrayeb, J. (1987). Human immunodeficiency virus: the eighth gene. *AIDS Res. Human Retroviruses*, **3**, 33–9

133. Miller, R. H. (1988). Human immunodeficiency virus may encode a novel protein on the genomic DNA plus strand. *Science*, **239**, 1420–2

134. Stevens, J. G., Wagner, E. K., Devi-Rao, G. B., Cook, M. L. and Feldman, L. T. (1987). RNA complementary to a herpesvirus alpha-gene mRNA is prominent in latently infected neurons. *Science*, **235**, 1056–9

135. Kindy, M. S., McCormack, J. E., Buckler, A. J., Levine, R. A. and Sonenshein, G. E. (1987). Independent regulation of transcription of the two strands of the c-myc gene. *Molec. Cell. Biol.*, **7**, 2857–62

136. Weber, J. N., Clapham, P. R., Weiss, R. A., Parker, D., Roberts, C., Duncan, J., Weller, I., Carne, C., Tedder, R. S., Pinching, A. J. and Cheingsong-Popov, R. (1987). Human immunodeficiency virus infection of two cohorts of homosexual men: neutralising sera and association of anti-gag antibody with prognosis. *Lancet*, **1**, 119–22

137. Walker, B. D., Chakrabarti, S., Moss, B., Paradis, T. J., Flynn, T., Durne, A. G., Blumberg, R. S., Kaplan, J. C., Hirsch, M. S. and Schooley, R. T. (1987). HIV-specific cytotoxic T-lymphocytes in seropositive individuals. *Nature*, **328**, 345–8

138. Plata, F., Autran, B., Martins, L. P., Wain-Hobson, S., Raphael, M., Mayaud, C., Denis, M., Guillon, J.-M. and Debre, P. (1987). AIDS virus-specific cytotoxic T-lymphocytes in lung disorders. *Nature*, **328**, 348–51

139. Walker, B. D., Flexner, C., Paradis, T. J., Fuller, T. C., Hirsch, M. S., Schooley, R. T. and Moss, B. (1988). HIV-I reverse transcriptase is a target for cytotoxic T-lymphocytes in infected individuals. *Science*, **240**, 64–6

140. Smith, T. F., Srinivasan, A., Schochetman, G., Marcus, M. and Myers, G. (1988). The phylogenetic history of immunodeficiency viruses. *Nature*, **333**, 573–5

141. Hahn, B. H., Shaw, G. M., Taylor, M. E., Redfield, R. R., Markham, P. D., Salahuddin, S. Z., Wong-Staal, F., Gallo, R. C., Parks, E. S. and Parks, W. P. (1986). Genetic variation in HTLV-III/LAV over time in patients with AIDS or at risk for AIDS. *Science*, **232**, 1548–53

142. Devare, S. G., Srinivasan, A., Bohan, C. A., Spira, T. J., Curran, J. W. and Kalyanaraman, V. S. (1986). Genomic diversity of the acquired immunodeficiency syndrome retroviruses is reflected in alteration of its translation products. *Proc. Natl. Acad. Sci. USA*, **83**, 5718–22

143. Willey, R. L., Rutledge, R. A., Dias, S., Folks, T., Theodore, T., Buckler, C. E. and Martin, M. A. (1986). Identification of conserved and divergent domains within the envelope gene of the acquired immunodeficiency syndrome retrovirus. *Proc. Natl. Acad. Sci. USA*, **83**, 5038–42

144. Starcich, B. R., Hahn, B. H., Shaw, G. M., McNeely, P. D., Modrow, S., Wolf, H., Parks, E. S., Parks, W. P., Josephs, S. F., Gallo, R. C. and Wong-Staal, F. (1986). Identification and characterization of conserved and variable regions in the envelope gene of HTLV-III/LAV, the retrovirus of AIDS. *Cell*, **45**, 637–48

145. Alizon, M., Wain-Hobson, S., Montagnier, L. and Sonigo, P. (1986). Genetic variability of the AIDS virus: nucleotide sequence analysis of two isolates from African patients. *Cell*, **46**, 63–74

146. Coffin, J. M. (1986). Genetic variation in AIDS viruses. *Cell*, **46**, 1–4

147. Cheng-Meyer, C., Homsy, J., Evans, L. A. and Levy, J. A. (1988). Identification of human immunodeficiency virus sub-types with distinct patterns of sensitivity to serum neutralization. *Proc. Natl. Acad. Sci. USA*, **85**, 2815–19

148. Weiss, R. A., Clapham, P. R., Weber, J. N., Dalgleish, A. G., Lasky, L. A. and Berman, P. W. (1986). Variable and conserved neutralization antigens of human immunodeficiency virus. *Nature*, **324**, 572–5

149. Palker, T. J., Matthews, T. J., Clark, M. E., Cianciolo, G. J., Randall, R. R., Langlois, A. J., White, G. C., Safai, B., Snyderman, R., Bolognesi, D. P. and Haynes, B. F. (1987). A conserved region at the COOH terminus of human immunodeficiency virus gp120 envelope protein contains an immunodominant epitope. *Proc. Natl. Acad. Sci. USA*, **84**, 2479–83

150. Ho, D. D., Sarngadharan, M. G., Hirsch, M. S., Schooley, R. T., Rota, T. R., Kennedy, R. C., Chanh, T. C. and Sato, V. L. (1987). Human immunodeficiency virus neutralizing antibodies recognize several conserved domains on the envelope glycoproteins. *J. Virol.*, **61** 2024–8

151. Ho, D. D., Kaplan, J. C., Rackauskas, I. E. and Gurney, M. E. (1988). Second conserved domain of gp120 is important for HIV infectivity and antibody neutralization. *Science*, **239**, 1021–3
152. Matthews, T. J., Langlois, A. J., Robey, W. G., Chang, N. T., Gallo, R. C., Fischinger, P. J. and Bolognesi, D. P. (1986). Restricted neutralization of divergent human T-lymphotropic virus type III isolates by antibodies to the major envelope glycoprotein. *Proc. Natl. Acad. Sci. USA*, **83**, 9709–13
153. Tersmette, M., DeGoede, R. E. Y., Al, B. J. M., Winkel, I. N., Gruters, R. A., Cuypers, H. T., Huisman, H. G. and Miedema, F. (1988). Differential syncytium-inducing capacity of human immunodeficiency virus isolates: frequent detection of syncytium-inducing isolates in patients with acquired immunodeficiency syndrome (AIDS) and AIDS-related complex. *J. Virol.*, **62**, 2026–32
154. Evans, L. A., Moreau, J., Odehouri, K., Legg, H., Barboza, A., Cheng-Meyer, C. and Levy, J. A. (1988). Characterization of a nonocytopathic HIV-2 strain with unusual effects on CD4 expression. *Science*, **240**, 1522–25
155. Kong, L. I., Lee, S.-W., Kappes, J. C., Parkin, J. S., Decker, D., Hoxie, J. A., Hahn, B. H. and Shaw, G. M. (1988). West African HIV-2-related human retrovirus with attenuated cytopathicity. *Science*, **240**, 1525–9
156. Cheng-Mayer, C., Seto, D., Tateno, M. and Levy, J. A. (1988). Biologic features of HIV-I that correlate with virulence in the host. *Science*, **240**, 80–2
157. Greenaway, P. J. and Farrar, G. H. (1987). Prospects for an AIDS vaccine. *PHLS Microbiol. Dig.*, **4**, 26–30
158. Chakrabarti, S., Robert-Guroff, M., Wong-Staal, F., Gallo, R. C. and Moss, B. (1986). Expression of the HTLV-III envelope gene by a recombinant vaccinia virus. *Nature*, **320**, 535–7
159. Hu, S.-L., Kosowski, S. G. and Dalrymple, J. M. (1986). Expression of AIDS virus envelope gene in recombinant vaccinia viruses. *Nature*, **320**, 537–40
160. Zarling, J. M., Morton, W., Moran, P. A., McClure, J., Kosowski, S. G. and Hu, S.-L. (1986). T-cell responses to human AIDS virus in macaques immunized with recombinant vaccinia viruses. *Nature*, **323**, 344–46
161. Zarling, J. M., Eichberg, J. W., Moran, P. A., McClure, J., Sridhar, P. and Hu, S.-L. (1987). Proliferative and cytotoxic T-cells to AIDS virus glycoproteins in chimpanzees immunized with a recombinant vaccinia virus expressing AIDS virus envelope glycoproteins. *J. Immunol.*, **139**, 988–90
162. Hu, S.-L., Fultz, P. N., McClure, H. M., Eichberg, J. W., Thomas, E. K., Zarling, J. M., Singhal, M. C., Kosowski, S. G., Swenson, R. B., Anderson, D. C. and Todaro, G. (1987). Effect of immunization with a vaccinia-HIV env recombinant on HIV infection of chimpanzees. *Nature*, **328**, 721–23
163. Zagury, D., Leonard, R., Fouchard, M., Reveil, B., Bernard, J., Ittele, D., Cattan, A., Zirimwabagabo, L., Kalumbu, M., Justin, W., Salaun, J.-J. and Goussard, B. (1987). Immunization against AIDS in humans. *Nature*, **326**, 249–50
164. Zagury, D., Bernard, J., Cheynier, R., Desportes, I., Leonard, R., Fouchard, M., Reveil, B., Itelle, D., Lurhuma, Z., Mbayo, K., Wane, J., Salaun, J. J., Goussard, B., Dechazal, L., Burny, A., Nara, P. and Gallo, R. C. (1988). A group specific anamnestic immune reaction against HIV-1 induced by a candidate vaccine against AIDS. *Nature*, **332**, 728–31
165. Pyle, S. W., Bess, J. W., Robey, W. G., Fischinger, P. J., Gilden, R. V. and Arthur, L. O. (1987). Purification of 120,000 dalton envelope glycoprotein from culture fluids of human immunodeficiency virus (HIV) infected H9 cells. *AIDS Res. Human Retroviruses*, **3**, 387–400
166. Pyle, S. W., Dubois, G. C., Robey, W. G., Bess, J. W., Fischinger, P. J. and Arthur, L. O. (1988). Purification and characterization of the external envelope glycoprotein from two human immunodeficiency virus type 1 variants, HTLV-III B and HTLV-III RF. *J. Virol.*, **62**, 2258–64
167. Zweig, M., Schowalter, S. D., Bladen, S V., Gilden, R. V., Arthur, L. O., Robey, W. G., Nara, P. L. and Fischinger, P. J. (1988). Partial purification of native HIV transmembrane protein gp41: generation of polyclonal and monoclonal antibodies. *AIDS Res. Human Retroviruses*, **4**, 51–62
168. Putney, S. D., Mathews, T. J., Robey, W. G., Lynn, D. L., Robert-Guroff, M., Mueller, W.

T., Langlois, A. J., Ghrayeb, J., Petteway, S. R., Weinhold, K. J., Fischinger, P. J., Wong-Staal, F., Gallo, R. C. and Bolognesi, B. P. (1986). HTLV-III/LAV neutralising antibodies to an *E. coli* produced fragment of the virus envelope. *Science*, **234**, 1392–5

169. Samuel, K. P., Seth, A., Zweig, M., Showalter, S. D. and Papas, T. S. (1988). Bacterial expression and characterization of nine polypeptides encoded by segments of the envelope gene of human immunodeficiency virus. *Gene*, **64**, 121–34
170. Steimer, K. S., Puma, J. P., Power, M. D., Powers, M. A., George-Nascimento, C., Stephans, J. C., Levy, J. A., Sanchez-Pescador, R., Luciw, P. A., Barr, P. J. and Hallewell, R. A. (1986). Differential antibody responses of individuals infected with AIDS-associated retroviruses surveyed using the viral core antigen p25 gag expressed in bacteria. *Virology*, **150**, 283–90
171. Dowbenko, D. J., Bekk, J. R., Benton, C. V., Groopman, J. E., Nguyen, H., Vetterlein, D., Capon, D. J. and Lasky, L. A. (1985). Bacterial expression of the acquired immunodeficiency syndrome retrovirus p24 gag protein and its use as a diagnostic reagent. *Proc. Natl. Acad. Sci. USA*, **82**, 7748–52
172. Tanese, N., Sodroski, J., Haseltine, W. A. and Goff, S. P. (1986). Expression of reverse transcriptase activity of human T lymphotropic virus type III (HTLV III/LAV) in *Escherichia coli. J. Virol.*, **59**, 743–5
173. Farmerie, W. G., Loebb, D. D., Casavant, N. C., Hutchison, C. A., Edgell, M. H. and Swanstrom, R. (1987). Expression and processing of the AIDS virus reverse transcriptase in *Escherichia coli. Science*, **236**, 305–8
174. Arya, S. K. and Gallo, R. C. (1986). Three novel genes of human T lymphotropic virus type III: immune reactivity of their products with sera from acquired immune deficiency syndrome patients. *Proc. Natl. Acad. Sci. USA*, **83**, 2209–13
175. Aldovini, A., Debouck, C., Feinberg, M. B., Rosenberg, M., Arya, S. K. and Wong-Staal, F. (1986). Synthesis of the complete transactivation gene product of human T-lymphotropic virus type III in *Escherichia coli*: demonstration of immunogenicity *in vivo* and expression *in vitro*. *Proc. Natl. Acad. Sci. USA*, **83**, 6672–6
176. Graves, M. C., Lim, J. J., Heimer, E. P. and Kramer, R. A. (1988). An 11KDa form of human immunodeficiency virus protease expressed in *Escherichia coli* is sufficient for enzymatic activity. *Proc. Natl. Acad. Sci. USA*, **85**, 2449–53
177. Goh, W. C., Sodroski, J. G., Rosen, C. A. and Haseltine, W. A. (1987). Expression of the art gene protein of human T-lymphotropic virus type III (HTLV-III/LAV) in bacteria. *J. Virol.*, **61**, 633–7
178. Le Grice, S. F. J., Beuck, V. and Mous, J. (1987). Expression of biologically active human T-cell lymphotropic virus type III reverse transcriptase in *Bacillus subtilis. Gene*, **55**, 95–103
179. Barr, P. J., Steimer, K. S., Sabin, E. A., Parkes, D., George-Nascimento, C., Stephans, J. C., Powers, M. A., Gyenes, A., Van Nest, G. A., Miller, E. T., Higgins, K. W. and Luciw, P. A. (1987). Antigenicity and immunogenicity of domains of the human immunodeficiency virus (HIV) envelope polypeptide expressed in the yeast *Saccharomyces cerevisiae. Vaccine*, **5**, 90–101
180. Adams, S. E., Dawson, K. M., Gull, K., Kingsman, S. M. and Kingsman, A. J. (1987). The expression of hybrid HIV:Ty virus-like particles in yeast. *Nature*, **329**, 68–70
181. Madisen, L., Travis, B., Hu, S. L. and Purchio, A. F. (1987). Expression of the human immunodeficiency virus gag gene in insect cells. *Virology*, **158**, 248–50
182. Rusche, J. R., Lynn, D. L., Robert-Guroff, M., Langlois, A. J., Lyerly, H. K., Carson, H., Krohn, K., Ranki, A., Gallo, R. C., Bolognesi, D. P., Putney, S. D. and Matthews, T. J. (1988). Humoral immune response to the entire human immunodeficiency virus envelope glycoprotein made in insect cells. *Proc. Natl. Acad. Sci. USA*, **84**, 6924–8
183. Lasky, L. A., Groopman, J. E., Fennie, C. W., Benz, P. M., Capon, D. J., Dowbenko, D. J., Nakamura, C. R., Nunes, W. M., Renz, M. E. and Berman, P. W. (1986). Neutralization of the AIDS retrovirus by antibodies to a recombinant envelope glycoprotein. *Science*, **233**, 209–12
184. Rekosh, D. S., Nygren, A., Flodby, P., Hammarskjold, M. L. and Wigzell, H. (1988). Coexpression of human immunodeficiency virus envelope proteins from tat and from a single simian virus 40 late replacement vector. *Proc. Natl. Acad. Sci. USA*, **85**, 334–8
185. Falkner, F. G., Fuerst, T. R. and Moss, B. (1988). Use of vaccinia virus vectors to study

the synthesis, intracellular localization and action of the human immunodeficiency virus transactivator protein. *Virology*, **164**, 450–7

186. Chanh, T. C., Dreesman, G. R., Kanda, P., Linette, G. P., Sparrow, J. T., Ho, D. D. and Kennedy, R. C. (1986). Induction of anti-HIV neutralizing antibodies by synthetic peptides. *EMBO J.*, **5**, 3065–71
187. Kennedy, R. C., Henkel, R. D., Pauletti, D., Allan, J. S., Lee, T. H., Essex, M. and Dreesman, G. R. (1986). Antiserum to a synthetic peptide recognises the HTLV-III envelope glycoprotein. *Science*, **231**, 1556–9
188. Van Regenmortel, M. H. V. (1986). Synthetic peptide vaccines and the prediction of epitopes in proteins. *Clin. Immunol. Newsl.*, **7**, 122–5
189. Zanetti, M., Sercarz, E. and Salk, J. (1987). The immunology of new generation vaccines. *Immunol. Today*, **8**, 18–25
190. Klausner, A. (1988). Adjuvants: a real shot in the arm for recombinant vaccines. *Bio/Technol.*, **6**, 773–7
191. Morein, B., Lovgren, K., Hoglund, S. and Sundquist, B. (1987). The ISCOM: an immunostimulating complex. *Immunol. Today*, **8**, 333–7
192. Morein, B. (1988). The iscom antigen-presenting system. *Nature*, **332**, 287–8
193. Delpeyroux, F., Chencincer, N., Lim, A., Malpiece, Y., Blondel, B., Crainic, R., Van Der Werf, S. and Streeck, R. E (1986). A poliovirus neutralization epitope expressed on hybrid hepatitis B surface antigen particles. *Science*, **233**, 472–5
194. Burdette, S. and Schwartz, R. S. (1987). Current concepts: Immunology. Idiotypes and idiotypic networks. *N. Engl. J. Med.*, **317**, 219–23
195. Koprowski, H. (1985). Unconventional vaccines: Immunisation with anti-idiotype antibody against viral diseases. *Cancer Res.* (Suppl.), **45**, 4689–90
196. Chanh, T. C., Dreesman, G. and Kennedy, R. C. (1987). Monoclonal anti-idiotypic antibody mimics the CD4 receptor and binds HIV. *Proc. Natl. Acad. Sci. USA*, **84**, 3891–5
197. Dalgleish, A. G., Thomson, B. J., Chanh, T. C., Mallkowsky, M. and Kennedy, R. C. (1987). Neutralisation of HIV isolates by anti-idiotypic antibodies which mimic the T4 (CD4) epitope: a potential AIDS vaccine. *Lancet*, **2**, 1047–9
198. Alter, H. J., Eichberg, J. W., Masur, H., Saxinger, W. C., Gallo, R., Macher, A. M., Lane, H. C. and Fauci, A. S. (1984). Transmission of HTLV/III infection from human plasma to chimpanzees: an animal model for AIDS. *Science*, **226**, 549–52
199. Gajdusek, D. C., Amyx, H. L., Gibbs, C. J., Asher, D. M., Yanagihara, R. T., Rodgers-Johnson, P., Brown, P. W., Sarin, P. S., Gallo, R. C., Malvish, A., Arthur, L. O., Gilden, R. V., Montagnier, L., Chermann, J.-C., Barre-Sinoussi, F., Mildvan, D., Mathur, U. and Leavitt, R. (1984). Transmission experiments with human T-lymphotropic retroviruses and human AIDS tissue. *Lancet*, **1**, 1415–16
200. Fultz, P. N., McClure, H. M., Swenson, R. B., McGrath, C. R., Brodie, A., Getchell, J. P., Jensen, F. C., Anderson, D. C., Broderson, J. R. and Francis, D. P. (1986). Persistent infection of chimpanzees with human T-lymphotropic virus type III/lymphadenopathy-associated virus: a potential model for acquired immunodeficiency syndrome. *J. Virol.*, **58**, 116–24
201. Goudsmit, J., Smit, L., Krane, W. J. A., Bakker, M., Van Der Noordaa, J., Gibbs, C. J., Epstein, L. G. and Gajdusek, D. C. (1987). IgG response to human immunodeficiency virus in experimentally infected chimpanzees mimics the IgG response in humans. *J. Infect. Dis.*, **155**, 327–31
202. Nara, P. L., Robey, W. G., Arthur, L. O., Asher, D. M., Wolff, A. V., Gibbs, C. J., Gajdusek, D. C. and Fischinger, P. J. (1987). Persistent infection of chimpanzees with human immunodeficiency virus: serological responses and properties of reisolated viruses. *J. Virol.*, **61**, 3173–80
203. Eichberg, J. W., Zarling, J. M., Alter, H. J., Levy, J. A., Berman, P. W., Gregory, T., Lasky, L. A., McClure, J., Cobb, K. E., Moran, P. A., Hu, S. L., Kennedy, R. C., Chanh, T. C. and Dreesman, G. R. (1987). T-cell responses to human immunodeficiency virus (HIV) and its recombinant antigens in HIV-infected chimpanzees. *J. Virol.*, **61**, 3804–8
204. Hu, S. L., Fultz, P. N., McClure, H. M., Eichberg, J. W., Thomas, E. K., Zarling, J., Singhal, M. C., Kosowski, S. G., Swenson, R. B., Anderson, D. C. and Todaro, G. (1987). Effect of immunization with a vacinia-HIV env recombinant on HIV infection of chimpanzees. *Nature*, **328**, 721–3

205. Zarling, J. M., Eichberg, J. M., Moran, P. A., McClure, J., Sridhar, P. and Hu, S. (1987). Proliferative and cytotoxic T-cells to AIDS virus glycoproteins in chimpanzees immunized with a recombinant vaccinia virus expressing AIDS virus envelope glycoproteins. *J. Immunol.*, **139**, 988–90
206. Arthur, L. O., Pyle, S. W., Nara, P. L., Bess, J. W., Gonda, M. A., Kelliher, J. C., Gilden, R. V., Robey, W. G., Bolognesi, D. P., Gallo, R. C. and Fischinger, P. J. (1987). Serological responses in chimpanzes inoculated with human immunodeficiency virus glycoprotein (gp120) sub-unit vaccine. *Proc. Natl. Acad. Sci. USA*, **84**, 8583–7
207. Kanki, P. J., Alroy, J. and Essex, M. (1985). Isolation of T-lymphotropic retrovirus related to HTLV-III/LAV from wild caught African Green monkeys. *Science*, **230**, 951–4
208. Fultz, P. N., McClure, H. M., Anderson, D. C., Swenson, R. B., Anand, R. and Srinivasan, A. (1986). Isolation of a T-lymphotropic retrovirus from naturally infected sooty mangabey monkeys (*Cercocebus atys*). *Proc. Natl. Acad. Sci. USA*, **83**, 5286–90
209. Murphey-Corb, M., Martin, L. N., Rangan, S. R. S., Baskin, G. B., Gormus, B. J., Wolf, R. H., Andes, W. A., West, M. and Montelaro, R. C. (1986). Isolation of an HTLV-III-related retrovirus from macaques with simian AIDS and its possible origin in asymptomatic mangabeys. *Nature*, **321**, 435–7
210. Benveniste, R. E., Arthur, L. O., Tsai, C.-C., Sowder, R., Copeland, T. D., Henderson, L. E. and Oroszlan, S. (1986). Isolation of a lentivirus from a macaque with lymphoma: comparison with HTLV-III/LAV and lentiviruses. *J. Virol.*, **60**, 483–90
211. Desrosiers, R. C. and Letvin, N. L. (1987). Animal models for acquired immunodeficiency syndrome. *J. Infect. Dis.*, **9**, 438–46
212. Schneider, J. and Hunsmann, G. (1988). Simian lentiviruses – the SIV group. *AIDS*, **2**, 1–9
213. Homma, T., Kanki, P. J., King, N. W., Hunt, R. D., O'Connell, M. J., Letvin, N. L., Daniel, M. D., Desrosiers, R. C., Yang, C. S. and Essex, M. (1984). Lymphoma in macaques: association with virus of human T-lymphotropic family. *Science*, **225**, 716–18
214. Kannagi, M., Kiyotaki, M., Desrosiers, R. C., Reimann, K. A., King, N. W., Waldron, L. M. and Letvin, N. L (1986). Humoral immune repones to T-cell tropic retrovirus, simian T-lymphotropic virus type III, in monkeys with experimentally induced acquired immune deficiency-like syndrome. *J. Clin. Invest.*, **78**, 1229–36
215. Chalifoux, L. V., Ringler, D. J., King, N. W., Sehgal, P. K., Desrosiers, R. C., Daniel, M. D. and Letvin, N. L. (1987). Lymphadenopathy in macaques experimentally infected with the simian immunodeficiency virus SIV. *Am. J. Pathol.*, **128**, 104–10
216. Daniel, M. D., Letvin, N. L., Sehgal, P. K., Hunsmann, G., Schmidt, D. K., King, N. W. and Desrosiers, R. C. (1987). Long-term persistent infection of macaque monkeys with the simian immunodeficiency virus. *J. Gen. Virol.*, **68**, 3183–9
217. Harbour, D. A., Williams, P. D., Gruffydd-Jones, T. J., Burbridge, J. and Pearson, G. R. (1988). Isolation of a T-lymphotropic lentivirus from a persistently leucopenic domestic cat. *Vet. Rec.*, **122**, 84–6
218. Overbaugh, J., Donahue, P. R., Quackenbush, S. L., Hoover, E. A. and Mullins, J. I. (1988). Molecular cloning of a feline leukemia virus that induces fatal immunodeficiency disease in cats. *Science*, **239**, 906–10
219. Katzenstein, D. A., Sawyer, L. A. and Quinnan, L. V. (1988). Issues in the evaluation of AIDS vaccines. *AIDS*, **2**, 151–5
220. Newmark, P. (1988). Receeding hopes of AIDS vaccines. *Nature*, **333**, 699
221. Barnes, D. M. (1988). AIDS vaccine trial expanded. *Science*, **239**, 457
222. Coles, P. (1988). AIDS vaccine trials to begin in Geneva. *Nature*, **333**, 792
223. Anon (1988). Britain begins first trials of AIDS vaccine. *New. Sci.*, **118**(1611), 26
224. Anon (1988). First trial of blocking antibody dispels safety fears. *New. Sci.*, **119**(1620), 33

14
Prospects for the development of a vaccine for schistosomiasis

M. G. TAYLOR and G. WEBBE

Schistosomiasis is endemic in 75 developing countries and some 200 million people are probably infected, with a further 500–600 million being exposed to infection. The disease has widespread distribution in Africa and the Middle East (*Schistosoma haematobium* and *S. mansoni*) and in the Western hemisphere (Brazil, Venezuela, Surinam and certain Caribbean islands) for *S. mansoni*. In the Far East, China the Philippines and Indonesia are endemic areas of *S. japonicum* and limited foci have also been recorded in the Mekong basin and now in Malaysia (*S. mekongi* and *S. japonicum*, respectively). Other species of schistosomes which infect humans include *S. intercalatum* (West Africa) and *S. mattheei* (South Africa). Schistosomiasis is predominantly an infection of rural and agricultural communities with some peri-urban distribution in many countries. Usually poor-quality housing, substandard hygienic practices and a complete absence of sanitary facilities exist in these places. Children are an important reservoir source of infection as they contaminate fresh water through indiscriminate urination, while pollution of water with faeces as the result of inadequate sewage disposal is a critical factor in maintaining transmission of *S. mansoni* and *S. japonicum*. Schistosomiasis is an occupational hazard for fishermen, peasant farmers and agricultural workers in developing countries, but other activities may also result in water-contact and transmission, including domestic, recreational and religious practices. During the past decade many programmes for developing water resources have been established in endemic areas, with a pronounced concomitant increase in prevalence and intensity of schistosomiasis. The development of man-made lakes and new irrigation schemes in endemic areas are important factors in the continuing spread of infection. Transmission is being established in new areas such as Sao Tome and Principe, Niger and Oman, while previously unexposed populations are migrating into endemic agricultural areas and schistosomiasis is being acquired for the first time with some clinical consequences[1].

EPIDEMIOLOGY

The adult worms may live for 20–30 years but the mean duration of lifespan is probably much shorter (3–8 years)[2]. Each worm pair, according to the species of schistosome, produces 300 to more than 3000 eggs a day. As is the case with most helminths, the schistosomes do not multiply in the definitive host and in terms of host–parasite populations this means that the infection process produces, or tends to produce, an over-dispersed distribution of parasites within the host population, in which most individuals carry very few parasites and a small proportion are heavily infected. In schistosomiasis, even if the proportion of those with infection of high intensity is low, morbidity may be appreciable. The pathology of infection in humans may be profoundly influenced by different patterns of exposure to cercariae, partly because of differences in immunological responses. Recent advances in knowledge through epidemiological, pathological and quantitative necropsy studies have established that egg output accurately reflects intensity of infection (worm burden) which is measured in the field either as eggs per gram of faeces (*S. mansoni, S. japonicum*) or eggs per unit volume of urine (*S. haematobium*). Egg output appears to be independent of the age of the host or the schistosomes, and is closely related to the number of worm pairs the host carries. The hatchability of eggs may decrease, however, with the age of the host. Age–intensity curves are similar to age–prevalence curves, but fall more sharply with age. The two indices, prevalence and intensity, are thus related and, generally, populations with high prevalence of infection tend to have high intensity. A direct linear relationship appears to exist between intensity of infection and clinical disease. The linear relationship of hepatosplenic disease to intensity has been derived for *S. mansoni* from data obtained in Puerto Rico, Brazil and St Lucia[3]. This correlation is, however, less positive for similar data obtained in Kenya and other African areas, and further studies are indicated. Thus most infected individuals in a population harbour few parasites and only a small proportion are heavily infected, being responsible for excreting the bulk of eggs and causing most of the contamination in the environment. In one example, 6% of the population was found to excrete 50% of the eggs[4]. Such information may be of direct relevance to developing new kinds of control strategies, including targeted or selected treatment of the heavily infected[5]. This approach might be highly effective in preventing disease in high-risk groups, but its value in controlling transmission is uncertain[6]. Egg-counting techniques have been refined with the introduction of quality control procedures[7,8]. Immunodiagnosis has also advanced, and recent studies have clarified the meaning of the epidemiological indices, incidence, prevalence and intensity of infection, and their implications in control programmes. Considerable interest also continues in epidemiological models of schistosome transmission and their relevance to control strategy[9]. Further progress will, however, depend on greater use of recorded data and consideration of seasonal variation in transmission, immune phenomena and differences in the epidemiological characteristics of endemic situations.

PROGRESS IN CONTROL

Progress in controlling schistosomiasis during the past 30 years has been substantial in some countries (e.g. China and Japan) but relatively slow compared with other communicable infections. It is believed that this is in part because of the inadequacy of available control methods for large-scale use, and in part due to the failure to appreciate the public health significance of schistosomiasis earlier and, therefore, to give it appropriate priority in public health programmes. It is considered necessary to establish the relative importance of schistosmiasis to other health problems, since such analyses are essential for public health planning and to the rational allocation of resources for this purpose. Certain parasitic diseases may constitute a serious economic burden in developing countries, and further research should be undertaken to measure their economic significance and the economic benefits that might result from their control[10].

CONTROL OF TRANSMISSION

Specific measures such as snail control and chemotherapy generally have little or no impact on health problems other than schistosomiasis, and thus are likely to be charged directly to a schistosomiasis health budget. Non-specific control measures involving water supply, sanitation and general improvement of the environment and living conditions are less dramatic, but they have wider social and medical benefits, and their costs can be shared by public health and community development budgets. The effective use of specific snail control measures brings about a slow reduction in the prevalence and intensity of infection, and then a reduction in morbidity. The use of chemotherapy, however, has a direct impact on the disease and can quickly reduce its prevalence and intensity and then its transmission[11]. During the 1960s the use of molluscicides was the only reliable approach to the control of schistosomiasis. During the next decade it became apparent that integrated methods directed against different links in the life-cycle were the best means of achieving rapid control. Integrated methods can assure rapid and effective control of transmission. Where funds are limited, however, disease prevention may still be obtained by applying a single control approach through selected or targeted chemotherapy. The choice must be determined by local conditions.

From a strategic point of view the World Health Organization has endorsed a global plan of action to reduce morbidity[12]. Control programmes should aim to achieve a reduction in prevalence and intensity that is great enough to make the disease of minimal public health importance in relation to other endemic diseases, and such reductions may be possible with current technology[13]. Where schistosomiasis is not a clear priority, however, the high cost of drugs, molluscicides and other methods may deter control operations. Thus, it is imperative to develop less costly technology. The availability of new efficient drugs, and the advances made in epidemiological knowledge, have resulted in much optimistic thinking that different drug delivery systems can now be used exclusively for control purposes in many situations. Clearly, however, much more information is required on the relative merits of such regimens as mass treatment (treatment of an entire community), selected population chemotherapy (examination of the community, followed by treatment of infected individuals), and targeted chemotherapy (treatment of high-risk groups only after diagnosis). What are the effects on transmission of treating only high-risk groups? How does treatment affect acquired immunity, and should this effect be considered in formulating treatment policy? When is the best time to apply chemotherapy to stop transmission and how frequently should it be used? The development of schistosome resistance to individual compounds and cross-resistance to others must also be monitored, along with long-term drug effects if periodic campaigns are to be used in a maintenance strategy[6].

Chemotherapy will unquestionably play a vital role in reducing the severity of disease and contamination in the environment, and will assist in the control of transmission. It must be recognized, however, that with a few notable exceptions, experience in the use of drugs for large-scale population-based chemotherapy or targeted treatments is very limited, and the proposed delivery systems have as yet not been adequately tested. Further, inadequate attention has been given to optimal chemotherapy delivery systems and the constraints imposed by underlying epidemiological and economic factors in devising them and in ensuring adequate financial resources for continuity[14]. Comparison with other endemic disease control programmes shows that those which relied exclusively on chemotherapy had difficulties after some years, either because of the development of drug resistance in the parasite, or because of relaxation in surveillance when the incidence of infection was substantially reduced.

The WHO Expert Committee of 1978[15] distinguished three phases of schistosomiasis control operations: first, definition of the goals of the programme in the light of the priority accorded the problem, epidemiological evaluation, the design of a feasible control strategy and the allocation of resources; second, active intervention using the chosen strategy and achieving substantial reducton in endemicity; and third, protracted maintenance of control measures with corresponding reduction in the increments of control inputs. Experience in long-term maintenance control operations is very limited, and the cost-effectiveness of the particular method, or of an integrated strategy, should be expressed in terms of the time-scale involved in achieving a particular goal. The scale and periodicity of control inputs during the maintenance phase will differ from those applied in the initial intensive phase of intervention, and cost-effectiveness data should be carefully assessed in relation to their magnitude and timing and the possible duration involved. Thus, adequate provision must be made for a long period of sustained effort and recurrent expenditure.

Measures must be identified and applied that will result in effective control and achieve predictable goals in short-, medium- and long-term periods. The available data suggest that in many cases chemotherapy may be the most cost-effective short-term method of reducing prevalence, incidence and intensity of schistosomiasis, at least for *S. mansoni* and possibly for *S. haematobium*[16]. The introduction of praziquantel in recent years as a safe and very effective treatment for all schistosome species, and usually given as a single dose, has further strengthened optimism about the possibility of control based on different chemotherapy delivery systems. Consequently, there is a widely held view that adequate tools for the successful control of schistosomiasis are indeed now available, and that there is little need to search for alternatives. This opinion has, however, been challenged and further, it has been indicated that although much may be achieved with chemotherapy, it has known present limitations and potential future problems[17]. The limitations of chemotherapy as a control method have certainly been underestimated. Although there is commonly an overall reduction in the prevalence and intensity of infection soon after large-scale chemotherapy operations, reinfection in areas of intense transmission can often be extremely rapid and children, in particular, may regain up to 40% of their pretreatment egg count within a year[18,19], and even when chemotherapy is supplemented with molluscicides[20]. It is thought that two factors may contribute towards this disappointing result: older children and adults apparently develop an immunity to reinfection in the face of continued exposure. Younger children, however, remain susceptible and may, therefore, become heavily and rapidly reinfected[21,22]; further, the constraints that regulate parasite numbers in foci of intense transmission may include not only transmission factors, but also various heterogeneously expressed processes that function at the level of the individual host, so that some individuals are predisposed to heavy infections[23]. It is believed that chemotherapy is likely to be less effective in such circumstances than in situations in which transmission factors are limiting[17].

Obviously, the nature of the different constraints that determine reinfection intensities after treatment require much greater investigation[24]. Certainly in areas of high transmission, reinfection after treatment is so rapid that treatment of many individuals in the younger age group must be carried out at frequent intervals, and indefinitely. There will therefore be a need for long-term resource provision in order to undertake parasitological examinations and requisite treatments. In so many endemic areas, schistosomiasis control inevitably competes for funds with many other public health issues, some of which have higher priority. There is therefore a need to continue the search for alternative, effective and cheap control methodology. Development of safe and effective vaccines preventing infection and disease would provide the most effective approach to control. Epidemiological observations bode well for the eventual deployment of a useful vaccine in the control of schistosomiasis, and encouraging progress is now being made in the development of defined antigen vaccines.

THE FOUNDATIONS OF VACCINE RESEARCH

In the early 1960s, when Smithers, Terry and colleagues[24] began their now-classical series of experiments on immunity to *S. mansoni*, schistosome immunology was in its infancy. Von Lichtenberg, Warren and others were beginning to unravel the complex immunopathogenesis of schistosomiasis, and already many attempts had been made to develop reliable immunodiagnostic tests. In the area of 'protective' immunity there was some circumstantial evidence that both humans and animals could naturally acquire resistance to reinfection, but the mechanisms involved were completely unknown. Also, there was clear evidence that rhesus monkeys could develop resistance to reinfection with *S. mansoni*, *S. japonicum* and *S. haematobium*, but the conditions under which this would happen had not been carefully defined, and nothing at all was known of the mechanisms involved. There was no convenient laboratory model for studying protective immunity at this time, because attempts to demonstrate resistance to reinfection in rodents had given contradictory results and, likewise, attempts to induce resistance by injecting crude schistosome extracts gave inconsistent, generally negative results.

Because of the perceived difficulties with the rodent models, Smithers and Terry at first concentrated on the *S. mansoni*/rhesus monkey model. They were able to show (see reviews in refs. 25 and 26) that this species would be reliably protected against an otherwise-lethal challenge infection by prior exposure to 1000 normal cercariae given 16 weeks previously. Since the worms of the initial exposure continued to produce eggs during the period when the challenge was eliminated, it was inferred that immunity was directed against the larval stages of the challenge, and that the adult worms of the 'immunizing' infections were somehow protected against the immunity which they had themselves engendered. This was seen to be an example of the 'concomitant immunity' first described by the tumour immunologists, in which an animal with a growing tumour could nevertheless be resistant to further tumour implants. Evidence that it was the adult stage of the immunizing infection (rather than the migrating larval stages) which was the main stimulus to immunity came from the long interval elapsing between cercarial exposure and the development of solid immunity. More direct proof of this came from the demonstration that monkeys could be protected against challenge by surgical implantation by adult worms, even of a single sex, the latter point indicating that *eggs* were not necessary for the induction of immunity; indeed immunization with large numbers of live eggs did not protect monkeys against challenge.

The survival of the adult worms in their intravascular site in the immunized monkeys was clearly an immunological phenomenon of great interest, particularly as schistosomes were known to be very long-lived in the human host, too. A clue to the possible mechanisms involved came from the observation made during the worm transplantation experiments, when it was noticed that worms derived from mouse donors initially had difficulty in adapting to their new monkey hosts (there was a long interval before resumption of egg-laying) compared to worms transplanted from monkey donors. It was suggested that this might be because they had already acquired mouse 'host antigens', and that this phenomenon might act in normal infections to provide 'immunological camouflage', with the schistosomes 'masquerading as host', and thus enabling their long-term survival in the immunized host.

Studies in which rhesus monkeys were immunized with red blood cells (RBC) from one host species and then transplanted with adult worms from the same host species showed that worms were killed by antibody-mediated destruction of their tegument, presumably against acquired, host antigens. This confirmation of the 'host antigen' theory stimulated a great deal of subsequent work which defined closely the types of antigens which could be acquired, including blood group glycolipids and histocompatibility glycoproteins. Subsequently, many other mechanisms, in addition to the acquisition of host antigens, seemingly involved in the survival of schistosomes in the immunized host were described, and it is still not clear which of them is mainly responsible (see reviews in refs. 22 and 28).

IN VITRO MODELS

The original work on 'host antigens' was greatly facilitated by the development of *in vitro* techniques for the production and culture of schistosomula by Stirewalt, Clegg and others, and it was these developments which also led to the first great growth phase of study on the immune mechanisms involved in 'protective' immunity (reviewed in ref. 29). The original stimulus for the development of the *in vitro* technology came from the impossibility of carrying out detailed studies on protective immune mechanisms in the rhesus monkey, which was at the time the only standardized laboratory model. Since the rhesus monkey work had strongly indicated that it was the larval stages which were the targets of immune attack, the first experiments[30] employing the *in vitro* approach involved the culture of schistosomula (produced by the *in vitro* penetration of rodent skin) in the presence of serum from immune rhesus monkeys. It was found that the parasites were killed by antibody and complement-mediated destruction of their tegument. Successful 'lethal antibody' attack could, however, be prevented by the culture of the newly transformed schistosomula for 4 days in the presence of RBC. Since this procedure was shown to result in the collateral acquisition of RBC host antigens by the parasites, it was inferred that it was the acquisition of host antigens which protected the parasite from lethal antibody attack. At first it was believed that the development of 'lethal antibody' could explain the development of protective immunity by rhesus monkeys, but further investigations showed that the presence of high titres of lethal antibody *in vivo* did not in fact guarantee immunity to challenge.

The search for other *in vitro* killing systems with more *in vivo* relevance therefore began. A large volume of high-quality immunological work ensued, and it was this that really established protective immunity in schistosomiasis as a highly productive research area. The results of all this work were that a large number of different *in vivo* killing mechanisms were described, some of which were subsequently shown to be important *in vivo*, and that a great deal was learned of relevance to immunology in general. In particular, novel forms of ADCC involving eosinophils, neutrophils, monocytes and platelets acting in concert with anaphylactic antibody classes were discovered, and there is now accumulating evidence of the participation of some of these mechanisms, *in vivo*, in man as well as animals (see review in ref. 31).

Description of these novel ADCC systems commenced in the mid-1970s with several groups working independently, using a variety of experimental systems: Butterworth and colleagues in Kenya were employing cells and sera from experimentally immunized baboons and infected humans; Dean and colleagues derived their materials from infected rats and guinea pigs; Capron and colleagues carried out most of their investigations using the rat model. Butterworth and colleagues soon found that it was feasible to obtain eosinophils at a high degree of purity from humans, and showed that schistosomula could be killed by eosinophils acting together with antibody. Later, they produced evidence that the expression of effective immunity to reinfection in treated children may be mediated by this ADCC mechanism, or, on the other hand, rendered ineffective by the occurrence of antibodies which block the same mechanism[31].

In this context there is now incontrovertible evidence that at least some individuals in *S. mansoni* and *S. haematobium* endemic areas develop, at around the time of adolescence, high levels of resistance to schistosome infection, as judged by their faecal egg counts[32-35]. Interestingly, this resistance survives chemotherapeutic removal of the 'immunizing' infections, and in some *S. haematobium* cases is a 'sterile' immunity, rather than concomitant immunity. In these respects, immunity in the human thus closely resembles naturally acquired immunity to bovine schistosomes[36]. There are clear indications that this resistance is a manifestation of specific acquired immunity, and that it may be mediated by antibody-dependent, cell-mediated mechanisms subject to modulation by the development of blocking antibodies induced by carbohydrate epitopes expressed by egg polysaccharides, which are cross-reactive with 'protective' glycan epitopes on schistosomula glycoproteins[31,37,38]. There is, however, some recent experimental evidence which would cast doubt on the *in vivo* relevance of the participation of blocking antibodies in the modulation of protective immunity[39]. Very recently, other studies on immunity in humans exposed to *S. mansoni* in Brazil[40] have, for the first time, given a clear indication of which particular antigens are involved in protection, IgG responses to a 37 kd antigen seemingly being associated with resistance in this study. Clearly, such studies on human immune responsiveness indicate the feasibility of inducing protective immunity tc schistosomes, as well as giving various leads in terms of vaccine design and development.

IN VIVO MODELS

During the same period, several groups of workers were making very full use of rat models to carry out *in vivo* investigations on mechanisms of immunity to *S. mansoni*. This work has proved to be of enormous value in unravelling the complexities of protective immunity to *S. mansoni* (reviewed in ref. 41). First of all, it was shown by the use of thymectomized and athymic rats that the development of resistance to reinfection was thymus-dependent. Then, evidence was gathered from a range of studies (passive transfers, irradiation and reconstitution, isotype suppression) that immunity to reinfection was primarily antibody-mediated. *In vitro* assays using eosinophils showed that the earliest cytotoxic antibodies developed were of the IgG2a subclass, but that later on in the course of the primary infection IgE was mainly responsible for cytotoxic attack on the schistosomula, acting in concert with macrophages, eosinophils or platelets. Receptors for IgE were demonstrated for the first time by Capron's group on all these cell types, and this work was the first demonstration of the direct participation of anaphylactic antibody isotypes in cytotoxicity reactions. *In vivo* confirmation that these mechanisms were actually responsible for the expression of immunity came from the close parallel between the appearance of such antibodies in the serum and the time course of development of immunity to reinfection, from passive transfer experiments using pools of serum specifically depleted of these isotypes and from the fact that the various effector cell types obtained from immune rats, which expressed the respective isotypes on their surface, could adoptively transfer immunity to normal recipients. Various regulatory molecules were implicated in ADDC in the rat model, and indeed a significant role for blocking antibodies in schistosome immunity was first discovered in this model. Significantly, all the major cytotoxic mechanisms directed against schistosomula in the rat model have now also been shown to exist in schistosomiasis in man. This fact has amply confirmed the great utility of the rat model, and has increased confidence that this model can reliably be used as a primary screen to evaluate potentially protective purified antigens[31,41].

IRRADIATED VACCINE MODELS

The other major animals models which have advanced our understanding of immune mechanisms in schistosomiasis are the mouse and the rat immunized with highly irradiated cercariae. Earlier 'mouse models' employed non-irradiated (i.e. normal) cercariae to study resistance to reinfection, but they were perceived to give inconsistent results, with many workers failing to demonstrate any significant resistance. It was also obvious that, in this small animal, 'immunization' with normal bisexual infections caused severe pathological complications, and this raised the possibility that non-specific organ or tissue changes might in some way contribute to the observed resistance, a suspicion that received ample confirmation by subsequent more formal studies (see e.g. refs. 42 and 43). In the late 1960s, work involving immunization with irradiation-attenuated, or heterologous, normal cercariae demonstrated that, using several different animal models (e.g. rhesus monkeys, sheep and cattle, mice) short-lived larval infections could reliably induce significant levels of resistance to challenge infection with normal cercariae. This showed that, although the adult worms might well be the main source of protective antigens in the concomitant immunity induced by normal infections, the larval stages also expressed potent 'protective' antigens. This led not only to the development of effective live, irradiation-attenuated vaccines for use against bovine schistosomiasis[36,44], but also to effective ways of immunizing some species of primates against human schistosomes by relatively non-pathogenic means, thus facilitating investigations of immune mechanisms (see e.g. Harrison *et al.*[45]) and, for the first time, to the development of a reliable way of immunizing rodents without the use of pathogenic infections with normal cercariae. These mouse models (Minard *et al.*[46] and Bickle *et al.*[47]) have been particularly widely used for 'mechanistic' studies, and for studies designed to identify 'protective' antigens for testing in defined antigen vaccines. Neither type of study was practical in the primate model.

The irradiated vaccine/mouse model also combined the great advantages of the mouse as a subject for experimental immunology, with the advantages of the mouse as a fully permissive host of *S. mansoni*. Use of highly irradiated *S. mansoni* vaccines in mice soon showed that the resistance conferred by such vaccination could be transferred by parabiosis[48], and evidence that it was immunologically based, with the involvement of antibody, came from the demonstration that athymic nude mice and isotype-suppressed mice failed to develop resistance after vaccination with irradiated organisms[49]. In subsequent investigations[50], studies on the species specificity of this resistance showed that significant levels of resistance against *S. mansoni* challenge were developed by mice exposed to highly irradiated cercariae of the homologous species, whereas vaccination with *S. bovis*, *S. haematobium*, or *S. japonicum* failed to confer significant levels of resistance, thus confirming the specificity of the immunizing procedure, and providing more evidence of its likely mediation by specific immune mechanisms. More formal proof of the immune basis of this resistance at first proved difficult in the mouse model, because attempts to transfer resistance to naive recipients by injection of serum and of spleen or lymph node cells from donor mice vaccinated with highly irradiated cercariae were largely unsuccessful, although significant levels of resistance could be transferred to mice by injection of serum from rabbits exposed to irradiated cercariae[50]. Passive transfer of immunity using homologous sera from irradiated–vaccinated donors was, however, subsequently achieved[51], and a key finding was that passive transfer was much more effective when the serum was injected at the time when the schistosomula were migrating through the lungs. This implication of the lung stage parasites as a target for immune attack was consistent with the passive transfer experiments using rabbit serum[50], in which comparable levels of resistance were conferred by injection of rabbit serum at the time of challenge, or 5–6 days later. Attrition of the lung or early post-lung stages in this model had originally been suggested as a possibility by Bickle and Ford[52], who had studied changes in the surface antigenicity and susceptibility to *in vitro* killing during development of schistosomula, and had shown that serum from mice vaccinated with highly irradiated cercariae did recognize the surface of lung stage schistosomula. Although lung stage schistosomula were nevertheless shown to be totally resistant to both eosinophil and complement-mediated, antibody-dependent killing systems, *in vitro*, quantitative histology and autoradiographic tracking techniques in mice (reviewed in ref. 43) confirmed *in vivo* that immune attrition can occur at the lung stage.

IDENTIFICATION OF THE PARASITE STAGES INVOLVED IN IMMUNITY

Use of this mouse model also provided important insights into which stages of the parasites were responsible for inducing immunity, i.e. which parasite stages expressed the 'protective' antigens. Thus, quantitative histology on the migration of highly irradiated immunizing infections showed that optimal resistance was stimulated by larvae which survived up to the lung stage[53], and this was confirmed by using chemotherapy to abbreviate irradiated infections[54]. Interestingly, it was found that exposure of the cercariae to irradiation profoundly altered the pattern of resistance induction following chemotherapy, because whereas optimal resistance following drug termination of unirradiated infections occurred by day 2 post-infection (PI), optimal levels of resistance following the irradiation infection did not occur until day 8 PI. It appeared, therefore, that irradiation delayed the presentation of 'protective' antigens to the host following chemotherapy, but that 'protective' antigens did normally appear early during schistosomular development.

Recently, irradiated vaccines have also been used in studies on immune mechanisms in the rat and the guinea pig[63], as may be illustrated by the following account of some of our own work on the rat model. In line with results from the mouse model, it was found that significant immunity to *S. mansoni* could be induced in Fischer rats by a single, percutaneous infection with cercariae exposed to irradiation doses as high as 80 krad, indicating that post-skin stages are not an absolute requirement for the induction of resistance. However, as the irradiation dose was decreased from 80 to 40 to 20 krad, so the levels of resistance increased, and it was shown that rats injected with irradiated lung schistosomula were as resistant as those exposed to a complete, unirradiated infection, demonstrating that lung-stage schistosomula were particularly immunogenic[55].

Although passive transfer of immunity had proved difficult in the mouse model, it was readily demonstrated that serum from rats immunized with unirradiated, or 20 or 40 krad-irradiated cercariae, which died predominantly in the liver, lungs and skin, respectively, were all capable of passively protecting naive recipients against infection[56]. The level of immunity in the recipients, although substantially lower than that of the multiply immunized donors, was of the same order as was previously demonstrated following a single immunization with 0, 20 or 40 krad-irradiated cercariae. Thus, the resistance induced in rats by infection with normal cercariae, or by vaccination with irradiation-attenuated cercariae seemed to be primarily mediated by humoral immune factors. As in the mouse model, these experiments again pinpointed the lung stage schistosomula as targets of immunity, because time-course passive transfer experiments showed that serum from vaccinated rats (VRS) was significantly protective if transferred within 7 days PI, being equally effective if transferred 12 h before, or up to 6 days PI, but ineffective at 8 or 10 days PI. Thus, schistosomula of up to 7 days of age were susceptible to VRS-dependent elimination, while 8–10-day-old parasites were refractory. Since the donors of VRS had been exposed to 20 krad-irradiated cercariae, almost all of which persisted and eventually died in the lungs, it appeared that VRS recognized and mediated the elimination of the parasite stage to which the donors were predominantly exposed (the lung stage). However, 40 VRS, taken from rats exposed to 40 krad-irradiated cercariae, which died almost exclusively at the skin stage, was equally effective when transferred on day 0 or days 5–7 PI, confirming the inference from work on the mouse model that the protective antigens expressed by skin and lung schistosmula share antigenic determinants with target antigens possessed by lung and/or post-lung schistosomula.

These experiments demonstrated that lung/post-lung schistosomula were susceptible to serum-dependent elimination, but did not exclude the possibility that this post-lung attrition was incapable of improving on attrition of a cercarial challenge that would normally have already occurred in the skin. When the migration of challenge parasites was investigated in vaccinated rats, however, it was found that although the peak recovery of lung schistosomula in vaccinated rats was delayed by 1 day, it was equal in magnitude to the peak recovery in normal rats, whereas as early as 7 days PI, there was a significant reduction in the number of liver-stage schistosomula and this reduction remained constant until at least 21 days PI, despite the recruitment of more parasites from the lungs. Total recoveries from the lungs and liver indicated that no attrition of the challenge occurred until day 8, but that this attrition was complete by day 10. Elimination of the parasites therefore occurred at the time when they became insusceptible to the effects of immune serum (7–10 days), suggesting that elimination occurred rapidly after target recognition. Alternatively, the parasites may have been damaged at any point between days 0 and 7, but died later, at a critical point in their development and/or migration. However, it was shown that the worm recovery of naive recipients of 7-day post-challenge lung schistosomula from vaccinated donors was not reduced compared with the recovery of parasites which had been derived from non-vaccinated rats. Also, as a control for any effect mediated by opsonizing antibody on the surface of these lung parasites, 7-day lung schistosomula derived from unimmunized rats were incubated in serum from these vaccinated donors prior to injection into naive recipients, but again these parasites were not subject to elimination. Since there was no evidence of irreversible damage to the parasites or attrition in the skin or lungs until at least day 7, when the parasites begin to lose their susceptibility to immune serum, it was concluded that target antigen recognition, putative parasite damage, and elimination, all occurred rapidly after day 7 in the lungs or, more likely, en route to the liver. A quite different picture is painted by the great majority of *in vitro* studies, which have consistently shown that, together with a decline in antigenicity, or even despite persistent antigenicity, schistosomula became intrinsically resistant to attack after skin penetration, schistosomula recovered from lungs and liver between 5 and 12 days PI being found to be totally resistant to immune attack. However, it has recently been reported by Pearce and James[57] that 2–2½-week PI liver stage worms are transiently susceptible in their mouse macrophage-mediated *in vitro* cytotoxicity assay.

THE ROLE OF HUMORAL FACTORS IN THE IRRADIATED VACCINE MODELS

Because of the high efficacy of passive transfer systems in the rat, this model was used to investigate the roles of different antibody isotypes by immunoabsorption of IgG, IgG2a and IgG2c, and by heating at 56°C to remove IgE[58]. The results confirmed previous demonstrations of the importance of IgE in the resistance acquired by rats immunized with unattenuated cercariae[41], but IgE was shown to be unimportant in the resistance transferred by serum from rats vaccinated with highly irradiated cercariae. In contrast, the removal of 75% of the IgG2a led to almost complete abrogation of the resistance transferred with untreated VRS, and the pure IgG2a eluate conferred comparable protection on recipient rats to that transferrable by whole VRS, or the ammonium sulphate-precipitable fraction of VRS. When antigens recognized by VRS and serum from rats infected with unattenuated cercariae (CIS) were compared by immunoprecipitation of surface antigens it was found that exactly the same antigens were precipitated by VRS and CIS. Thus, the anti-schistosomula responses of rats infected by normal or irradiated cercariae were very similar, and differences in the mechanisms of resistance observed were likely to be due to differences in the antibody isotypes and/or effector cells involved, rather than differences in their antigenic specificity.

Since these experiments had suggested a key role for antibody, but had left open the possible participation of complement, subsequent experiments were carried out to determine the extent of C′ involvement in passively and actively immunized rats, and in actively immunized mice[59]. To do this the roles of C′ at various stages of parasite migration were investigated by administering CoF and anti-CoF antibody. In the rat model, roles for C′ could be demonstrated in both acquired and innate immunity. C′ was shown to play an important role in innate immunity, being more involved later in larval migration (days 8–13 PI) than at earlier times (days 0–8). Furthermore, the specific component of immunity conferred by immune serum transferred at the lung migration stage also required C′ for optimal expression, again supporting the notion that both innate and acquired immunity act primarily against the lung stage schistosomula. Furthermore, although decomplementation at earlier stages of parasite migration (<day 3 PI) did cause some reduction in innate immunity, there was no evidence of any effect on the levels of resistance actively-induced by exposure to irradiated cercariae, suggesting that, while C′ may play a role in innate immunity during the skin migration phase, specific C′-mediated attrition does not occur during this time.

Despite strong evidence for roles for C′ in both acquired and innate immunity in rats, no similar roles for C′ could be detected in mice, since in experiments examining the role of C′ up to day 15 PI, no variations in worm recovery were demonstrated after treatment with CoF, despite a 99% reduction in serum C3 levels. This corroborated previous findings in vaccinated mice[49] which suggested that C′ is not a limiting factor in immunity in mice vaccinated with irradiated cercariae.

THE ROLE OF CELLULAR IMMUNITY IN THE IRRADIATED VACCINE MODELS

Experiments were carried out to determine the possible contribution of cellular immunity in vaccinated rats, using the 'late' passive transfer model, which involved the transfer of immune serum 5–7 days PI. In this way the mechanisms of antibody-dependent elimination of post-lung stages could be analysed, without possible contributions from non-specific, or specific but antibody-independent mechanisms, or mechanisms acting against pre-lung stages. In this work[60], immunity was investigated in congenitally athymic (Nu/Nu) rats, irradiated rats, and in mast cell-depleted rats. It was shown that Nu/Nu rats failed to develop significant resistance following vaccination with irradiated cercariae, but that Nu/Nu recipients of serum from vaccinated Fischer rats manifested resistance comparable to heterozygous controls, suggesting that T cells were required in the induction of resistance but were not involved in the efferent arm of antibody-dependent elimination.

Radiosensitive cell types, including eosinophils, basophils, neutrophils, lymphocytes and mast cells, were apparently not essential for the antibody-dependent elimination of lung or post-lung stages, since irradiated (700–750 rad) recipients of VRS were as resistant as unirradiated controls, despite greater than 85% reductions in total blood leucocyte counts after irradiation. Also, depletion of 90% of tissue mast cells by treatment with compound 48/80 had no significant effect on the attrition of a challenge infection in rats rendered immune either with irradiated cercariae or by transfer of VRS. However, there was a significant increase in worm recovery in unimmunized and mast cell-depleted or irradiated rats, indicating that mast cells and perhaps other radiosensitive cell types may be involved in *innate* resistance.

In a later study using the same 'late' passive transfer system in rats, Vignali *et al.*[80] studied the reactions around lung schistosomula in immune serum recipients, with a view to establishing whether parasite trapping occurred in the lungs, and to investigate the cellular composition of any reactions around trapped parasites. They found that VRS elicited an accelerated, enhanced cellular reaction around the parasites, confirming the antigenicity of the lung stage schistosomula. Comparison of the numbers of parasite-associated foci and total parasite counts at days 12 and 16 indicated that the schistosomula were held up in the lungs of passively immunized rats, and many more free parasites were found in the lungs of unirradiated, NRS recipients than passively immunized rats, at day 8 PI, corroborating the impression that parasites were rapidly enveloped by granulomata in rats receiving immune serum. Examination of the cellular composition of the foci in unirradiated animals revealed a predominantly mononuclear response, which was equally composed of lymphocytes and macrophages. In irradiated rats, however, fewer lymphocytes were present, and in both irradiated and unirradiated rats, eosinophils accounted for only 1–3% of the cells in the foci, and were usually remote from the parasites, which argued against their role in specific immunity.

In similar studies in mice, the effects of whole-body irradiation on the immunity actively induced by 20 krad irradiated cercariae were investigated[61]. Immunized mice irradiated with 650 or 525 rad manifested comparable levels of resistance to unirradiated, immunized mice, in spite of marked reductions in blood leucocytes (>90%) and platelets (>85%), and despite an abrogation of DTH responses to schistosomular antigens. Histopathological comparison of lung sections from irradiated and unirradiated mice 7 days post-challenge showed that cellular reactions ('foci') around parasites were essentially similar in size and cellular composition, except that, in irradiated mice, eosinophils were scarce both in the foci and in lung tissue in general. Neither presumed immune complex mediated (type III) hypersensitivity (as determined by footpad swelling, 5 h after injection of antigen), nor serum levels of anti-schistosmula extract antibody (as determined by ELISA), were affected by the irradiation, and in addition, the patterns of ^{125}I-labelled schistosomula surface antigens immunoprecipitated with serum from irradiated and unirradiated mice were essentially similar. Nevertheless, subsequent studies (Vignali *et al.*, unpublished) using *in vivo* depletion of T cell subsets with cytotoxic rat McAbs clearly demonstrated that involvement of $CD4^+$T cells, since immunity could be completely abolished with these reagents, whereas $CD8^+$T cell depletion was without effect. Interestingly, other workers showed that abrogation of immunity by $CD4^+$T cell depletion happened only when depletion occurred at the skin stage of migration of the challenge (rather than the lung or post-lung stages), suggesting that only during the skin stage were $CD4^+$T cells essential for the expression of immunity[62]. It was also shown that the requirement for $CD4^+$T cells could be overcome by multiple vaccination, a result consistent with the previous demonstration[51] that mouse serum from multiply vaccinated, but not singly vaccinated, donors, contains passively protective antibodies. The importance of the skin as a site of immune attrition in mice is also supported by the results of a detailed series of experiments by McLaren and colleagues (reviewed in ref. 63). For example, histological evidence has been found that schistosomula became trapped in subdermal foci comprising eosinophils and macrophages. Furthermore, use of a cytotoxic rat monoclonal antibodies directed against mouse neutrophils at the time of challenge significantly depleted the cutaneous reaction around the challenge parasites, and also the level of resistance expressed as determined from worm recoveries[63].

IDENTIFICATION OF THE 'PROTECTIVE' ANTIGENS

All the early work on concomitant immunity to *S. mansoni* and on *in vitro* cytotoxicity was consistent with the idea that it was the young schistosomula which were the targets of immune attack, and various groups therefore started to try to identify the target antigens on this parasite stage. One of the most frequently used approaches, first described in a 1979 paper[64], was radiolabelling of schistosomular surface proteins: it seemed likely from the *in vitro* work on immune mechanisms that it was the surface of the parasites which was the target of immune attack. It was soon shown that a restricted set of protein antigens could be radiolabelled reproducibly, and beginning in 1981[65] several groups of researchers went on to determine, by immunoprecipitation techniques, which of these were antigenic in man and animals. Because of the difficulty in obtaining sufficient quantities of these antigens for biochemical purification, indirect approaches were used, such as the development of monoclonal or polyclonal antibodies (see reviews in refs. 27 and 66–68).

Smith *et al.*, in 1982[69], were the first to describe the production of mouse hybridoma cell lines producing monoclonal antibodies (McAbs) specific for schistosome antigens, usng spleen cells from a mouse vaccinated with irradiated *S. mansoni* cercariae and challenged with normal cercariae. Both McAbs described were of the IgM isotype, and both were capable of C′-mediated *in vitro* killing of schitosomula. The McAb demonstrating the highest levels of *in vitro* cytotoxicity was also shown to be effective *in vivo* in passive transfer of immunity to mice. Both McAbs recognized the surface of skin-transformed schistosomula, and male and female adult worms and miracidia, and were shown to be species-specific. The molecular weight of the antigen recognized by the passively protective McAb was 155 kd in both adult and schistosomular extracts; the presence of larger quantities of this molecule in adults was exploited to provide an adequate supply of antigen for preliminary immunization tests in mice and monkeys[70]. A variable but statistically significant protection was observed, and this was the first indication of the protective potential of defined antigen vaccines in schistosomiasis. Subsequently, many other candidate vaccine antigens have been described, and what follows is an account of several currently promising examples.

GP38 (reviewed in ref. 71)

In 1982 Grzych *et al.* described a rat hybridoma line secreting a *S. mansoni* IgG2a McAb which caused high levels of rat eosinophil-mediated cytotoxicity *in vitro* and also had the ability to passively immunize rats *in vivo*. The McAb bound to antigens of molecular weight 38 000 and >15 000 on the surface of schistosomula of <24 h post-transformation, and these antigens were also recognized by serum from infected humans and animals. The protective epitope was also found on the 115 kd molecule in adult metabolic products, and was thus conceivably involved in inducing concomitant immunity. A second McAb was also produced which recognized the same 38 kd antigen, but demonstrated no *in vitro* killing activity. Indeed, this IgG2c McAb inhibited both *in vitro* eosinophil-dependent killing of schistosomula and the *in vivo* passive transfer of immunity by the protective IgG2a McAb.

Further analysis showed that the 38 kd antigen was a glycoprotein but although GP38 seemed in many respects a good candidate for a potential vaccine, it was capable of inducing ‘blocking’ antibodies, and furthermore the sensitivity of the protective epitope to periodate treatment and the inability of the IgG2a McAb to immunoprecipitate *in vitro* translation products from parasite mRNA showed that the epitope was carbohydrate. Therefore, Grzych and colleagues developed an alternative approach to vaccine development based on the production of anti-idiotype antibodies, by showing that immunization of rats with a monoclonal anti-idiotype antibody (AB2) raised against the protective IgG2a McAb (AB1) led to a high degree of protection to challenge infection in recipient rats. A similar protection could be obtained by passive transfer of serum (AB3) from rats immunized with AB2.

Although encouraging, these results remained of limited application for vaccination against the human disease. Further studies were therefore concerned with the biochemical characterization of the protective epitope, and were aided by the chance discovery that *S. mansoni* shares this epitope with its snail host and indeed various other aquatic molluscs. In fact, immunization with the blood protein of the keyhole limpet (KLH) protected rats against *S. mansoni* infection and elicited anti-38 kd antibodies which could passively protect rats; deglycosylation of KLH abolished these properties. The availability of commercially purified KLH will obviously greatly facilitate the detection of the cross-reactive carbohydrate structure, and knowledge of the precise structure of this protective KLH oligosaccharide may allow the production of synthetic oligosaccharides bearing the protective epitope but lacking the blocking epitopes.

P28 (reviewed in ref. 71)

In a directed search for protective antigens which would be suitable for gene cloning, Balloul and colleagues separated components of *S. mansoni* adult worms by preparative SDS-PAGE and electroelution into distinct fractions. Three of these induced an antibody response in rats, but only one antiserum, directed against a 28 kd fraction, immunoprecipitated an antigen from surface-labelled schistosomula as well as from cell free translation productions of adult worm or schistosomular mRNA. This fraction induced significant levels of immunity in rats and mice, and use of the specific antiserum led to the isolation of a cDNA clone corresponding to a protective 28 kd antigen. Immunization of rats and hamsters with the fusion protein in alum induced significant protection. The full cDNA sequence of this antigen was determined and the molecular weight of the polypeptide calculated to be 28 000, suggesting there was no post-translational processing. Interestingly, cross-reactive epitopes were found, not only in at least two other human schistosome species (*S. japonicum* and *S. haematobium*), but also in the cattle parasite *S. bovis*. This has encouraged us to undertake immunization experiments in cattle, which have already demonstrated the good immunogenicity of the recombinant P28 expressed in either *E. coli* or yeast. More recently, significant protection of baboons against *S. mansoni* has also been achieved[31].

Computer-assisted comparisons later identified P28 as a subunit of glutathione (GSH) transferase, with significant homologies with both the α and μ families of mammalian GSH transferases[72]. It was also demonstrated that P28 produced from cDNA in both *E. coli* and yeast can be purified by GSH sepharose affinity chromatography and is a GSH transferase identical in subunit molecular weight, structure and substrate specificity to the major GSH transferase isoenzyme isolated from homogenates of *S. mansoni*. Immunogold electron microscopy showed that the native molecule was present in the tegument, cytons and the protonephridia of adult worms and, in addition, the head glands of schistosomula. In spite of the homology between P28 and the mammalian enzymes it was encouraging, from the point of view of vaccine development, to find that there was no significant immunological cross-reactivity between the schistosome and mammal GSH transferases.

Sj26 (see Smith *et al.*[73])

In independent studies on *S. japonicum*, carried out at the same time as those on P28, Mitchell and colleagues investigated antibody responses to adult worm antigens in the mouse strain WEHI 129/J, which is relatively resistant to primary infection with *S. japonicum*. In contrast to susceptible mouse strains, mice of the resistant strain were high responders to an antigen of molecular weight 26 000. Clones corresponding to this antigen were identified in a cDNA library in λgt11, and the full sequence of the antigen was determined. On the basis of its amino acid sequence and some additional properties, Sj26 was identified as a glutathione-S-transferase. Vaccination of mice with the β-galactosidase/Sj26 fusion protein induced significant protection. As GSH transferases are cytosolic enzymes, it was suggested that the protective effect induced by vaccination was a consequence of antibody binding to and inhibiting the form of the enzyme which might be expressed in the parasite gut, thereby neutralizing the enzyme's postulated vital detoxifying activities.

P97

James, Sher and colleagues have made particularly effective use of the *S. mansoni* irradiated vaccine mouse model to identify protective immune responses, with a view to developing new immunization methods employing non-living preparations (reviewed in refs. 74 and 75). Their conclusions were that this immmunity is both T and B cell-dependent, and involves a cell-mediated response requiring the participation of lymphocyte-activated macrophages as effector cells. The latter hypothesis was based on the identification of an inbred mouse strain (P) which failed to develop immunity and possessed unique defects in macrophage activation. That the P-strain mouse defects in vaccine-induced resistance and cell-mediated immune responses were related was suggested by the close association observed between the two recessively inherited traits in the progeny of crosses with highly resistant C57BL/6 mice. Also, macrophages from responder mice, but not from P strain mice, activated by lymphokine exposure *in vitro* or *in vivo*, could kill 3 h schistosomula and 2–3-week-old juvenile worms. Thus, the timing of parasite susceptibility to macrophage killing *in vitro* was consistent with the early and late stages of resistance already described *in vivo*[57]. For P mice the defect in macrophage larvicidal activity appeared to result from a deficiency in the capacity of their T cells to produce γ-INF when exposed to antigen, and also in the reduced ability to the macrophages to respond to this lymphokine.

An immunization protocol using non-living antigens was then designed with the intention of inducing specific CMI. It was found that injection of crude, freeze–thaw preparations of schistosomula with BCG sensitized for CMI, including specific DTH, lymphokine production, and macrophage activation, and induced up to 70% resistance to challenge, whereas intravenous immunization with the same antigens failed to induce either CMI or resistance. Characterization of the protective antigens involved showed that they were not stage-specific, being present in cercariae, 3h schistostomula, and adult worms and mice immunized with crude extracts with BCG developed minimal antibody responses to surface antigen but did produce antibody to a single internal protein of molecular weight 97 000. Upon gel filtration the protective activity separated in a high molecular weight fraction containing the same molecule.

Two cDNA clones expressing products reactive with a McAb against P97 were then identified, and from the deduced amino acid sequence it was inferred that P97 was paramyosin. In agreement with this, when paramyosin was isolated from adult worms, antibodies to P97 were shown to react with it, as well as with a known paramyosin from molluscan muscle. This work was taken an interesting step further by Matsumoto and colleagues[76], who examined the localization of this protective antigen in the parasites using gold-labelled anti-paramyosin antibodies. These antibodies bound to the contents of the non-filamentous membrane-bound elongate bodies in the tegument and cytons, and paramyosin was also observed in the oesophageal lining, which is contiguous with the tegument and which contains elongate bodies similar to those in the tegument.

The localization of paramyosin in a non-filamentous, membrane-bound form in non-muscle tissue was a novel and quite unexpected result, because paramyosin is usually organized into the core structure of the thick filaments, where it probably forms a scaffold into which cortical myosin molecules attach. The presence of this protein in the elongate bodies of the schistosome tegument and cytons suggests that it may be a secretory product of this tissue, which may explain its role in protective immunity. The fact that paramyosin does not occur in vertebrates suggests that autoimmune reactions to a P97-based vaccine would be minimal.

Schistosomular-specific antigens

Although, as described above, encouraging progress has been made in vaccination experiments with several antigens which are each shared by several stages of the schistosome life cycle, there is also considerable interest in that group of antigens specific to the schistosomular stages[77,78]. Our own approach was based upon the finding that, whereas high levels of resistance to *S. mansoni* could be induced in mice by highly irradiated cercariae, which died by the lung stage, no resistance could be stimulated by single-sex infections with normal adult worms, or by injection of viable eggs. As one explanation for this might be the existence of a particularly potent set of stage-specific protective antigens in the schistosomular stages, Bickle and colleagues[77] sought such antigens by raising monoclonal antibodies from mice immunized with highly irradiated cercariae or with 'tegumental' extracts of schistosomula (previously shown to contain 'protective' antigens[79]) and testing these in passive transfer experiments. As a result of this work we became interested in two schistosomular surface antigens of molecular weight 32 000 and 16 000. The 32 kd antigen was shown to be present in the adult worm tegument, but was species-specific, not being present on *S. haematobium* or *S. japonicum* schistosomula. This was of interest because species-specific antigens may be important candidates as protective molecules; for example, the resistance induced by irradiated cercariae is species-specific. Also, since the 32 kd antigen was present in the adult worms and on the schistosomular surface, and was recognized by sera both from demonstrably immune animals and infected humans, it was suggested that it might be involved in the immunity reported to operate in the human population. The 16 kd schistosomular surface antigen was also species-specific but, in contrast to the 32 kd antigen, was not recognized by serum from chronically infected mice or from single-sex infected mice, but only by serum from mice vaccinated with irradiated cercariae, indicating that this antigen is not presented to the host by the adult worm or by the egg. Purification and testing of this antigen is now under way.

CONCLUSIONS

Despite the highly commendable successes achieved by certain national control programmes, schistosomiasis remains a significant public health problem in numerous tropical and subtropical countries and, indeed, is spreading in many areas because of water resource developments and various other socioeconomic changes. Although several safe and effective antischistosomal drugs are now available, control remains difficult to maintain on a wide scale because of various logistical and financial constraints exacerbated by the rapidity of reinfection.

Although no vaccines are yet available, development work has reached a highly promising state, and there are several indications that effective vaccines will become available within the foreseeable future. Firstly, it has become clear that at least some residents in endemic areas develop an effective, immunologically based resistance to reinfection following repeated natural exposures. *In vitro* analyses of the mechanisms involved have provided considerable insights which have facilitated vaccine design and development. Secondly, reliable methods have been developed for inducing immunity in a wide range of animal models, and those models have proved susceptible to detailed *in vivo* and *in vitro* analyses which have greatly expedited vaccine development. Thirdly, live, attenuated vaccines have reached the stage of field evaluation in bovine schistosomiasis and their success has demonstrated that vaccines can provide a useful degree of protection under conditions of natural exposure to schistosomes. Finally, several promising candidate defined-antigen vaccines for human schistosomiasis have now been developed, and these are currently being evaluated in lower primates as a preliminary to possible clinical trials.

REFERENCES

1. Mott, K. E. (1987). Epidemiological considerations for development of a schistosome vaccine. *Acta. Tropica*, **44**(Suppl. 12), 12–20

2. Wilkins, H. A., Goll, P. H., Marshall, T. F. de C. and Moore, P. J. (1984). Dynamics of *Schistosoma haematobium* infection in a Gambian community. III. Acquisition and loss of infection. *Trans. Roy. Soc. Trop. Med. Hyg.*, **48**, 227–32
3. Jordan, P. (1977). Schistosomiasis – research to control. *Am. J. Trop. Med. Hyg.*, **26**, 877–86
4 Cook, J. A. A. (1974). A controlled study of morbidity of schistosomiasis mansoni in St. Lucian children, based on quantitative egg excretion. *Am. J. Trop. Med. Hyg.*, **23**, 625–33
5. Kloetzel, K. (1974). Selective chemotherapy for schistosomiasis mansoni. *Trans. Roy. Soc. Trop. Med. Hyg.*, **68**, 344
6. Webbe, G. (1986). Future research in schistosomiasis. *Méd. Chir. Dig.*, **15**, 121–3
7. Bartholomew, R. K. and Goddard, M. J. (1978). Quality control in laboratory investigations in *Schistosoma mansoni* in Saint Lucia, West Indies: a staff assessment scheme. *Bull. WHO*, **56**, 309–19
8. Goddard, M. J. (1980). A statistical procedure for quality control in diagnostic laboratories. *Bull. WHO*, **58**, 313–20
9. Fine, P. E. M. and Lehman, J. S. (1977). Mathematical models of schistosomiasis: report of a workshop. *Am. J. Trop. Med. Hyg.*, **26**, 500–4
10. Webbe, G. (1981). Schistosomiasis: some advances. *Br. Med. J.*, **283**, 1104–6
11. Jordan, P. and Webbe, G. (1982). *Schistosomiasis: Epidemiology, Treatment and Control.* (London: Heinemann), pp. 1–361
12. World Health Organization (1985). The control of schistosomiasis. *Tech. Rep. Ser.*, No. 728, Geneva
13. Webbe, G. (1987). Treatment of schistosomiasis. *Europ. J. Clin. Pharmacol.*, **32**, 433–6
14. Prescott, N. M. (1987). The economics of schistosomiasis chemotherapy. *Parasitol. Today*, **3**, 11–16
15. World Health Organization (1980). Epidemiology and control of schistosomiasis. *Tech. Rep. Ser. No.* **643**
16. Hoffman, D. B. Jr., Lehman, J. S. Jr., Scott, V. C., Warren, K. S. and Webbe, G. (1979). Control of schistosomiasis. Report of a workshop. *Am. J. Trop. Med. Hyg.*, **28**, 249–59
17. Butterworth, A. E., Wilkins, H. H., Capron, A. and Sher, A. (1987). The control of schistosomiasis – is a vaccine necessary? *Parasitol. Today*, **3**, 1–3
18. Polderman, A. M. and Manshande, J. P. (1981). Failure of targeted mass treatment to control schistosomiasis. *Lancet*, **1**, 217–18
19. Anon (1987). Report of an independent evaluation mission on the national bilharzia control program in Egypt, 1985 (abridged version), *Trans. Roy. Soc. Trop. Med. Hyg.*, **81**(Suppl.), 1–57
20. Kloetzel, K. and Schuster, N. H. (1987). Repeated mass treatment of schistosomiasis mansoni: experience in hyperendemic areas of Brazil, I. Parasitological effects and morbidity *Trans. Roy. Soc. Trop. Med. Hyg.*, **81**, 365–70
21. Butterworth, A. E., Capron, M., Cordingley, J. S., Dalton, P. R., Dunne, D. W., Kariuki, H. C., Kimani, G., Koech, D., Mugambi, M., Ouma, J. H., Prentice, M. A., Richardson, B. A., Arap Siongok, T. K., Sturrock, R. F. and Taylor, D. W. (1985). Immunity after treatment of human schistosomiasis mansoni. II. Identification of resistant individuals, and analysis of their immune responses. *Trans. Roy. Soc. Trop. Med. Hyg.*, **79**, 393–408
22. Clarke, V. de V. (1966). Evidence of the development in man of acquired resistance to infection of schistosoma. *Suppl. Centr. African Med. J.*, **12**(Suppl. 1), 1–30
23. Anderson, R. M. and Medley, G. F. (1985). Community control of the helminth infections of man by mass and selective chemotherapy. *Parasitology*, **90**, 629–60
24. Butterworth, A. E. and Hagan, P. (1987). Immunity in schistosomiasis. *Parasitol. Today*, **3**, 11–16
25. Smithers, S. R. and Terry, R. J. (1969). The immunology of schistosomiasis. *Adv. Parasitol.*, **7**, 41–93
26. Smithers, S. R. (1968). Immunity to blood helminths. In Taylor, A. E. R. (ed.), *Proceedings of the 6th Symposium of the British Society for Parasitology – Immunity to Parasites*, pp. 55–56 (Oxford: Blackwell Scientific Publications)
27. Simpson, A. J. G. and Smithers, S. R. (1985). Schistosomes: surface, egg and circulating antigens. In Parkhouse, R. M. E. (ed.), *Current Topics in Microbiology and Immunology*, Vol. 120, pp. 205–39 (Berlin: Springer-Verlag)

28. Pearce, E. J. and Sher, A. (1987). Mechanisms of immune evasion in schistosomiasis. *Contr. Microbiology Immunol.*, **8**, 219–32
29. McLaren, D. J. (1980). *Schistosoma mansoni*: the parasite surface in relation to host immunity. In Brown, K. N. (ed.), *Tropical Medicine Research Studies*, Vol. I, pp. 1–229 (Chichester: John Wiley)
30. Clegg, J. A. and Smithers, S. R. (1972). The effects of immune rhesus monkey serum on schistosomula of *Schistosoma mansoni* during cultivation *in vitro*. *Int. J. Parasitol.*, **2**, 79–98
31. Capron, A., Dessaint, J. P., Capron, M., Ouma, J. H. and Butterworth, A. E. (1987). Immunity to schistosomes: progress toward vaccine. *Science*, **238**, 1065–72
32. Butterworth, A. E. (1987). Potential for vaccines against human schistosomiasis. In Mahmoud, A. A. F. (ed.), *Schistosomiasis: Baillière's Clinical Tropical Medicine and Communicable Diseases, International Practice and Research*, Vol. 2, pp. 465–83. (London: Baillière Tindall)
33. Wilkins, H. A. (1987). The epidemiology of schistosome infections in man. In Rollinson, D. and Simpson, A. J. G. (eds), *The Biology of Schistosomes: from Genes to Latrines*, pp. 379–97. (London: Academic Press)
34. Hagan, P. (1987). The immune response to schistosome infections. In Rollinson, D. and Simpson, A. J. G. (eds), *The Biology of Schistosomes: from Genes to Latrines*, pp. 295–320. (London: Academic Press)
35. Anderson, R. M. (1987). Determinants of infection in human schistosomiasis. In Mahmoud, A. A. F. (ed.), *Schistosomiasis: Baillière's Clinical Tropical Medicine and Communicable Diseases, International Practice and Research*, Vol. 2, pp. 279–300. (London: Baillière Tindall)
36. Taylor, M. G. (1987). Schistosomes of domestic animals: *Schistosoma bovis* and other animal forms. In Soulsby, E. J. L. (ed.), *Immune Responses in Parasitic Infections: Immunology, Immunopathology and Immunoprophylaxis*, Vol. 2, pp. 50–90. (Boca Raton: CRC Press)
37. Dunne, D. W. and Bickle, Q. D. (1987). Identification and characterisation of a polysaccharide-containing antigen from *Schistosoma mansoni* eggs which cross reacts with the surface of schistosomula. *Parasitology*, **44**, 255–68
38. Dunne, D. W., Bickle, Q. D., Butterworth, A. E. and Richardson, B. A. (1987). The blocking of human antibody-dependent, eosinophil mediated killing of schistosomula by monoclonal antibodies which cross-react with a polysaccharide-containing egg antigen. *Parasitology*, **94**, 269–80
39. Bickle, Q. D. and Andrews, B. J. (1988). Characterisation of *Schistosoma mansoni* monoclonal antibodies which block *in vitro* killing: failure to demonstrate blockage of immunity *in vivo*. *Parasite Immunol.*, **10**, 151–68
40. Dessein, A. J., Begley, M., Demeure, C., Caillol, D., Fueri, J., dos Reis, M. G., Andrade, Z. A., Prata, A. and Bina, J. C. (1988). Human resistance to *Schistosoma mansoni* is associated with IgG reactivity to a 37 kDa larval surface antigen. *J. Immunol.*, **140**, 2727–36
41. Capron, M. and Capron, A. (1986). Rats, mice and men – models for immune effector mechanisms against schistosomiasis. *Parasitol. Today*, **2**, 69–75
42. Dean, D. A. (1983). A review. *Schistosoma* and related genera: acquired resistance in mice. *Exp. Parasitol.*, **55**, 1–104
43. Wilson, R. A. (1987). Cercariae to liver worms: development and migration in the mammalian host. In Rollinson, D. and Simpson, A. J. G. (eds), *The Biology of Schistosomes: from Genes to Latrines*, pp. 115–146. (London: Academic Press)
44. Taylor, M. G., Hussein, M. F. and Harrison, R. A. (1989). Baboons, bovines and bilharzia vaccines. In Macpherson, C. N. L. and Craig, P. S. (eds), *Parasitic Worms, Zoonoses, and Human Health in Africa, a Festschrift for Professor G. S. Nelson* (London: Unwin Hyman) (In press)
45. Harrison, R. A., Bickle, Q. D., Kiare, S., James, E. R., Andrews, B. J., Sturrock, R. F., Taylor, M. G. and Webbe, G. (1989). Immunisation of baboons with attenuated schistosomula of *Schistosoma haematobium*: levels of protection induced by immunization with 20 Krad and 60 Krad irradiated larvae. *Trans. Roy. Soc. Trop. Med. Hyg.*, **82** (In press)
46. Minard, P., Dean, D. A., Jacobson, R. H., Vannier, W. E. and Murrell, K. D. (1978). Immunisation of mice with cobalt-60 irradiated *Schistosoma mansoni* cercariae. *Am. J. Trop. Med. Hyg.*, **27**, 76–86

47. Bickle, Q. D., Tayor, M. G., Doenhoff, M. J. and Nelson, G. S. (1979). Immunisation of mice with gamma-irradiated, intramuscularly injected schistosomula of *Schistosoma mansoni*. *Parasitology*, **79**, 209–22
48. Dean, D. A., Bukowski, M. A. and Clark, S. S. (1981). Attempts to transfer the resistance of *Schistosoma mansoni*-infected and irradiated cercariae-immunised mice by means of parabiosis. *Am. J. Trop. Med. Hyg.*, **30**, 113–20
49. Sher, A., Hieny, S., James, S. L. and Asofsky, R. (1982). Mechanisms of protective immunity against *Schistosoma mansoni* infection in mice vaccinated with irradiated cerariae. II. Analysis of immunity in hosts deficient in T lymphocytes, B lymphocytes, or complement. *J. Immunol.*, **128**, 1880–4
50. Bickle, Q. D., Andrews, B. J., Doenhoff, M. J., Ford, M. J. and Taylor, M. G. (1985). Resistance against *Schistosoma mansoni* induced by highly irradiated infections: studies on species specificity of immunisation and attempts to transfer resistance. *Parasitology*, **90**, 301–12
51. Mangold, B. L. and Dean, D. A. (1986). Passive transfer with serum and IgG antibodies of irradiated cercariae-induced resistance against *Schistosoma mansoni* in mice. *J. Immunol.*, **136**, 2644–8
52. Bickle, Q. D. and Ford, M. J. (1982). Studies on surface anigenicity and susceptibility to antibody-dependent killing of developing schistosomula using sera from chronically infected mice and mice vaccinated with irradiated cercariae. *J. Immunol.*, **128**, 2101–6
53. Mastin, A. J., Bickle, Q. D. and Wilson, R. A. (1983). *Schistosoma mansoni*: migration and attrition of irradiated and challenge schistosomula in the mouse. *Parasitology*, **87**, 87–102
54. Bickle, Q. D. and Andrews, B. J. (1985). Resistance following drug attenuation (Ro11-3128 and Oxamniquine) of early *Schistosoma mansoni* infections in mice. *Parasitology*, **90**, 325–38
55. Ford, M. J., Bickle, Q. D. and Taylor, M. G. (1984a). Immunisation of rats against *Schistosoma mansoni* using irradiated cercariae, lung schistosomula and liver-stage worms. *Parasitology*, **89**, 327–44
56. Ford, M. J., Bickle, Q. D., Taylor, M. G. and Andrews, B. J. (1984b). Passive transfer of resistance and site of immune-dependant elimination of the challenge infection in rats vaccinated with highly irradiated cercariae of *Schistosoma manson*. *Parasitology*, **89**, 461–82
57. Pearce, E. J. and James, S. L. (1986). Post lung stage schistosomula of *Schistosoma mansoni* exhibit transient susceptibility to macrophage-mediated cytotoxicity *in vitro* that may relate to late phase killing *in vivo*. *Parasite Immunol.*, **8**, 513–27
58. Ford, M. J., Dissous, C., Pierce, R. J., Taylor, M. G., Bickle, Q. D. and Capron, A. (1987a). The isotypes of antibody responsible for the 'late' passive transfer of immunity in rats vaccinated with highly irradiated cercariae. *Parasitology*, **94**, 509–22
59. Vignali, D. A. A., Bickle, Q. D., Taylor, M. G., Tennent, G. and Pepys, M. B. (1988). Comparison of the role of complement in immunity to *Schistosoma mansoni* in rats and mice. *Immunology*, **63**, 55–61
60. Ford, M. G., Bickle, Q. D. and Taylor, M. G. (1987b). Immunity to *Schistosoma mansoni* in congenitally athymic, irradiated and mast cell depleted rats. *Parasitology*, **94**, 313–26
61. Vignali, D. A. A., Bickle, Q. D. and Taylor, M. G. (1988a). Studies on immunity to *Schistosoma mansoni in vivo*: whole-body irradiation has no effect on vaccine-induced resistance in mice. *Parasitology*, **96**, 49–61
62. Kelly, E. A. B. and Colley, D. G. (1988). *In vivo* effects of monoclonal anti-L3T4 antibody on immune responsiveness of mice infected with *Schistosoma mansoni*. *J. Immunol.*, **140**, 2727–45
63. McLaren, D. J. and Smithers, S. R. (1987). The immune response to schistosomiasis in experimental hosts. In Rollinson, D. and Simpson, A. J. G. (eds), *The Biology of Schistosomes: from Genes to Latrines*, pp. 233–263. (London: Academic Press)
64. Ramasamy, R. (1979). Surface proteins on schistosomula and cercariae of *Schistosoma mansoni*. *Int. J. Parasitol.*, **9**, 491–3
65. Dissous, C., Dissous, C. and Capron, A. (1981). Isolation and characterization of surface antigens from *Schistosoma mansoni* schistosomula. *Molec. Biochem. Parasitol.*, **3**, 215–25
66. Simpson, A. J. G. (1987). Schistosome molecular biology. In Rollinson, D. and Simpson, A. J. G. (eds), *The Biology of Schistosomes: from Genes to Latrines*, pp. 147–161. (London: Academic Press)

67. Kelly, C. (1987). Molecular studies of schistosome immunity. In Rollinson, D. and Simpson, A. J. G. (eds), *The Biology of Schistosomes: from Genes to Latrines*, pp. 265–293. (London: Academic Press)
68. Knight, M., Simpson, A. J. G., Bickle, Q. D., Hagan, P., Moloney, A., Wilkins, A. and Smithers, S. R. (1986). Adult schistosome cDNA libraries as a source of antigens for the study of experimental and human schistosomiasis. *Molec. Biochem. Parasitol.*, **18**, 235–53
69. Smith, M. A., Clegg, J. A., Snary, D. and Trejdosiewicz, A. J. (1982). Passive immunisation of mice against *Schistosoma mansoni* with an IgM monoclonal antibody. *Parasitology*, **84**, 83–91
70. Smith, M. A. and Clegg, J. A. (1985). Vaccination against *Schistosoma mansoni* with purified surface antigens. *Science*, **227**, 535–8
71. Dissous, C., Balloul, J. M., Pierce, R. and Capron, A. (1987). Protective antigens of schistosomes. In Mahmoud, A. A. F. (ed.), *Schistosomiasis: Baillière's Clinical Tropical Medicine and Communicable Diseases, International Practice and Research*, Vol. 2, pp. 267–277. (London: Baillière Tindall)
72. Taylor, R. B., Vidal, A., Torpier, G., Meyer, D. J., Roitsch, C., Balloul, J. M., Southan, C., Sondermeyer, P., Premble, S., Lecocq, J.-P., Capron, A. and Ketterer, B. (1988). The glutathione transferase activity and tissue distribution of a cloned Mr 28K protective antigen of *Schistosoma mansoni*. *EMBO J.*, **7**, 465–72
73. Smith, D. B., Davern, K. M., Board, P. G., Till, W. U., Garcia, E. G. and Mitchell, G. F. (1986). Mr 26,000 antigen of *Schistosoma japonicum* recognised by resistant WEHI 129/J mice is a parasite glutathione S-transferase. *Proc. Natl. Acad. Sci. USA*, **83**, 8703–7
74. James, S. L. (1986). Activated macrophages and effector cells of protective immunity to schistosomiasis. *Immunol. Res.*, **5**, 139–48
75. James, S. L., Pearce, E. J., Lanar, D. and Sher, A. (1987). Induction of cell-mediated immunity as a strategy for vaccination against *Schistosoma mansoni*. *Acta Tropica*, **44**(Suppl. 12), 50–4
76. Matsumoto, Y., Perry, G., Levine, R. J., Blanton, R., Mahmoud, A. A. F. and Aikawa, M. (1988). Paramyosin and actin in schistosomal teguments. *Nature*, **333**, 76–8
77. Bickle, Q. D., Andrews, B. J. and Taylor, M. G. (1986). *Schistosoma mansoni*: characterisation of two protective monoclonal antibodies. *Parasite Immunol.*, **8** 95–107
78. Cioli, D., Liberti, P. and Festucci, A. (1987). Stage-specific schistosome antigens. *Acta Tropica*, **44**(Suppl. 12), 70–4
79. Ford, M. J., Taylor, M. G. and Bickle, Q. D. (1987). Re-evaluation of the potential of *Fasciola hepatica* antigens for immunisation against *Schistosoma mansoni* infection. *Parasitology*, **94**, 327–36
80. Vignali, D. A. A., Klaus, S. N., Bickle, Q. D. and Taylor, M. G. (1989). Histological examination of the cellular reactions around schistosomula of *Schistosoma mansoni* in the lungs of sublethally irradiated and unirradiated, immune and control rats. *Parasitology*, **98**, 57–65

15
Recombinant vaccinia virus vaccines

G. L. SMITH

INTRODUCTION

Vaccinia virus made a major contribution to world medicine as the live vaccine used to eradicate smallpox. Although smallpox vaccination has been discontinued, in the future vaccinia virus might be reused as a live vaccine but against other medical or veterinary pathogens. This possibility arises due to advances in molecular genetics that enable the construction of vaccinia virus recombinants which express antigens derived from other pathogens. Inoculation of animals with such live recombinant viruses results in simultaneous synthesis of the foreign antigen and presentation of it to the host's immune system. This provides an effective and inexpensive means of stimulating specific immune responses that may confer protection against challenge with the pathogen from which the foreign antigen was derived. Moreover, the great experience gained during the mass producton and administration of vaccinia virus as the live smallpox vaccine could be applied during future vaccination campaigns using vaccinia recombinants directed against other pathogens. To increase the safety of vaccinia virus as a live vaccine, research is focusing on vaccinia virus molecular biology and particularly on the genes that influence vaccinia virus virulence. The resulting information will facilitate the construction of attenuated vaccinia strains which retain their immunogenicity but which do not cause vaccination-related complications. This chapter discusses the development of vaccinia virus recombinants, their potential application as new live vaccines and the pros and cons of such an approach.

VACCINIA VIRUS BIOLOGY

Vaccinia virus is an orthopoxvirus that is serologically related to, and distinct from, both cowpox virus and variola virus[1]. Although Jenner introduced a poxvirus isolated from a cow (probably cowpox) for vaccination against smallpox[2], vaccinia virus subsequently became established as the orthopoxvirus used for this purpose. The time of introduction of vaccinia virus and its origin remain obscure, but it is apparent from comparative genome analyses that vaccinia did not arise as a product of recombination between cowpox and variola[3].

Orthopoxviruses, of which vaccinia is the prototype, are large and complex. Unlike most DNA viruses which replicate in the nucleus of the host cell, poxviruses have evolved to replicate in the cytoplasm[1]. This requires additional complexity since the cellular nucleic acid polymerases, which can be utilized by viruses within the nucleus, are not available for poxvirus transciption and DNA replication. In consequence, poxviruses provide their own DNA polymerase and a multi-subunit RNA polymerase. Vaccinia virus also contains many other virus-coded enzymes involved in nucleic acid metabolism. Several of these have been purifed from virus particles and their biochemical activities have proved useful to the molecular biologist[4].

Particle structure

Vaccinia virus particles are of two types. Both contain at least one lipid envelope and are infectious, but they differ antigenically and in the composition of the external envelope[5]. The virus particle most commonly used in the laboratory is purified from cytoplasmic extracts of infected cells and usually comprises greater than 90% of infectious progeny. It contains one envelope synthesized *de novo* within infected cells. The second particle type is released from infected cells and possesses an additional lipid envelope derived from Golgi membrane in which several virus glycoproteins are embedded. These extra proteins account for the altered antigenicity and are involved in the more rapid penetration of particles into host cells[6]. With these exceptions the two particle types are the same.

Overall virion dimensions are 200 nm by 300 nm with an oval or brick-shaped structure. There is no icosahedral or helical symmetry. Inside the lipid envelope a biconcave core is associated with two lateral bodies which fit into the concavities. Purified particles contain more than 100 proteins[7] including some 15 enzymes. The composition of particles by mass is 90% protein, 5% lipid, 3.2% DNA, and there are also trace amounts of RNA and spermidine.

Genome structure

The virus genome is a linear double-stranded DNA molecule of 185 kilobase pairs (kb) (Figure 1). It has a composition of 66% adenine plus thymine (A:T) and is non-infectious when stripped of associated proteins. At the termini the DNA strands are linked by a hairpin loop into a continuous polynucleotide chain[8]. This hairpin structure is characteristic of chromosomal telomeres and can exist in two inverse and complementary forms termed flip and flop[9]. Similar structures are also found at the termini of parvovirus genomes. The genome contains inverted terminal repeats (ITR) of 10 kb within which there are blocks of tandemly repeated sequences adjacent to

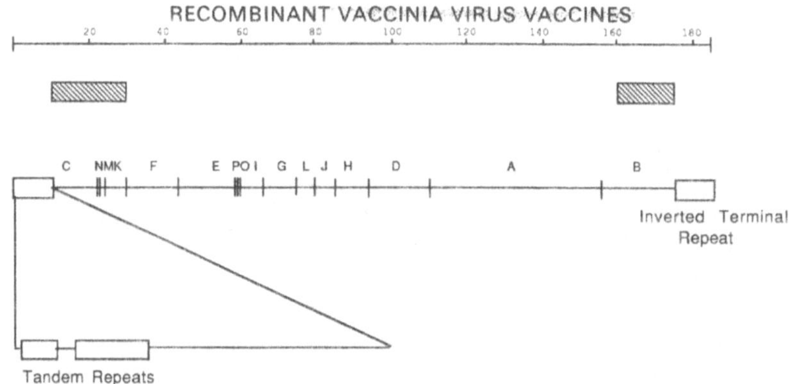

Figure 1 Structure of the vaccinia virus genome. The positions of Hind III restriction sites within the 185 kb, linear, double-stranded genome are shown. One inverted terminal repeat (ITR) is enlarged to show the blocks of tandem repeats adjacent to the terminal hairpin. Hatched boxes indicate the regions of the genome adjacent to the ITRs that may be non-essential for virus replication in tissue culture

the hairpin. There are also three genes within the ITR which are therefore diploid. The size of the ITR and the composition of adjacent internal sequences are variable among orthopoxviruses[3]. The latter regions are also non-essential for replication *in vitro* and contain genes which influence virus pathogenicity and host range. These will be discussed further in considering virus attenuation (below). In contrast the central regions of orthopoxvirus genomes show a high degree of conservation and encode many genes essential for virus replication. The nucleotide sequence of approximately one half of the vaccinia genome has been determined[10-24] and further analysis is in progress. Overall the genes are closely packed with little intervening non-coding sequences. The genes have contiguous protein coding sequences without introns, consistent with a lack of splicing of vaccinia mRNAs.

Gene expression

Vaccinia genes are transcribed by the virus-coded RNA polymerase and not RNA polymerase II of the host cell[25]. This explains why the genome is non-infectious when deproteinized. In addition, since the virus RNA polymerase does not recognize promoters from other unrelated viruses or cells, vaccinia promoters are necessary to drive expression of foreign genes by vaccinia virus recombinants[26-28]. Vaccinia genes can be arranged into three groups which are temporally controlled. Early genes are transcribed immediately after infection by the virus-associated RNA polymerase and *de novo* protein synthesis is not required for this process. Late genes are transcribed after the onset of virus DNA replication and prior expression of early genes is necessary. The third group of genes is constitutively expressed throughout infection. Generally early genes code for enzymes involved in replication, e.g. DNA and RNA polymerase and thymidine kinase (TK). Late genes code for most of the virus structural proteins.

Gene expression is controlled principally at the transcriptional level, although more subtle translational controls may exist. These processes are being intensely investigated and an understanding of them will enable more efficient expression of foreign genes in vaccinia virus recombinants. Nucleotide sequencing and mutagenesis of vacinia promoters has identified regions necessary for either early or late gene expression. Early promoters are very A:T-rich and sequences as short as 32 nucleotides upstream from the RNA start site function efficiently as early promoters[29-31]. Conserved motifs within these short sequences have been proposed based upon mutagenesis studies and homology with other early promoters[30,32]. Several early transcription factors have been identified. A 130 kd virion component binds upstream of early RNA start sites[33], and 77 kd and 87 kd polypeptides which possess DNA-dependent ATPase activity are also required for early transcription[34,35]. Termination of early transcription is mediated by the virus-coded capping enzymes which recognize the sequence UUUUUNU in nascent RNA, and which direct termination 50–70 nucleotides downstream of this sequence[36-38].

Late transcription initiates at or near a conserved motif TAAAT(G) that is present in all late promoters which have so far been identified[12,39]. This motif, which is essential[39-42], and sequences of only 15 bp upstream of it, function as late promoters. Late mRNAs are very heterogeneous in length resulting from a lack of discrete transcriptional termination at the 3′ end. In addition there are 5′ poly-A sequences that are added by a discontinuous transcriptional mechanism and which are not encoded in the virus DNA[42-47]. How these sequences influence translation of late mRNAs is unknown. Late genes code for some of the most abundant virus proteins and the promoters from these genes are consequently of interest for increased expresion of foreign genes (see below).

CONSTRUCTION OF VACCINIA VIRUS RECOMBINANTS

Vaccinia recombinants are constructed in two steps because (a) it is not practicable to directly manipulate the whole vaccinia genome, due to its large size and lack of infectivity and (b) expression of foreign genes is dependent upon vaccinia promoters. Therefore, the first stage in the construction of recombinant vaccinia viruses is to clone the foreign gene downstream of a vaccinia promoter within a plasmid vector. In the second step this chimeric gene is transferred into the vaccinia genome by homologous recombination in virus-infected cells that are transfected with the plasmid[27,48,49]. Plasmid vectors, termed insertion vectors, have been specifically designed to construct vaccinia recombinants expressing foreign genes[27,50-54]. The design of these plasmids determines the quantitative and temporal expression of the foreign gene, the site of insertion within the virus genome and the mechanism used to isolate the recombinant virus. They have the properties illustrated in Figure 2.

A vaccinia promoter is positioned upstream of several unique restriction endonuclease sites so that the transcriptional but not translational initiation site of the vaccinia promoter is retained. Foreign genes containing their own translation initiation and termination codons may then be conveniently

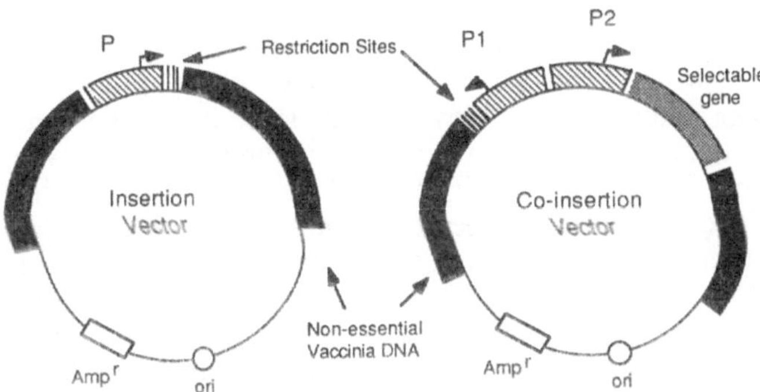

Figure 2 Plasmid insertion vectors. Two types of plasmid that are suitable for construction of vaccinia virus recombinants expressing foreign genes are shown. Hatched boxes indicate vaccinia promoters, filled boxes vaccinia DNA taken from a non-essential genomic location, and cross lines unique cloning sites. The plasmid antibiotic resistance marker and origin of DNA replication are also shown

inserted downstream of the vaccinia promoter. Some insertion vectors have been designed to create fusion proteins by retaining the vaccinia ATG codon upstream of the restriction sites[54]. More recent insertion vectors contain a second vaccinia promoter driving expression of a gene that aids isolation of the recombinant virus[50,53,54].

Vaccinia virus DNA taken from a region of the genome that is non-essential for virus replication is used to flank the promoter and restriction sites. This enables the site-specific insertion of the foreign gene into the virus genome by homologous recombination in virus-infected cells. The vaccinia TK gene is a commonly used site for insertion of foreign DNA because the resultant TK negative (TK^-) viruses may be genetically selected[27]. However, many other sites have been identified, particularly within the variable, non-essential regions adjacent to the ITRs or within the ITRs themselves[27,48,55–57]. Although these sites are non-essential for replication *in vitro* they may influence the replication or dissemination of the virus *in vivo*.

The methods used to generate and select recombinant vaccinia viruses fall into two groups, based upon the type of virus used to infect the host cells:

1. If replication-competent viruses are used, techniques are required to subsequently select or distinguish the recombinant viruses since the frequency of homologous recombination produces recombinants at only 0.1–1.0% of total progeny virus;
2. alternatively, if replication-defective viruses are used, such as conditional lethal mutants, the progeny virus may be predominantly or exclusively recombinant if the conditions chosen prevent replication of the parental virus.

If replication-dependent viruses are used, cells are infected and then transfected with the plasmid vector. The recombinants are subsequently isolated from the total progeny virus by genetic selection, visual or immunological detection, or identification by DNA hybridization. Genetic selection may involve either the inactivation of an endogenous vaccinia gene, e.g. TK[27], or insertion and expression of selectable marker genes, e.g. herpes simplex virus (HSV) TK in vaccinia virus TK$^-$ mutants[26,48], neomycin resistance[52], or *E. coli* xanthine–guanine phosphoribosyltransferase (gpt)[53,54]. The latter is particularly versatile since it may be used in most cell lines and does not require mutagenic compounds but only mycophenolic acid (to block purine metabolism) xanthine and hypoxanthine. Visual detection of recombinants has been obtained by expressing β-galactosidase, which produces a blue colour from its substrate X-gal[50] or luciferase from the firefly *Photinus pyralis* which emits light in the presence of luciferin[58]. Other types of visual selection are rescue of a small plaque phenotype to large plaques controlled by the 14 kd envelope protein[59], and loss of ability to bind chicken erythrocytes, controlled by the vaccinia haemagglutinin. Immunological detection of recombinant plaques is possible if an antibody specific for the expressed antigen is available[60]. Finally it is possible to detect the foreign DNA with specific DNA probes[48]. In the case of genetic selection of TK$^-$ viruses, detection of the foreign gene by DNA hybridization is also necessary, since spontaneous TK$^-$ viruses arise in the presence of the selective drug bromodeoxyuridine.

The use of conditional lethal mutants for the construction of recombinant viruses was introduced as a means of overcoming the problem that only a low proportion of progeny virus is recombinant. Temperature-sensitive and drug-dependent mutants have been used[61,62]. Cells are infected under non-permissive conditions so that only an abortive infection may be established. These cells are then transfected with wild-type (WT) virus DNA and a plasmid insertion vector. Recombinant genomes are formed by homologous recombination between these transfected DNAs and are then transcribed, replicated and packaged into progeny virus by *trans*-acting enzymes provided by the conditional lethal mutant. In this way the majority of progeny virus is recombinant and selective methods are unnecessary.

Properties of recombinant vaccinia viruses

The most important feature of recombinant vaccinia viruses is the retention of infectivity so that live infections may be established in cultured cells or in animals. This property contrasts with some other virus vectors such as simian virus 40, which, due to its icosahedral particle structure and small genome (5.2 kb), can accommodate additional genes only after deletion of endogenous DNA and is consequently replication-defective. Poxviruses have large genomes with more flexibility in the amount of DNA that may be packaged. Twenty-five kilobases of foreign DNA has been inserted into vaccinia without compensatory deletion[63]. Moreover, large regions (up to 21 kb) of the vaccinia genome are non-essential for replication *in vitro*[64], so that if necessary at least 46 kb of foreign DNA could be accommodated in a replication-competent vaccinia virus recombinant. This provides ample capacity for inclusion and expression of multiple different foreign genes or multiple copies of the same gene[64]. The significance of this for polyvalent vaccines is discussed below. Recombinant poxviruses are stable provided that the foreign gene is not inserted into the variable regions of the virus genome adjacent to the ITRs. Duplicate copies of foreign DNA might be stably inserted provided that each copy is separated by an essential vaccinia gene, so that any products of homologous recombination between the duplicated copies produce non-viable virus. However, defective genomes generated in this way could possibly be packaged together with replication-competent, helper genomes.

Expression of foreign genes

Vaccinia virus has been widely used as an expression vector for genes from diverse origins[49,65]. The major requirements are that the gene should have contiguous proein coding sequences without introns, that it should not contain the early transcriptional termination signal TTTTTNT and that the first ATG codon at the 5′ end of the gene should be the one which initiates translation of the desired open reading frame. If genes containing introns are to be expressed it is necessary to obtain a cDNA copy since vaccinia will not splice out these introns. The presence of TTTTTNT within the gene may be overcome by expressing the gene from a late vaccinia promoter so that the signal is no longer recognized. For example, expression of human papilloma virus type 16 L1 gene (which contains three early termination signals) from the late 4b promoter, increased expression levels by approximately 10-fold compared with the 7.5K early/late promoter[66]. Additional ATG codons between the RNA start site and the real translational initiation codon are also a problem. Some expression may still be obtained, particularly if translation terminates before the authentic ATG, but it is reduced in comparison with situations in which there is only a single ATG codon[47]. In these cases it may be necessary to remove the upstream ATG codons by Bal31 exonuclease or olignucleotide-directed mutagenesis.

The sequence around the ATG initiating translation of vaccinia early mRNAs closely mimics the consensus sequence proposed by Kozak for eukaryotic mRNAs. For late vaccinia mRNAs, although the DNA sequence predicts the present of T at the −3 position in most cases, the addition of 5′ poly-A means a purine is present at the −3 position. Consequently there is currently no reason to believe that foreign genes containing Kozak consensus sequences around their ATG codons are translated less efficiently than other vaccinia genes. However, for late mRNAs the function of the 5′ poly-A sequence and its influence on translation remain unknown. Differences in levels of expression of foreign genes are primarily controlled by the vaccinia promoter chosen, and those from major late structural proteins such as 11K and 4b have given the highest levels of expression.

In the great majority of cases foreign proteins expressed by vaccinia recombinants have been correctly post-translationally processed, migrate to the predicted subcellular location and have the predicted antigenicity. Glycoproteins may migrate to the cell surface at either the apical or basal membrane[67], or to the nuclear membrane, e.g. some herpesvirus glycoproteins[68–70], or may be excreted from the cell, e.g. hepatitis B virus surface antigen (HBsAg)[71–73]. Some other proteins, e.g. influenza nucleoprotein or polyoma virus structural proteins, migrate to the nucleus[74,94]. The extent of glycosylation is similar to that of the glycoprotein in its normal environment. Specific examples where differences occur are influenza haemagglutinin (HA)[74] and glycoprotein H (gH) of HSV and human cytomegalovirus (HCMV)[70]. In the case of HA the greater extent of glycosylation probably reflects a lack of influenza virus-encoded neuraminidase to trim terminal sialic acid. Incorrect processing and transport of proteins have also been reported in a few cases[70,75,76]. In these instances it is usual for both incorrect processing and aberrant transport to occur, suggesting these events are linked.

APPLICATIONS AS VACCINES

Much of the interest in recombinant vaccinia viruses stems from their potential application as new live vaccines. The broad host range of vaccinia in man and animals enables the use of vaccinia-based vaccines in both medical and veterinary practice. There are many examples of successful immunization of experimental animals (and a few cases in man) with vaccinia virus recombinants expressing foreign antigens[60,61,68–104]. The virus can be administered by dermal scarification or intradermal injection (analogous to smallpox vaccination) and causes a local lesion which heals in 1–2 weeks. Viruses have also been administered by intraperitoneal or intravenous injection and by oral ingestion of infected food[100]. In the majority of cases specific imunological responses to the foreign antigen have been stimulated. These have been both cell-mediated and humoral, reflecting the live nature of the vaccine. Some examples of these immune responses and factors which influence their type and magnitude are given below.

Antibody responses

Primary vaccination has usually resulted in synthesis of antibody against both the foreign antigen and vaccinia proteins. However, considerable variations in the level of antibody have been observed even when different foreign antigens are expressed from the same vaccinia promoter and, therefore, probably at similar levels. In these cases the different immune responses are most likely reflections of the variable intrinsic immunogenicity of the antigens. The location of the antigen within an infected cell, or whether it is secreted in a soluble or particulate form, are also relevant factors. Generally, glycoproteins expressed on the cell surface have proved good immunogens, with a few exceptions[84,90], and antigens within the cytoplasm or nucleus may be less immunogenic. However, no absolute generalizations are possible. The rabies virus glycoprotein has proved to be an exceptionally potent immunogen capable of stimulating high levels of neutralizing antibody in addition to cytotoxic T lymphocytes (CTL)[61,78]. Antibody responses are mostly serum IgG but local secretory IgA has also been produced if the vaccinia virus is administered onto a mucous membrane[85,101].

Revaccination of an immune animal with the same recombinant virus can give rise to increases in antibody titres to both vaccinia virus and the foreign antigen. More importantly, revaccination with a different recombinant virus expressing an antigen to which the animal is immunologically naive, can stimulate antibody to the new antigen despite existing immunity to vaccinia virus[64]. Although this is so, the level of antibody produced is reduced compared to primary vaccination. Nonetheless, this demonstrates that vaccination with vaccinia recombinants need not be considered as strictly a single event. Vaccination of humans with recombinant vaccinia viruses, purposeful or accidental, has also produced antibody responses to the foreign antigen even when the vaccinee has previously received smallpox vaccination[102,103]. In the case of a recombinant vaccinia virus expressing the human immunodeficiency virus (HIV) envelope protein gp160, revaccination and administration of autologous, virus-infected cells has boosted antibody levels to this antigen[104]. Vaccinia virus recombinants expressing several foreign antigens have simultaneously stimulated antibody to all these antigens, demonstrating the practicality of polyvalent vaccinia-based vaccines[64].

Cellular immune responses

Live vacines are often efficient at stimulating cell-mediated immune responses as well as antibody. Therefore, it was hoped that vaccinia recombinants would stimulate T-cell responses to foreign antigens. This has proved to be true for vaccinia recombinants expressing antigens at the cell surface and 'internally' within the cytoplasm or nucleus[78,84,95,105-116]. Indeed, the use of vaccinia vectors has helped to establish that 'internal' virus antigens may be efficiently recognized by CTL, and in some cases are the major target antigens. These viruses are proving to be versatile immunological tools to determine which virus antigens are recognized by, or stimulate, CTL[116-118] and have also demonstrated that recognition of some virus antigens is dependent upon major histocompatibility complex (MHC) haplotype[108].

Most of the recombinant vaccinia viruses that have been used for studies of antigen recognition by T cells have utilized the early/late 7.5K vaccinia promoter to express the foreign antigen. This has proved fortuitous, since it is now recognized that vaccinia virus sometimes interferes with antigen presentation to T cells, and that this interference is more profound when the foreign antigen is expressed from a late vaccinia promoter[110,118]. The interference is neither universal nor absolute but appears to be antigen-dependent. Nonetheless, the failure of T cells to recognize or be primed by antigens expressed late in vaccinia-infected cells would be of major significance in the design of recombinant vaccinia vaccines that need to stimulate T-cell immunity. As mentioned above, it is sometimes necessary to express antigens from late and not early vaccinia promoters.

One hypothesis to explain this partial lack of antigen presentation in association with class I MHC antigens, is that the proteolytic degradation of antigens into peptides is blocked late in vaccinia infection. This idea is supported by the recent demonstration that for some antigens that are expressed in vaccinia-infected cells but are not recognized by CTL, the blockage in recognition may be overcome by expressing unstable, rapidly degraded forms of the antigen[118]. The mechanism by which vaccinia prevents antigen breakdown is uncertain, but the identification of a family of vaccinia proteins with homology to serine protease inhibitors (serpins) (G. L. Smith, unpublished data) raises the fascinating possibility that these proteins are responsible. If this is so, it is likely that presentation of vaccinia antigens is also blocked by the same mechanism and, therefore, that the serpins may be a means by which the virus evades the immune surveillance of the host.

Despite this partial interference in antigen presentation to T cells, vaccinia recombinants have often effectively stimulated T cells against foreign antigens in humans and animals.

Protection against disease

Vaccinia virus recombinants have protected experimental animals against many diseases including those caused by influenza[77], hepatitis B virus (HBV)[119], HSV[72,79], rabies[61], vesicular stomatitis[60], Friend's murine leukaemia (F-MuLV)[84], respiratory syncytial virus (RSV)[85–87], polyoma[95], parainfluenza[98] and measles[99]. There are also many other cases where immune responses to foreign antigens have been observed but protection not tested or obtained. In some cases vaccination induced protection despite the lack of neutralizing antibody in the vaccinated animals[84,119]. These animals had been immunologically primed so that a rapid antibody response resulted following re-exposure to the foreign antigen during challenge, and there may also have been a T cell response.

Immunization with vaccinia recombinants has also prevented formation of tumours induced by viruses or other agents[84,95,120]. Vaccination of rodents with recombinant viruses expressing polyoma virus large or middle T antigen prevented subsequent polyoma-induced tumours. In addition, immunization of animals possessing established tumours caused regression and clearance[95]. Malignant melanoma has also been prevented by immunization with a vaccinia recombinant expressing melanoma-associated antigen[120]. However, in this case the antigen expressed by vaccinia is a natural host protein and the possibility of inducing autoimmune disease must be considered. Despite this the concept of using vaccinia recombinants as anti-tumour agents is an exciting development.

Several groups of researchers are attempting to construct vaccines for HIV based upon vaccinia recombinants[82,83]. Despite good expression of HIV gp160 and immunogenicity, protection of chimpanzees was not obtained in one trial[121]. However, the animal model for HIV is poor and the dose of challenge virus difficult to compare to the *in vivo* situation. Nonetheless immune respones to gp160 have been obtained in humans, and the long-term efficacy of such an approach is under evaluation[104].

Rabies may become the first pathogen to be controlled by vaccinia recombinants. This is partly because the rabies glycoprotein is exceptionally immunogenic and a wide range of experimental animals have been protected by immunization with these recombinants, but also because animals (foxes) can be effectively immunized by ingestion of virus-infected food[100]. This permits immunization of wild animals by scattering of virus-infected bait, and a field trial to test the efficacy of this approach is in progress in Europe. Whether virus left in the open will cause accidental infections in humans is being considered.

IMPROVEMENTS TO VACCINA-BASED VACCINES

Experimental vaccination of animals has so far only been performed with the first generation of vaccinia recombinants in which the expression of foreign antigens and their immunogenicity have not been optimized. If vaccinia recombinants are to find widespread application as new vaccines, improvements in expression and immunogenicity are needed. In addition, improvements to the safety of vaccinia virus as a vaccine are necessary to overcome the complications sometimes associated with vaccination.

Expression may be improved by increasing the level of transcription or translation, or increasing the gene copy number. Since transcription is dependent on poxvirus promoters considerable effort has been put into the isolation of stronger promoters. The genes coding for the major structural components of the virus have been mapped and their promoters used. The late 11K and 4b promoters have given levels of expression approximately four-fold greater than those obtained by the widely used 7.5K promoter. Although a step in the right direction, this level of increase has been somewhat disappointing, since these promoters are likely to be the strongest vaccinia promoters to have evolved naturally, and the antigens expressed from them are not visible as major components of infected cell protein as has been found with the insect baculovirus expression vectors. However, two other approaches are providing more optimistic results. One method uses a hybrid vaccinia virus–T7 RNA polymerase system for expression of target genes[122,123]. Two vaccinia virus recombinants are constructed; one contains the bacteriophage T7 RNA polymerase gene downstream of a vaccinia promoter, and the second contains the target gene downstream of a T7 promoter. Co-infection of cells with these two viruses yields greater amounts of foreign antigen than produced from conventional vaccinia promoters, but unfortunately it was not possible to co-express the T7 RNA polymerase and T7 promoter in the same virus reducing the potential usefulness as a vaccine.

Another promising approach utilizes a very strong promoter derived from cowpox virus, but which is also functional in vaccinia-infected cells. During the late phases of cowpox infection a cytoplasmic A-type inclusion body is formed that is composed predominantly of a single virus protein[46]. The promoter from the gene encoding this protein is extremely strong and foreign genes expressed from it are visible as Coumassie-stained bands in extracts of total infected cell protein.

Another way of increasing expression is to produce multiple gene copies. The most extreme example of this concerns an endogenous vaccinia gene encoding ribonucleotide reductase (RR). In the presence of hydroxyurea, gene amplification of the small subunit of RR occurs to overcome the toxicity of this drug[124]. However, the tandemly repeated amplified copies are unstable if the selective pressure of the drug is withdrawn. Similarly, tandem repeats of foreign genes are unstable unless they are separated by essential vaccinia genes.

The effects of optimizing translation of foreign genes may prove to be of minor significance compared to transcriptional effects. However, the presence of 5′ poly-A sequences on late mRNAs makes this uncertain, and a rigorous investigation of the role of sequences between the 5′ end of the mRNA and AUG codon and around the AUG codon of early and late vaccinia mRNAs is being undertaken.

Improvements in antigen immunogenicity are more difficult to achieve. However, several relevant factors have been identified, including the location of the antigen within the cell, whether the antigen is soluble or particulate and whether T helper and T cytotoxic epitopes are present on the protein. The route of inoculation and MHC type may also be important. The importance of antigen location was demonstrated by experiments comparing the immunogenicity of recombinant viruses that expresed an antigen from the blood form stage of the malarial parasite *Plasmodium falciparum*. The natural secreted form of the antigen was poorly immunogenic, but immunogenicity was greatly improved by the anchoring of the antigen on the cell surface[93]. In another study the immunogenicity of the major antigenic determinant of foot and mouse disease virus (FMDV) VP1 was compared when expressed as an amino terminal fusion with β-galactosidase, or when fused to the core protein of HBV, which spontaneously forms a particulate structure[125]. In the former case the product was a soluble cytoplasmic protein and only very low levels of antibody were induced to VP1. In contrast, the FMDV epitope expressed on the surface of HBV core particles was highly immunogenic, inducing levels of immunity surpassed only by whole FMDV particles. T helper epitopes present on the HBV core protein, the particular nature of the antigen, and high epitope density probably all influenced this enhanced immunogenicity.

The importance of the route of inoculation of virus has also been demonstrated. For protection against respiratory infections induced by influenza virus or RSV, the presence of local secretory IgA antibody was necessary to prevent nasal infection, although serum IgG could prevent viral pneumonia[85,86,101]. Local IgA antibody was only induced by local administration of vaccine. As a further example, dermal scarification of a vaccinia recombinant expressing F-MuLV gp85 envelope conferred protection against Friend virus leukaemia to both male and female mice[84]. However, intraperitoneal injection of the virus induced much better protection in males than females. This latter study also illustrated the influence of MHC type upon protection.

A recent approach to increase immunogenicity is to co-express lymphokines such as interleukin 2 (IL-2) or γ-interferon by vaccinia recombinants[55,126]. Although the effects of expressing these genes on immunogenicity have not yet been adequately analysed, expression of IL-2 markedly attenuated the virus (see below).

Safety and attenuation

A major criticism of the reuse of vaccinia virus as a vaccine is the absolute safety of the virus. Indeed the eradication of smallpox was welcomed not only as the end of a greatly feared disease, but also as the end of the need for vaccination with vaccinia virus and the vaccine-related complications that could ensue. As with other live vaccines, immunization with vaccinia virus creates a small risk of vaccine-related complications. The frequency and types of these complications have been carefully studied by several groups, but probably the most comprehensive study was performed in the USA in 1968[127]. A total of 14.2 million vaccinations resulted in 512 complications and nine deaths. Complications were 10-fold more common in cases of primary rather than secondary vaccination, and approximately 20% occurred in contacts of vaccinees. Eczema and immunodeficiency were recognized as contraindications to vaccination; nonetheless many of the complications occurred in patients with these conditions. While more rigorous screening of patients would undoubtedly have reduced vaccine-related disease, there were also less predictable neurological complications, such as post-vaccinial encephalitis, that occurred in healthy individuals. European studies have implicated the strain of vaccinia as being a major factor in the frequency of this condition.

Against this background the resistance to the idea of reintroducing vaccinia is at first understandable. However, as with all vaccines there is a balance between the benefit from, and risks of, vaccination. For diseases that carry high mortality or morbidity, such as smallpox, AIDS, HBV (with resultant hepatocellular carcinoma) and malaria, the benefit from protective immunization would seem to greatly outweigh the low risk from vaccination. Nonetheless, there is a clear need to develop more attenuated strains of vaccinia virus, and considerable effort and progress is being made in this direction.

The large genome of vaccinia virus includes many genes dispensable for growth in tissue culture in addition to genes essential for virus propagation. Many of these non-essential genes are clustered in variable regions of the virus genome adjacent to the ITR, but others are scattered throughout the genome. It is partly due to the development of vaccinia recombinants and the search for non-essential loci into which foreign genes may be inserted that these non-essential genes have been identified. Some of the functions of these genes are to help the virus to replicate better in unfavourable environments. Two examples of such genes are the vaccinia growth factor (VGF)[56] and TK[128]. VGF is a secreted protein, with homology to epidermal growth factor, that interacts with cells around the focus of virus infection and stimulates these quiescent cells to proliferate. Actively dividing cells have a greater metabolic activity and are better able to support virus replication. This protein is at least partly responsible for the dermal hyperplasia characteristic of poxvirus pathology. TK increases the intracellular levels of DNA precursors, which in turn aids virus replication. In quiescent dermal or neurological cells these intracellular nucleotide pools may be low. Other non-essential virus genes control host range[24], or may enable the virus to escape from the host's immune surveillance (serpin genes).

Deletion of several non-essential genes profoundly influences vaccinia virus biology. The host range gene that is essential for growth in human cells[24] has important implications for the use of vaccinia virus recombinants in veterinary medicine, since viruses lacking these gene would prevent the accidental transmission of the virus to humans. This would be valuable for vaccination of wild animals against rabies by leaving virus-containing bait. How such a deletion would influence the immunogenicity of the recombinant virus remains to be established.

Attenuation of vaccinia in animals has resulted from deletion or inactivation of the following virus genes: TK[128], VGF[56], haemagglutinin[55] and 14K envelope proein[129]. In addition, deletion of large non-essential regions near the left-hand ITR also greatly reduces virus virulence[129]. TK^- viruses have decreased ability to disseminate to, or replicate in, internal organs or brain[128]. This may be particularly relevant to the least predictable complication of vaccination, post-vaccinal encephalitis. Any reduction in the ability of the virus to spread, cause viraemia or replicate in neural tissue is likely to reduce the incidence of this condition. Despite the fact that TK^- viruses are attenuated, most animal protection studies and inoculation of humans have used TK^- recombinant vaccinia viruses. Probably immune responses would have been greater if viruses with wild-type pathogenesis had been used. The VGF gene also influences virus virulence. Removal of this gene, which is present in each ITR, results in reduction of virus-induced hyperplasia and virus replication in dermal tissue[56]. Virus glycoproteins that influence virulence are the 14K envelope antigen that is involved in virus entry and membrane fusion[130] and the haemagglutinin which is present on extracellular virus[6,55]. It is very probable that other virus genes will influence virulence. Other virus gycoproteins present on the extracellular virus particles and the vaccinia serpin genes may be good candidates. In the latter case, deletion of serpin genes may have the dual benefits of reducing virulence and increasing immunogenicity. Restoration of antigen presentation to T cells might increase immunogenicity, but also render virus-infected cells more sensitive to the host's immune system and thereby restrict virus growth. Serpin-deficient viruses may also become less able to infect, and be disseminated by, circulating macrophages because the abundant proteasese of these cells would no longer be inhibited.

IL-2 expression has also caused attenuation of vaccinia virus[55,126]. Originally expressed in vaccinia as a means to increase immunogenicity, it was observed that this protein attenuated the virus, particularly in immunosuppressed hosts. Whereas vaccinia viruses lacking this gene produce progressive fatal infections in nude mice, recombinants expressing this gene are tolerated and cleared by these animals. The use of vaccinia virus is contraindicated in populations where HIV or other immunosuppressive agents are endemic, since generalized or progressive vaccinia infections can result[131]. Co-expression of IL-2 or other lymphokines might change this.

The generation of attenuated forms of vaccinia virus is therefore possible. What remains to be evaluated is how the various types of attenuation influence immunogenicity. A suitable balance between safety, through attenuation, and efficacy, through immunogenicity, must be reached.

Although the reuse of vaccinia virus as a live vaccine is only one of several approaches to vaccine development, it has several advantages. The virus can simultaneously express, and immunize against, several foreign antigens providing multiple benefit from a single vaccination. The virus is easy and cheap to mass-produce, and can be stored and transported without refrigeration. It can be rapidly administered to large populations by relatively unskilled personnel in field conditions. The virus stimulates both antibody and T cell responses and can be re-administered to booster existing immunity or to deliver new antigens. The virus can be used in both human and veterinary medicine. Lastly, the virus can be attenuated to varying degrees from wild-type virus to viruses that establish only abortive infections in human cells. The prospects for this type of live vaccine remain exciting.

ACKNOWLEDGMENTS

I thank Mrs M. Wright and Mrs H. Wilson for typing the manuscript, and Dr S. Kerr for artwork and critical reading of the manuscript.

REFERENCES

1. Moss, B. (1985). Replication of poxviruses. In Fields, B. N., Chanock, R. M. and Roizman, B. (eds), *Virology*, pp. 658–703. (New York: Raven Press)
2. Jenner, E. (1798). *An inquiry into the causes and effects of the variolae vaccinae, a disease discovered in some regions of western counties of England, particularly Gloucestershire, and known by the name of cowpox.* (Reprinted by Cassel, London, in 1896)
3. Mackett, M. and Archard, L. E. (1979). Conservation and variation in the orthopoxvirus genome structure. *J. Gen. Virol.*, **45**, 658–702
4. Moss, B. (1981). End labelling of RNA with capping and methylating enzymes. In Chirikjian, J. G. and Papas, T. S. (eds), *Gene Amplification and Analysis*, Vol 2, pp. 254–66 (Elsevier: North Holland)
5. Boulter, E. A. and Appleyard, G. (1973). Differences between the extracellular and intracellular forms of poxvirus and their implications. *Prog. Med. Virology*, **16**, 86–108
6. Payne, L. G. (1980). Significance of extracellular enveloped virus in the *in vitro* and *in vivo* dissemination of vaccinia. *J. Gen. Virol.*, **50**, 98–100
7. Oie, M. and Ichihashi, Y. (1981). Characterization of vaccinia polypeptides. *Virology*, **113**, 263–76
8. Geshelin, P. and Berns, K. I. (1974). Characterization and localization of the naturally occurring cross-links in vaccinia virus DNA. *J. Mol. Biol.*, **88**, 785–96
9. Baroudy, B. M., Venkatesan, S. and Moss, B. (1982). Incompletely base-paired flip-flop terminal loops link the two strands of the vaccinia genome into one uninterrupted polynucleotide chain. *Cell*, **18** 315–24
10. Pluicienniczak, A., Schroeder, E., Zettlemeissl, G. and Streeck, R. E. (1985). Nucleotide sequence of a cluster of early and late genes in a conserved segment of the vaccinia virus genome. *Nucl. Acids Res.*, **13** 985–98
11. Broyles, S. and Moss, B. (1986). Homology between RNA polymerases of poxviruses, prokaryotes and eukaryotes: nucleotide sequence and transcriptional analysis of vaccinia virus genes encoding 147 kDa and 22 kDa subunits. *Proc. Natl. Acad. Sci. USA*, **83**, 3141–5
12. Rosel, J. L., Earl, P. L., Weir, J. P. and Moss, B. (1986). Conserved TAAATG sequence at the transcriptional and translational start sites of vaccinia virus late genes deduced by structural and functional analysis of the HindIII H genome fragment. *J. Virol.*, **60**, 436–49
13. Niles, E. G., Condit, R. C., Caro, P., Davidson, K., Matusick, L. and Seto, J. (1986). Nucleotide sequence and genetic map of the 16-kb vaccinia virus HindIII D fragment. *Virology*, **153**, 96–112
14. Weinrich, S. L. and Hruby, D. E. (1986). A tandemly-orientated late gene cluster within the vaccinia virus genome. *Nucl. Acids Res.*, **14**, 3003–16

15. Rosel, J. and Moss, B. (1985). Transcriptional and translational mapping and nucleotide sequence of a vaccinia virus gene encoding the precursor of the major core polypeptide 4b. *J. Virol.*, **56**, 830–8
16. Venkatesan, S., Gershowitz, A. and Moss, B. (1982). Complete nucleotide sequence of two adjacent early vaccinia virus genes located within the inverted terminal repetition. *J. Virol.*, **44**,. 637–46
17. Shida, H. (1986). Nucleotide sequence of the vaccinia virus haemagglutinin gene. *Virology*, **150**, 451–62
18. Hirt, P., Hiller, G. and Wittek, R. (1986). Localization and fine structure of a vaccinia virus gene encoding an envelope antigen. *J. Virol.*, **58**, 757–64
19. Earl, P. L., Jones, E. V. and Moss, B. (1986). Homology between DNA polymerases of poxviruses, herpesviruses and adenoviruses: nucleotide sequence of the vaccinia virus DNA polymerase gene. *Proc. Natl. Acad. Sci. USA*, **83**, 3659–63
20. Schmitt, J. F. C. and Stunnenberg, H. G. (1988). Sequence and transcriptional analysis of the vaccinia virus HindIII I fragment. *J. Virol.*, **62**, 1889–97
21. Rodriguez, J. F. and Esteban, M. (1987). Mapping and nucleotide sequence of the vaccinia virus gene that encodes a 14 kDa fusion protein. *J. Virol.*, **61**, 3550–4
22. Tamin, A., Villarreal, E. C., Weinrich, S. L. and Hruby, D. E. (1988). Nucleotide sequence and molecular genetic analysis of the vaccinia virus HindIII N/M region encoding the genes responsible for resistance to α-amanitin. *Virology*, **165**, 141–50
23. Boursnell, M. E. G., Foulds, I. J., Campbell, J. I. and Binns, M. A. (1988). Non-essential genes in the vaccinia HindIII K fragment: a gene related to serine protease inhibitors and a gene related to the 37K vaccinia major envelope antigen. *J. Gen. Virol.*, **69**, 2995–3003
24. Gillard, S. D., Spehner, D., Drillien, R. and Kirn, A. (1986). Localization and sequence of a vaccinia virus gene required for multiplication in human cells. *Proc. Natl. Acad. Sci. USA*, **83**, 5573–7
25. Puckett, C. and Moss, B. (1983). Selective transcription of vaccinia virus genes in template-dependent extracts of infected cells. *Cell*, **35**, 441–8
26. Mackett, M., Smith, G. L. and Moss, B. (1982). Vaccinia virus: a selectable eukaryotic cloning and expression vector. *Proc. Natl. Acad. Sci. USA*, **79**, 7415–19
27. Mackett, M., Smith, G. L. and Moss, B. (1984). General method for the production and selection of infectious vaccinia virus recombinants expressing foreign genes. *J. Virol.*, **49**, 857–64
28. Cochran, M. A., Mackett, M. and Moss, B. (1985). Eukaryotic transient expression system dependent on transcription factors and regulatory DNA sequences of vaccinia virus. *Proc. Natl. Acad. Sci. USA*, **82**, 19–23
29. Cochran, M. A., Puckett, C. and Moss, B. (1985). *In vitro* mutagenesis of the promoter region of a vaccinia virus gene: evidence for tandem early and late regulatory signals. *J. Virol.*, **54**, 30–7
30. Weir, J. P. and Moss, B. (1987). Determination of the promoter region of an early vaccinia virus gene encoding thymidine kinase. *Virology*, **158**, 206–10
31. Coupar, B. E. H., Boyle, D. B. and Both, G. W. (1987). Effect of *in vitro* mutations in a vaccinia virus early promoter region monitored by herpes simplex virus thymidine kinase expression in recombinant vaccinia virus. *J. Gen. Virol.*, **68**, 2299–309
32. Vassef, A. (1987). Conserved sequences near the early transcriptional start sites of vaccinia virus. *Nucl. Acids Res.*, **15**, 1427–43
33. Yuen, L., Davison, A. J. and Moss, B. (1987). Early promoter-binding factor from vaccinia virus virions. *Proc. Natl. Acad. Sci. USA*, **84**, 6069–73
34. Broyles, S. S., Yuen, L., Shuman, S. and Moss, B. (1988). Purification of a factor required for transcripion of vaccinia virus early genes. *J. Biol. Chem.*, **263**, 10754–60
35. Broyles, S. S. and Moss, B. (1988). DNA-dependent ATPase activity associated with vaccinia virus early transcription factor. *J. Biol. Chem.*, **263**, 100761–5
36. Rohrmann, G., Yuen, L. and Moss, B. (1986). Transcription of vaccinia virus early genes by enzymes isolated from vaccinia virions terminates at a downstream regulatory sequence. *Cell*, **46**, 1029–35
37. Yuen, L. and Moss, B. (1986). Multiple 3′ ends of mRNA encoding vaccinia virus growth factor occur within a series of repeated sequences downstream of T clusters. *J. Virol.*, **60**, 320–3

38. Schuman, S., Broyles, S. S. and Moss, B. (1987). Purification and characterization of a transcription termination factor from vaccinia virions. *J. Biol. Chem.*, **262**, 13272–80
39. Hanngi, M., Banwarth, W. and Stunnenberg, H. G. (1986). Conserved TAAAT motif in vaccinia virus late promoters: overlapping TATA box and site of transcription. *EMBO J.*, **5**, 1071–6
40. Bertholet, C., Stocco, P., van Meir, E. and Wittek, R. (1986). Functional analysis of the 5′ flanking sequence of a vaccinia virus late gene. *EMBO J.*, **5**, 1951–7
41. Weir, J. P. and Moss, B. (1987). Determination of the transcriptional regulatory region of a late vaccinia virus gene. *J. Virol.*, **61**, 75–80
42. Wright, C. F. and Moss, B. (1987). *In vitro* synthesis of vaccinia virus late mRNA containing a 5′ poly (A) leader sequence. *Proc. Natl. Acad. Sci. USA*, **84**, 8883–7
43. Bertholet, C., van Meir, E., ten Heggeler-Bordier, B. and Wittek, R. (1987). Vaccinia virus produces late mRNAs by dicontinuous synthesis. *Cell*, **50**, 153–62
44. Schwer, B., Visca, P., Vos, J. C. and Stunnenberg, H. G. (1987). Discontinuous transcription or RNA processing of vaccinia virus late mRNA results in a 5′ poly A leader. *Cell*, **50**, 163–9
45. Schwer, B. and Stunnenberg, H. G. (1988). Vaccinia virus late transcripts generated *in vitro* have a poly(A) head. *EMBO J.*, **7**, 1183–90
46. Patel, D. D. and Pickup, D. J. (1987). Messenger RNAs of a strongly-expressed late gene of cowpox virus contain 5′-terminal poly(A) sequences. *EMBO J.*, **6**, 3787–94
47. De Magistris, L. and Stunnenberg, H. G. (1988). Cis-acting sequences affecting the length of the poly (A) head of vaccinia virus late transcripts. *Nucl. Acids. Res.*, **16**, 3141–56
48. Panicali, D. and Paoletti, E. (1982). Construction of poxviruses as cloning vectors: insertion of the thymidine kinase gene from herpes simplex virus into the DNA of infectious vaccinia virus. *Proc. Natl. Acad. Sci. USA*, **79**, 4927–31
49. Mackett, M. and Smith, G. L. (1986). Vaccinia virus expression vectors. *J. Gen. Virol.*, **67**, 2067–82
50. Chakrabarti, S., Brechling, K. and Moss, B. (1985). Vaccinia virus expression vector: co-expression of beta-galactosidase provides visual selection of recombinant virus plaques. *Mol. Cell Biol.*, **5**, 3403–9
51. Boyle, D. B., Couper, B. E. H. and Both, G. W. (1985). Multiple-cloning-site plasmids for the rapid construction of recombinant poxviruses. *Gene*, **35**, 169–77
52. Franke, C. A., Rice, C. M., Strauss, J. H. and Hruby, D. E. (1985). Neomycin resistance as a dominant selectable marker for selection and isolation of vaccinia virus recombinants. *Mol. Cell. Biol.*, **5** 1918–24
53. Boyle, D. B. and Coupar, B. E. H. (1988). A dominant selectable marker for the construction of recombinant poxviruses. *Gene*, **65**, 123–8
54. Falkner, F. G. and Moss, B. (1988). *Escherichia coli* gpt gene provides dominant selection for vaccinia virus open reading frame expression vectors. *J. Virol.*, **62**, 1849–54
55. Flexner, C., Hugin, A. and Moss, B. (1987). Prevention of vaccinia virus infection in immunodeficient mice by vector-directed IL-2 expression. *Nature*, **330**, 259–61
56. Buller, R. M. L., Chakrabarti, S., Cooper, J. A., Twardzik, D. R. and Moss, B. (1988). Deletion of the vaccinia growth factor gene reduces virus virulence. *J. Virol.*, **62**, 866–74
57. Perkus, M. E., Panicali, D., Mercer, S. and Paoletti, E. (1986). Insertion and deletion mutants of vaccinia virus. *Virology*, **152**, 285–97
58. Rodriguez, J. F., Rodriguez, D., Rodriguez, J.-R., McGowan, E. B. and Esteban, M. (1988). Expression of the firefly luciferase gene in vaccinia virus: a highly sensitive gene marker to follow virus dissemination in tissues of infected animals. *Proc. Natl. Acad. Sci. USA*, **85**, 1667–71
59. Rodriguez, J. F. and Esteban, M. (1988). Plaque size phenotype as a selectable marker to generate vaccinia virus recombinants. *J. Virol.*, **63**, 997–1001
60. Mackett, M., Yilma, T., Rose, J. and Moss, B. (1985). Vaccinia virus recombinants: expression of VSV genes and protective immunization of mice and cattle. *Science*, **227**, 433–5
61. Kieny, M. P., Lathe, R., Drillien, R., Sphener, D., Skory, S., Schmitt, D., Wiktor, T., Koprowski, H. and Lecocq, J. P. (1984). Expression of rabies virus gycoprotein from a recombinant vaccinia virus. *Nature*, **312**, 163–6
62. Fathi, Z., Sridhar, P., Facha, R. F. and Condit, R. (1986). Efficient targeted insertion of an unselected marker into the vaccinia virus genome. *Virology*, **155** 97–105

63. Smith, G. L. and Moss, B. (1983). Infectious poxvirus vectors have capacity for at least 25,000 base pairs of foreign DNA. *Gene*, **25**, 21–8
64. Perkus, M. E., Piccini, A., Lipinskas, B. R. and Paoletti, E. (1985). Recombinant vaccinia virus: immunization against multiple pathogens. *Science*, **229**, 981–4
65. Flexner, C. and Moss, B. (1987). Vaccinia virus expression vectors. *Ann. Rev. Immunol.*, **5**, 305–24
66. Browne, H. M., Churcher, M. J., Stanley, M. A., Smith, G. L. and Minson, A. C. (1988). Analysis of the L1 gene product of human papillomavirus type 16 by expression in a vaccinia virus recombinant. *J. Gen. Virol.*, **69** 1263–73
67. Stephens, E. B., Compans, R. W., Earl, P. and Moss, B. (1986). Surface expression of viral glycoproteins is polarized in epithelial cells infected with vaccinia viral vectors. *EMBO J.*, **5** 237–45
68. Sullivan, V. and Smith, G. L. (1987). Expression and characterization of herpes simplex virus type 1 (HSV-1) glycoprotein G (gG) by recombinant vaccinia virus: neutralization of HSV-1 infectivity with anti-gG antibody. *J. Gen. Virol.*, **68** 2587–98
69. Sullivan, V. and Smith, G. L. (1988). The herpes simplex virus type 1 US7 gene product is a 66K glycoprotein and is a target for complement-dependent virus neutralization. *J. Gen. Virol.*, **69**, 859–67
70. Cranage, M. P., Smith, G. L., Bell, S. E., Hart, H., Brown, C., Bankier, A. T., Tomlinson, P., Barrell, B. G. and Minson, A. C. (1988). Identification and expression of a human cytomegalovirus glycoprotein with homology to the Epstein–Barr virus BXLF2 product, varicella-zoster virus gpIII, and herpes simples virus type 1 glycoprotein H. *J. Virol.*, **62**, 1416–22
71. Smith, G. L., Mackett, M. and Moss, B. (1983). Infectious vaccinia virus recombinants that express hepatitis B virus surface antigen. *Nature*, **302**, 490–5
72. Paoletti, E., Lipinskas, B. R., Samsonoff, C., Mercer, S. and Panicali, D. (1984). Construction of live vaccines using genetically engineered poxviruses: biological activity of vaccinia virus recombinants expressing the hepatitis B virus surface antigen and the herpes simplex virus glycoprotein D. *Proc. Natl. Acad. Sci. USA*, **81** 193–7
73. Cheng, K.-C. and Moss, B. (1987). Selective synthesis and secretion of particles composed of the hepatitis B virus middle surface protein directed by a recombinant vaccinia virus: induction of antibody to preS and S epitopes. *J. Virol.*, **61**, 1286–90
74. Smith, G. L., Levin, J., Palese, P. and Moss, B. (1987). Synthesis and cellular location of the ten influenza polypeptides individually expressed by recombinant vaccinia viruses. *Virology*, **160**, 336–45
75. Smith, G. L., Godson, N. G., Nussenzweig, V., Nussenzweig, R. S., Barnwell, J. and Moss, B. (1984). *Plasmodium knowlesi* sporozoite antigen: expression by infectious recombinant vaccinia virus. *Science*, **114**, 397–9
76. Smith, G. L., Cheng, K.-C. and Moss, B. (1986). Vaccinia virus: an expression vector for genes from parasites. *Parasitology*, **92S**, 109–18
77. Smith, G. L., Murphy, B. R. and Moss, B. (1983). Construction and characterization of an infectious vaccinia virus recombinant that expresses the influenza virus haemagglutinin and induces resistance to influenza virus infection in hamsters. *Proc. Natl. Acad. Sci. USA*, **80**, 7155–9
78. Wiktor, T. J., MacFarlan, R. I., Reagen, K. J., Dietzschold, B., Curtis, P. J., Wunner, W. H., Kieny, M.-P., Lathe, R., Lecocq, J.-P., Mackett, M., Moss, B. and Koprowswki, H. (1984). Protection from rabies by a vaccinia virus recombinant containing the rabies virus glycoprotein gene. *Proc. Natl. Acad. Sci. USA*, **81** 7194–8
79. Cremer, K., Mackett, M., Wohlenberg, C., Notkins, A. L. and Moss, B. (1985). Vaccinia virus recombinants expressing herpes simplex virus type 1 glyoprotein D prevents latent herpes in mice. *Science*, **228**, 737–40
80. Mackett, M. and Arrand, J. R. (1985). Recombinant vaccinia virus induces neutralizing antibodies in rabbits against Epstein-Barr virus membrane antigen gp340. *EMBO J.*, **4**, 3229–34
81. Cheng, K.-C., Smith, G. L. and Moss, B. (1986). Hepatitis B virus large surface protein is not secreted but is immunogenic when selectively expressed by recombinant vaccinia virus. *J. Virol.*, **60**, 337–44
82. Chakrabarti, S., Robert-Guroff, M., Wong-Staal, F., Gallo, R. C. and Moss, B. (1986).

Expression of HTLV-III envelope gene by recombinant vaccinia virus. *Nature*, **320**, 535–7

83. Hu, S.-K., Kosowski, S. G. and Dalrymple, J. M. (1986). Expression of the AIDS virus envelope gene in recombinant vaccinia viruses. *Nature*, **320**, 537–40
84. Earl, P. L., Moss, B., Morris, R. P., Wehrl, Y. K., Nihsio, J. and Chesebro, B. (1986). T-lymphocyte priming and protection against Friend leukaemia by vaccinia-retrovirus env gene recombinant. *Science*, **234**, 728–31
85. Olmsted, R. A., Elango, N., Prince, G. A., Murphy, B. R., Johnson, P. R., Moss, B., Chanock, R. M. and Collins, P. L. (1986). Expression of the F glycoprotein of respiratory syncytial virus by a recombinant vaccinia virus: comparisons of the individual contributions of the F and G glycoproteins to host immunity. *Proc. Natl. Acad. Sci. USA*, **83**, 7462–6
86. Elango, N., Prince, G. A., Murphy, B. R., Venkatesan, S., Chanock, R. M. and Moss, B. (1986). Resistance to human respiratory syncytial virus (RSV) infection induced by immunization of cotton rats with a recombinant vaccinia virus expressing the RSV G protein. *Proc. Natl. Acad. Sci. USA*, **83**, 1906–10
87. Wertz, G. W., Stott, E. J., Young, K. K., Anderson, K. and Ball, L. A. (1987). Expression of the fusion protein of human respiratory syncytial virus from recombinant vaccinia vectors and protection of vaccinated mice. *J. Virol.*, **61**, 294–301
88. Rice, C. M., Franke, C. A., Stauss, J. H. and Hruby, D. E. (1985). Expression of Sindbis virus structural proteins via recombinant vaccinia virus: synthesis, processing and incorporation into mature Sindbis virions. *J. Virol.*, **56**, 227–39
89. Cranage, M. P., Kouzarides, T., Bankier, A. T., Satchwell, S., Weston, K., Tomlinson, P., Barrell, B., Hart, H., Bell, S. E., Minson, A. C. and Smith, G. L. (1986). Identification of the human cytomegalovirus glycoprotein B gene and induction of neutralising antibodies via its expression in recombinant vaccinia virus. *EMBO J.*, **5**, 3057–63
90. Gilbert, J. H., Pedersen, N. C. and Nunberg, J. H. (1987). Feline leukemia virus envelope protein expression encoded by a recombinant vaccinia virus: apparent lack of immunogenicity in vaccinated animals. *Virus Res.*, **7**, 49–67
91. Andrew, M., Boyle, D., Coupar, B. E. H., Whitfield, P. L., Both, G. W. and Bellamy, A. R. (1987). Vaccinia virus recombinants expressing the SA11 rotavirus VP7 glycoprotein gene induce sero-specific neutralising antibodies. *J. Virol.*, **61**, 1054–60
92. Tomley, F. M., Mockett, A. P. A., Boursnell, M. E. G., Binns, M. M., Cook, J. K. A., Brown, T. D. K. and Smith, G. L. (1987). Expression of the infectious bronchitis virus spike protein by recombinant vaccinia virus and induction of neutralising antibodies in vaccinated mice. *J. Gen. Virol.*, **68**, 2291–8
93. Langford, C. J., Edwards, S. J., Smith, G. L., Moss, B., Kemp, D. J., Anders, R. F. and Mitchell, G. F. (1986). A plasmodium antigen secreted by recombinant vaccinia virus becomes immunogenic when converted into surface antigen. *Mol. Cell. Biol.*, **6**, 3191–9
94. Stomatos, N. M., Chakrabarti, S., Moss, B. and Hare, J. D. (1987). Expression of polyomavirus virion proteins by a vaccinia virus vector: association of VP1 and VP2 with the nuclear framework. *J. Virol.*, **61**, 516–25
95. Lathe, R., Kieny, M. P., Gerlinger, P., Clertant, P., Guizani, I., Cuzin, R. and Chambon, P. (1987). Tumour prevention and rejection with recombinant vaccinia virus. *Nature*, **326**, 878–80
96. Panicali, D., Davis, S. W., Weinberg, R. L. and Paoletti, E. (1983). Construction of live vaccines by using genetically engineered poxviruses: biological activity of recombinant vaccinia virus expressing the influenza virus hemagglutinin. *Proc. Natl. Acad. Sci. USA*, **80**, 5364–8
97. King, A. M. Q., Stott, E. J., Langer, S. J., Young, K. K.-Y., Ball, L. A. and Wertz, G. W. (1987). Recombinant vaccinia virus carrying the N gene of respiratory syncytial virus: studies of gene expression in cell culture and immune responses in mice. *J. Virol.*, **61**, 2885–90
98. Spriggs, M. K., Collins, P. C., Tierney, E., London, W. T. and Murphy, B. R. (1988). Immunization with vaccinia virus recombinants that express the surface glycoproteins of human parainfluenza type 3 (PIV3) protects patas monkeys against PIV3 infection. *J. Virol.*, **62**, 1293–6
99. Drillien, R., Sphener, D., Kirn, A., Giraudon, P., Buckland, R., Wild, F. and Lecocq, J.-P. (1988). Protection of mice from fatal measles encephalitis by vaccination with vaccinia

virus recombinants encoding either the hemagglutinin or the fusion protein. *Proc. Natl. Acad. Sci. USA*, **85**, 1252–6

100. Blancou, J., Kieny, M. P., Lathe, R., Lecocq, J. P., Pastoret, P. P., Soulebot, J. P. and Desmettre, P. (1986). Oral vaccination of the fox against rabies using a live recombinant vaccinia virus. *Nature*, **322**, 373–5
101. Small, P. A., Smith, G. L. and Moss, B. (1985). Intranasal vaccination with recombinant vaccinia containing influenza haemagglutinin prevents both influenza virus pneumonia and nasal infection: intradermal vaccination prevents only viral pneumonia. In Quinnan, G. V. (ed.). *Vaccinia Viruses as Vectors for Vaccine Antigens*, pp. 175–8. (New York: Elsevier)
102. Jones, L., Ristow, S., Yilma, T. and Moss, B. (1986). Accidental human vaccination with vaccinia virus expressing nucleoprotein gene. *Nature*, **319**, 543
103. Zagury, D., Leonard, R., Fouchard, M., Reveil, B., Bernard, J., Ittele, D., Cattan, R., Zirimwabagabo, L., Kalumbu, M., Justin, W., Saluan, J.-J. and Goussard, B. (1987). Immunization against AIDS in humans. *Nature*, **326**, 249–50
104. Zagury, D., Bernard, J., Cheynier, R., Desportes, I., Leonard, R., Fouchard, M., Reveil, B., Ittele, D., Lurhuma, Z., Mbayo, K., Wane, J., Salaun, J.-J., Goussard, B., Dechazal, L., Burny, A., Nara, P. and Gallo, R. C. (1988). A group specific anamnestic immune reaction against HIV-1 induced by a candidate vaccine against AIDS. *Nature*, **332**, 728–31
105. Zarling, J. M., Morton, W., Moran, P. A., McClure, J., Kosowski, S. G. and Hu, S.-L. (1986). T-cell responses to human AIDS virus in macaques immunized with recombinant vaccinia viruses. *Nature*, **323**, 344–6
106. Bennink, J. R., Yewdell, J. W., Smith, G. L., Moller, C. and Moss, B. (1984). Recombinant vaccinia virus primes and stimulates influenza virus haemagglutinin-specific cytotoxic T lymphocytes. *Nature*, **311**, 578–9
107. Bennink, J. R., Yewdell, J. W., Smith, G. L. and Moss, B. (1986). Recognition of cloned influenza virus haemagglutinin gene products by cytotoxic T lymphocytes. *J. Virol.*, **57**, 786–91
108. Bennink, J. R., Yewdell, J. W., Smith, G. L. and Moss, B. (1987). Anti-influenza virus cytotoxic T lymphocytes recognises the three viral polymerases and a nonstructural protein: responsiveness to individual viral antigens is major histocompatibility complex controlled. *J. Virol.*, **61**, 1098–102
109. Yewdell, J. W., Bennink, J. R., Smith, G. L. and Moss, B. (1985). Influenza A virus nucleoprotein is a major target antigen for influenza A virus cross-reactive cytotoxic T lymphocytes. *Proc. Natl. Acad. Sci. USA*, **82**, 1785–9
110. Yewdell, J. W., Bennink, J. R., Mackett, M., Lefrancois, L., Lyles, D. S. and Moss, B. (1986). Recognition of cloned vesicular stomatitis virus internal and external gene products by cytotoxic T lymphocytes. *J. Exp. Med.*, **163**, 1529–38
111. McMichael, A. J., Michie, C. A., Gotch, F. M., Smith, G. L. and Moss, B. (1986). Recognition of influenza virus nucleoprotein by human cytotoxic T lymphocytes. *J. Gen. Virol.*, **67**, 719–26
112. Gotch, F., McMichael, A., Smith, G. and Moss, B. (1987). Identification of viral molecules recognized by influenza-specific human cytotoxic T lymphocytes. *J. Exp. Med.*, **165**, 408–16
113. Coupar, B. E. H., Andrew, M. E., Both, G. W. and Boyle, D. B. (1986). Temporal regulation of influenza hemagglutinin expression in vaccinia. *Eur. J. Immunol.*, **16**, 1479–87
114. Andrew, M. E., Coupar, B. E. H., Ada, G. L. and Boyle, D. B. (1986). Cell-mediated immune response to influenza virus antigens expressed by vaccinia recombinants. *Microb. Pathogen.*, **1**, 443–52
115. Andrew, M. E., Coupar, B. E. H., Boyle, D. B. and Ada, G. L. (1987). The roles of influenza virus haemagglutinin and nucleoprotein in protection: analysis using vaccinia virus recombinants. *Scand. J. Immunol.*, **25**, 21–8
116. Bangham, C. R. M., Openshaw, P. J. M., Ball, L. A., King, A. M. Q., Wertz, G. M. and Askonas, B. A. (1986). Human and murine cytotoxic T cells to respiratory syncytial virus recognise the viral nucleocapsid (N), but not the major glycoprotein (G), expressed by vaccinia virus recombinants. *J. Immunol.*, **137**, 3973–7
117. Borysiewicz, L. K., Hickling, J. K., Graham, S., Sinclair, J., Cranage, M. P., Smith, G. L. and Sissons, J. G. P. (1988). Human cytomegalovirus specific cytotoxic T cell: relative frequency of stage specific CTL recognising the 72 kDa immediately early protein and glycoprotein B expressed by recombinant vaccinia viruses. *J. Exp. Med.*,**168**, 919–931

118. Townsend, A., Bastin, J., Gould, K., Brownlee, G., Andrew, M., Boyle, D. B., Chan, Y. S. and Smith, G. L. (1988). Defective presentation to class I restricted CTL in vaccinia infected cells is overcome by enhanced degradation of antigen. *J. Exp. Med.*,**168**, 1211–1224
119. Moss, B., Smith, G. L., Gerin, J. L. and Purcell, R. H. (1984). Live recombinant vaccinia virus protects chimpanzees against hepatitis B. *Nature*, **311**, 67–9
120. Estin, C. D., Stevenson, U. S., Plowman, G. D., Hu, S.-K., Sridhar, P., Hellstrom, I., Brown, J. P. and Hellstrom, K. E. (1988). Recombinant vaccinia virus against the human melanoma antigen p97 for use in immunotherapy. *Proc. Natl. Acad. Sci. USA*, **85**, 1052–6
121. Hu, S.-L., Fultz, P. N., McClure, H. M., Eichberg, J. W., Thomas, E. K., Zarling, J., Singhal, M. C., Kosowski, S. G., Swenson, R. B., Anderson, D. C. and Todaro, G. (1987). Effect of immunization with a vaccinia-HIV env recombinant on HIV infection of chimpanzees. *Nature*, **328**, 721–3
122. Fuerst, T. R., Niles, E. G., Studier, F. W. and Moss, B. (1986). Eukaryotic transient-expression system based upon recombinant vaccinia virus that synthesizes bacteriophage T7 RNA polymerase. *Proc. Natl. Acad. Sci. USA*, **83**, 8122–6
123. Fuerst, T. R., Earl, P. C. and Moss, B. (1987). Use of a hybrid vaccinia virus-T7 RNA polymerase system for expression of target genes. *Mol. Cell. Biol.*, **7**, 2538–44
124. Slabaugh, M., Roseman, N., Davis, R. and Mathews, C. (1988). Vaccinia virus-encoded ribonucleotide reductase: sequence conservation of the gene for the small subunit and its amplification in hydroxyurea resistant mutants. *J. Virol.*, **62**, 519–27
125. Clarke, B. E., Newton, S. E., Carroll, A. R., Francis, M. J., Appleyard, G., Syred, A. D., Highfield, P. E., Rowlands, D. J. and Brown, F. (1987). Improved immunogenicity of a peptide epitope after fusion to hepatitis B core protein. *Nature*, **330**, 381–4
126. Ramshaw, I. A., Andrew, M. E., Philips, S. M., Boyle, D. B. and Coupar, B. E. H. (1987). Recovery of immunodeficient mice from a vaccinia virus/IL-2 recombinant infection. *Nature*, **329**, 545–7
127. Lane, J. M., Ruben, F. L., Neff, J. M. and Millar, J. D. (1969). Complications of smallpox vaccination. 1968 Surveillance in the United States. *N. Engl. J. Med.*, **281**, 1201–8
128. Buller, R. M. L., Smith, G. L., Cremer, K., Notkins, A. L. and Moss, B. (1985). Decreased virulence of recombinant vaccinia virus expression vectors is associated with a thymidine kinase-negative phenotype. *Nature*, **317**, 813–15
129. Dallo, S. and Esteban, M. (1987). Isolation and characterization of attenuated mutants of vaccinia virus. *Virology*, **159** 408–22
130. Rodriguez, J. F., Paez, E. and Esteban, M. (1987). A 14,000-Mr envelope protein of vaccinia virus is involved in cell fusion and forms covalently linked trimers. *J. Virol.*, **61**, 395–404
131. Redfield, R. R., Wright, D. C., James, W. D., Jones, T. S., Brown, C. and Burke, M. D. (1987). Disseminated vaccinia in a military recruit with human immunodeficiency virus (HIV) disease. *N. Engl. J. Med.*, **316**, 673–6

Index